Women's Health in Gastroenterology

Editor

LAUREL R. FISHER

GASTROENTEROLOGY CLINICS OF NORTH AMERICA

www.gastro.theclinics.com

Consulting Editor
GARY W. FALK

June 2016 • Volume 45 • Number 2

ELSEVIER

1600 John F. Kennedy Boulevard • Suite 1800 • Philadelphia, Pennsylvania, 19103-2899
http://www.theclinics.com

GASTROENTEROLOGY CLINICS OF NORTH AMERICA Volume 45, Number 2
June 2016 ISSN 0889-8553, ISBN-13: 978-0-323-44614-3

Editor: Kerry Holland
Developmental Editor: Alison Swety

Gastroenterology Clinics of North America (ISSN 0889-8553) is published quarterly by Elsevier Inc., 360 Park Avenue South, New York, NY 10010-1710. Months of issue are March, June, September, and December. Business and Editorial Offices: 1600 John F. Kennedy Blvd., Suite 1800, Philadelphia, PA 19103-2899. Customer Service Office: 6277 Sea Harbor Drive, Orlando, FL 32887-4800. Periodicals postage paid at New York, NY and additional mailing offices. Subscription prices are $320.00 per year (US individuals), $100.00 per year (US students), $587.00 per year (US institutions), $350.00 per year (Canadian individuals), $720.00 per year (Canadian institutions), $445.00 per year (international individuals), $220.00 per year (international students), and $720.00 per year (international institutions). Foreign air speed delivery is included in all *Clinics* subscription prices. All prices are subject to change without notice. **POSTMASTER**: Send address changes to *Gastroenterology Clinics of North America*, Elsevier Health Sciences Division, Subscription Customer Service, 3251 Riverport Lane, Maryland Heights, MO 63043. **Telephone: 1-800-654-2452 (U.S. and Canada); 314-447-8871 (outside U.S. and Canada). Fax: 314-447-8029. E-mail: journalscustomerservice-usa@elsevier.com (for print support); journalsonlinesupport-usa@elsevier.com (for online support).**

Reprints. For copies of 100 or more, of articles in this publication, please contact the Commercial Reprints Department, Elsevier Inc., 360 Part Avenue South, New York, New York 10010-1710. Tel. 212-633-3874, Fax: 212-633-3820, E-mail: reprints@elsevier.com.

Gastroenterology Clinics of North America is also published in Italian by Il Pensiero Scientifico Editore, Rome, Italy; and in Portuguese by Interlivros Edicoes Ltda., Rua Commandante Coelho 1085, 21250 Cordovil, Rio de Janeiro, Brazil.

Gastroenterology Clinics of North America is covered in *MEDLINE/PubMed (Index Medicus), Excerpta Medica, Current Contents/Clinical Medicine, Science Citation Index, ISI/BIOMED,* and *BIOSIS*.

Contributors

CONSULTING EDITOR

GARY W. FALK, MD, MS
Professor of Medicine, Division of Gastroenterology, Hospital of the University of Pennsylvania, University of Pennsylvania Perelman School of Medicine, Philadelphia, Pennsylvania

EDITOR

LAUREL R. FISHER, MD
Professor of Clinical Medicine, Division of Gastroenterology, Department of Internal Medicine, University of Pennsylvania Health System, Philadelphia, Pennsylvania

AUTHORS

JOHN I. ALLEN, MD, MBA
Immediate Past-President: AGA, Professor of Medicine, Clinical Chief of Digestive Diseases, Yale University School of Medicine, New Haven, Connecticut

NOEMI BAFFY, MPH, MD
Division of Gastroenterology and Hepatology, Mayo Clinic, Scottsdale, Arizona

CAMERON BODY, MD
Internal Medicine Resident, Emory University School of Medicine, Atlanta, Georgia

DARREN M. BRENNER, MD, AGAF
Assistant Professor of Medicine and Surgery, Division of Gastroenterology, Northwestern University Feinberg School of Medicine, Chicago, Illinois

JENNIFER A. CHRISTIE, MD, FASGE
Director of Gastrointestinal Motility, Emory University School of Medicine, Atlanta, Georgia

ERICA COHEN, MD
Division of Gastroenterology, Cedars Sinai Medical Center, Los Angeles, California

SHEILA E. CROWE, MD, FRCPC, FACP, FACG, AGAF
Professor, Division of Gastroenterology, Department of Medicine, University of California San Diego, La Jolla, California

LINDA A. FEAGINS, MD
Associate Professor of Medicine, Division of Gastroenterology and Hepatology, VA North Texas Healthcare System, University of Texas Southwestern Medical Center, Dallas, Texas

ALISON FREEMAN, MD, MPH
Gastroenterology Fellow, Division of Gastroenterology, Department of Internal Medicine, University of Michigan Health System, Ann Arbor, Michigan

JEANNE-MARIE GIARD, MD, MPH
Division of Gastroenterology, Department of Medicine, University of California, San Francisco, San Francisco, California

LISA M. GLASS, MD
Staff Physician, Gastroenterology Section, Department of Internal Medicine, VA Ann Arbor Healthcare System; Clinical Lecturer, University of Michigan Health System, Ann Arbor, Michigan

LUCINDA A. HARRIS, MS, MD
Division of Gastroenterology and Hepatology, Mayo Clinic, Scottsdale, Arizona

MARGARET M. HEITKEMPER, RN, PhD
Department of Biobehavioral Nursing and Health Systems, School of Nursing, University of Washington, Seattle, Washington

SUNANDA V. KANE, MD, MSPH
Professor of Medicine, Division of Gastroenterology and Hepatology, Mayo Clinic, Rochester, Minnesota

UMA MAHADEVAN, MD
Professor of Medicine, Division of Gastroenterology, UCSF Center for Colitis and Crohn's Disease, San Francisco, California

RYAN A. McCONNELL, MD
Division of Gastroenterology, University of California, San Francisco, San Francisco, California

STACY MENEES, MD, MS
Assistant Professor, Division of Gastroenterology, Department of Internal Medicine, University of Michigan Health System, Ann Arbor, Michigan

LAURA A. PACE, MD, PhD
Division of Gastroenterology, Department of Medicine, University of California San Diego, La Jolla, California

OCTAVIA PICKETT-BLAKELY, MD, MHS
Director, Obesity, Nutrition and Celiac Disease Program; Assistant Professor of Medicine, Division of Gastroenterology and Hepatology, University of Pennsylvania, Philadelphia, Pennsylvania

FARZANA RASHID, MD
Assistant Professor of Medicine, Division of Gastroenterology and Hepatology, University of Pennsylvania, Philadelphia, Pennsylvania

COLLEEN M. SCHMITT, MD, MHS
Immediate Past-President: ASGE, Galen Medical Group, Chattanooga, Tennessee

MARMY SHAH, MD
Assistant Professor of Medicine, Division of Gastroenterology and Nutrition, Loyola University Medical Center, Maywood, Illinois

GRACE LI-CHUN SU, MD
Chief, Gastroenterology Section; Associate Chief of Medicine, Specialty Care and
Access, VA Ann Arbor Healthcare System; Professor of Medicine, University of Michigan
Medical School, Ann Arbor, Michigan

NORAH A. TERRAULT, MD, MPH
Division of Gastroenterology, Department of Medicine, University of California,
San Francisco, San Francisco, California

TRAM T. TRAN, MD, FAASLD, FACG
Liver Transplant, Cedars Sinai Medical Center, Los Angeles, California

SARAH B. UMAR, MD
Division of Gastroenterology and Hepatology, Mayo Clinic, Scottsdale, Arizona

LAURA UWAKWE, MD
Medical Resident, Department of Medicine, Drexel University College of Medicine,
Philadelphia, Pennsylvania

JASMINE K. ZIA, MD
Division of Gastroenterology and Hepatology, Department of Medicine, University of
Washington, Seattle, Washington

Contents

for the stomach. It also describes differences in upper GI motility signs and symptoms during each female hormonal stage (ie, menstrual cycle, pregnancy, perimenopause, menopause) for both healthy participants and those suffering from one of the aforementioned upper GI dysmotility conditions. More research still needs to be conducted to better understand sex differences in upper GI motility.

Diet is a risk factor in several medically important disease states, including obesity, celiac disease, and functional gastrointestinal disorders. Modification of diet can prevent, treat, or alleviate some of the symptoms associated with these diseases and improve general health. It is important to provide patients with simple dietary recommendations to increase the probability of successful implementation. These recommendations include increasing vegetable, fruit, and fiber intake, consuming lean protein sources to enhance satiety, avoiding or severely limiting highly processed foods, and reducing portion sizes for overweight and obese patients.

Many disorders of the gastrointestinal tract are common in pregnancy. Elevated levels of progesterone may lead to alterations in gastrointestinal motility which could contribute to nausea, vomiting, and/or GERD. Pregnancy-induced diarrhea may be due to elevated levels prostaglandins. This article reviews the normal physiologic and structural changes associated with pregnancy that could contribute to many of the common gastrointestinal complaints in pregnant patients. Additionally, the appropriate clinical and laboratory evaluations, other pathologic conditions that should be included in the differential, as well as the nonpharmacologic and pharmacologic therapies for each of these conditions is discussed.

For many women with inflammatory bowel disease (IBD), the illness coincides with their childbearing years. IBD increases the risk of pregnancy complications and adverse pregnancy outcomes. The multidisciplinary care team should emphasize the importance of medication adherence to achieve preconception disease control and maintain corticosteroid-free remission throughout pregnancy. Medication adjustments to reduce fetal exposure may be considered on an individualized basis in quiescent disease; however, any benefits of such adjustments remain theoretic and there is risk of worsening disease activity. Mode of delivery is determined by obstetric indications, except for women with active perinatal disease who should consider cesarean delivery.

Linda A. Feagins and Sunanda V. Kane

Ulcerative colitis and Crohn disease are chronic inflammatory diseases with typical onset in early adulthood. These diseases, therefore, can affect a woman throughout the many stages of her life, including menstruation, sexuality, pregnancy, and menopause. Unique health issues face women during these stages and can affect the course of their inflammatory bowel disease as well as treatment strategies and health maintenance. This article covers the non–pregnancy-related issues that are important in caring for women with inflammatory bowel disease. The topics of pregnancy and fertility are covered in a separate review.

Octavia Pickett-Blakely, Laura Uwakwe, and Farzana Rashid

Approximately 36% of adult women in the United States are obese. Although obesity affects women similarly to men in terms of prevalence, there seem to be gender-specific differences in the pathophysiology, clinical manifestations, and treatment of obesity. Obesity is linked to comorbid diseases involving multiple organ systems, including the gastrointestinal tract, like gastroesophageal reflux disease, fatty liver disease, and gallstones. This article focuses on obesity in women, specifically the impact of obesity on gastrointestinal diseases and reproductive health, as well as the treatment of obesity in women.

Lisa M. Glass and Grace Li-Chun Su

Primary biliary cirrhosis (PBC) is a liver-specific autoimmune disease that primarily affects women (female-to-male ratio, 10:1) between 40 and 60 years of age. Metabolic bone disease is a common complication of PBC, affecting 14% to 52% of patients, depending on the duration and severity of liver disease. The osteoporosis seen in PBC seems mainly due to low bone formation, although increased bone resorption may contribute. Treatment of osteoporosis consists primarily of antiresorptive agents. Additional large prospective, long-term studies in patients with PBC are needed to determine efficacy in improving bone density as well as reducing fracture risk.

Jeanne-Marie Giard and Norah A. Terrault

Cirrhosis is less frequent in women than in men, in large part due to the lower prevalence of hepatitis B, hepatitis C, and alcohol use in women. The most common causes of cirrhosis among women are hepatitis C, autoimmune etiologies, nonalcoholic steatohepatitis, and alcoholic liver disease. For most chronic liver diseases, the risk of progression to cirrhosis and rates of liver failure and hepatocellular carcinoma are lower in women than in men. Pregnancy is very infrequent in women with cirrhosis due to reduced fertility, but when it occurs, requires specialized management.

GASTROENTEROLOGY
CLINICS OF NORTH AMERICA

Preface

Women's Gastrointestinal Health in 2016: An Introduction to an Expanding Field in Gastroenterology

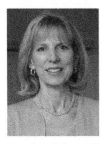

Laurel R. Fisher, MD
Editor

Several years ago, the *Gastroenterology Clinics of North America* released a publication devoted to Women's Issues, reflecting an early awareness of potential differences in women's gastrointestinal (GI) health and management. Since that time, our understanding of the effect of gender on our approach to GI diseases has increased substantially, and addressing the uniqueness of women's GI health has become an important goal in our profession. Increasingly, data have been sought to clarify differences between men and women in the pathophysiology of disease states, the variability in presentation, and the success in treatment and management of disease. A greater consciousness of gender differences in disease complications and an awareness of distinct features of female patients' perception of disease and health may contribute to optimizing women's GI health care.

The role of female gastroenterologists is central to the changing approach to women's health. While women outnumber men in medical school, there is not yet gender parity in numbers of GI fellows, and the percentage of female gastroenterologists remains strikingly low. With increasing frequency, fellowship programs include women's health training, and there is growing recognition that female leadership in GI Divisions and on the national stage can constructively shape the growth and direction of the field of gastroenterology.

The goal of this issue is to present GI diseases that affect women uniquely, such as pelvic floor problems and pregnancy-related disorders, and to examine common GI conditions that require a more considered approach in women, such as functional bowel disease or autoimmune processes. It will also address the position of women and female gastroenterologists in the health system as a whole. The progress and

Gastroenterol Clin N Am 45 (2016) xiii–xiv
http://dx.doi.org/10.1016/j.gtc.2016.03.001
0889-8553/16/$ – see front matter © 2016 Published by Elsevier Inc.

the challenges we have witnessed in the last decade are discussed in the last article of this issue by two eminent society leaders who provide inspiration and direction for future initiatives.

This issue, dedicated to Women's GI Health, is published at an exciting, transitional time in the future of our profession, as we adjust approaches for the assessment of disease in a large portion of our patient population, and as we address the challenges in practicing a more personalized medicine based on the uniqueness of specific populations.

Laurel R. Fisher, MD
Professor of Clinical Medicine
Division of Gastroenterology
Department of Internal Medicine
University of Pennsylvania Health System
3400 Civic Center Boulevard
Perelman Center for Advanced Medicine
7 South
Philadelphia, PA 19104, USA

E-mail address:
laurel.fisher@uphs.upenn.edu

Irritable Bowel Syndrome and Female Patients

Lucinda A. Harris, MS, MD[a,*], Sarah B. Umar, MD[a], Noemi Baffy, MPH, MD[a], Margaret M. Heitkemper, RN, PhD[b]

KEYWORDS

- Irritable bowel syndrome • Female gender • Diet • Treatment • Constipation
- Diarrhea

KEY POINTS

- Irritable bowel syndrome (IBS) is a predominantly female disorder characterized by abdominal pain or discomfort associated with altered bowel habit (diarrhea, constipation, or both) symptoms.
- Pathophysiology of IBS is heterogeneous and includes altered motility, visceral hypersensitivity, changes in gut permeability, immune activation, brain-gut dysregulation, autonomic nervous system dysfunction, and changes in gut microbiome, all of which may be mediated by gender-related differences.
- A confident IBS diagnosis can be made based on symptom criteria, exclusion of alarm features, recognition of female predominant overlap syndromes, and thoughtful use of bowel habit–based diagnostic work-up.
- Successful management of the female patients with IBS involves understanding female gender roles as well as establishment of active listening and a caring positive clinician-patient relationship.
- Treatment approach requires an assessment of lifestyle (diet, sleep, and exercise), gut-directed pharmacotherapy, and psychological therapies as indicated by IBS disease severity.

INTRODUCTION

Irritable bowel syndrome (IBS) is a common gastrointestinal (GI) disorder characterized by abdominal pain and discomfort that is associated with altered bowel function and that can involve diarrhea, constipation, or mixed bowel patterns. It is a chronic

Conflict of Interest: Consulting for Ironwood, Allergan (formerly Forest Pharmaceuticals), Valeant (formerly Salix and Commonwealth Laboratories), QoL Medical, Synergy Pharmaceuticals. Research for Rhythm Pharmaceuticals, Alvine Pharmaceuticals (L.A. Harris); None (S.B. Umar, N. Baffy, M.M. Heitkemper).
[a] Division of Gastroenterology & Hepatology, Mayo Clinic, 13400 East Shea Boulevard, Scottsdale, AZ 85259, USA; [b] School of Nursing, Biobehavioral Nursing and Health Systems, University of Washington, Seattle, WA, USA
* Corresponding author.
E-mail address: Harris.Lucinda@mayo.edu

Gastroenterol Clin N Am 45 (2016) 179–204
http://dx.doi.org/10.1016/j.gtc.2016.02.001
0889-8553/16/$ – see front matter © 2016 Elsevier Inc. All rights reserved.

disorder with a female predominance ranging from 2:1 to 4:1 depending on the clinical setting.[1] Worldwide the prevalence varies from 7% to 21%.[2] Female prevalence may also vary according to geographic location. In Asia the distribution seems to be fairly equal between men and women but in the United States, Israel, and Canada the disorder is twice as prevalent in women.[3] In veterans returning from the Gulf War, IBS is more prevalent in women than in men (3.7% vs 1.6%) and more often linked to depression, whereas men have a greater likelihood of having posttraumatic stress disorder (PTSD).[4] Female patients have more constipation and abdominal pain and male patients complain more of diarrhea.[5,6]

Although several pathophysiologic mechanisms have been put forth, including increased visceral sensation, alterations in intestinal motility and permeability, autonomic nervous system dysregulation, activation of GI immune function, brain-gut dysregulation, and alterations in the gut microbiome, sex hormones and psychosocial factors may also play a pathophysiologic role.[7,8] It is also notable that many of the comorbid conditions associated with IBS also have a female predominance; for example, fibromyalgia, chronic pelvic pain, migraine headache, and chronic fatigue syndrome, as well as other functional GI disorders such as functional dyspepsia.[8] This article focuses on how female gender influences the pathophysiology, diagnosis, management, and treatment of this common disorder and discusses the evidence and important controversies related to these areas.

PATHOPHYSIOLOGY

Table 1 summarizes the proposed mechanisms of IBS and emphasizes the heterogeneity of the disorder. Diet, gut (motility, visceral hypersensitivity), psychological

Table 1
Pathophysiology of IBS: site of defect and proposed mechanisms

Site of Defect	Proposed Problem/Defect
GI tract	Diet (food intolerance or sensitivity)
	Changes in microbiome (possibly antibiotics, dysbiosis)
	Immune mediated secondary to infection
	Altered motility
	Increased intestinal permeability
	Increased mast cells
	Effects of sex hormones
Genetic[a]	Abnormality in serotonin receptors
	Abnormality in sodium ion channel
	Defect in protein in immune response
	Altered bile acid metabolism
Psychological	Depression
	Anxiety
	Stress
	Coping
	Abuse: sexual, physical, verbal, early adverse life events
	Somatization
	Posttraumatic stress disorder
CNS	CNS processing of afferent gut signals
	Visceral hypersensitivity
	Sex hormones

Abbreviation: CNS, central nervous system.
[a] May only be present in a few individuals.

(somatization, anxiety, and depression), and genetic and central (eg, brain-gut signaling) factors have all been postulated to play a role in pathophysiology but may not all be present in each individual.[9–12] Likely there is interplay of genetic and environmental factors that influence the development of this disorder.[13] Recent research has emphasized immune-mediated factors, especially the effect of infection on the gut microbiome (postinfectious IBS) as well as intestinal dysbiosis (small intestinal bacterial overgrowth [SIBO]).[12] A recent review showed that female sex, in addition to severity of infection, and psychological distress at the time of infection are strong risk factors for developing postinfectious IBS.[14]

Although these factors may be important, it ignores the research on sex hormones (estrogen, progesterone, and testosterone) and how these too may influence the pathogenesis of this disorder.[8] **Table 2** summarizes the key points about the role of hormones in the pathophysiology of IBS. Much of this research has been done in animal models and not in humans. In many human studies the effects of the menstrual cycle and menopause have not been considered. Estrogen and progesterone receptors exist in the brain and the gut and therefore influence motility, visceral sensitivity, and autonomic processing. Evidence also points to estrogen receptors modifying gut permeability, which likely influences the microbiome in ways that are not yet appreciated. A better understanding of the role of female hormones in the pathogenesis of IBS may help the approach to diagnosis as well as possibly to drug development.

DIAGNOSIS
Female Patients: Social Considerations

In the literature on diagnosis there is little discussion of social considerations. Recognition of these factors could result in more directed questioning when diagnosing and treating patients with IBS. Appreciation of gender roles may help providers take better care of female patients. Within society there are certain expectations of women that influence how they behave as patients and what they reveal in the health care setting. Toner and Akman[35] identified several themes in women with IBS that clinicians should keep in mind when seeing patients: shame and bodily functions; bloating, physical appearance, and pleasing others; assertion and anger. Women are socialized to think that bodily functions are private and that losing control is shameful. This attitude may make them reluctant to disclose information and may necessitate more gentle probing about symptoms and response to treatment. Women are socialized to want to be thin and attractive.[36] However, clinicians often minimize the importance of this symptom and the degree to which bloating causes psychological as well as physical distress results in hypervigilance about these symptoms. If not taken seriously, patients develop further distress and more pain from bloating, which can also result in seeking care from multiple providers. Attention to this symptom is important to both history taking and ultimately the treatment plan. In addition, in Western society women are the primary caregivers and, as such, they are trained to please others and suppress their own needs. Many female patients are concerned that being assertive or angry or asking a lot of questions is not seen as socially acceptable. In an effort to be reassuring, providers may trivialize the patient's concerns and the patient in turn may self-silence (ie, not fully disclose her symptoms).[37] In a study of patients with inflammatory bowel disease (IBD) compared with patients with IBS, patients with IBS were less expressive about their needs.[38] Clinicians should be careful not to demean symptoms and take extra care to address patients' concerns so that symptoms, and even response to treatment, are fully understood.

Table 2
Actions of ovarian hormones and possible influences in the pathophysiology of IBS

Known Effects of Ovarian Hormones	Influences of Hormones in Pathophysiology of IBS
GI Motility	
• Transit ○ F<M (effect of E2, P4 on smooth muscle) ○ Menses: slower transit in luteal phase[15,a] ○ Pregnancy: NO slows proximal colon transit (E2 mediated)[16]	• Transit ○ F pt with IBS report C>D,[5] M pt with IBS D>C[6] ○ Menses: ovarian hormone levels low and F pt with IBS report more diarrhea[5] ○ F pt with IBS report greater severity of symptoms during menses
Visceral Hypersensitivity	
—	F pt with IBS at greater risk for somatic and visceral pain conditions[5,17]
• Peripheral/spinal pain processing ○ E2, P4 mediated (conflicting results in different species and different doses) ○ ERα and ERβ receptors modulate pain in DRG[18]	• Peripheral visceral pain processing in IBS ○ F pt with IBS: more abdominal pain and lower threshold for discomfort during CRD[21] ○ Premenopausal F pt with IBS with greater pain during menses (effects of low E2[22]) ○ Testosterone may have protective effects against pain[23] ○ E2 has both pronociceptive and antinociceptive effects (depending on model studied and NT system)[8]

• Central pain processing
 ○ Spinal cord: ERs in DRG[8]
  E2 may cause variable effects on hypersensitivity to pain depending on model studied and NT involved
 ○ Brain: ERs in amygdala[19]
  Increased E2 causes increased sensitivity to CRD; possible opioid effect[20]
	• Central visceral pain processing in IBS
	 ○ Increased visceral pain perception result of hypervigilance premenopausal F[24]
	  ■ Spinal cord studies: F pt with IBS show increase in electrical activity measured in spinal cord with harmful stimulation (mediated by sex hormones)[25,26]
	  ■ Brain fMRI studies: F pt with IBS with painful stimuli show greater activation of emotional pain processing (amygdala, insula, and cingulate cortex) and greater connectivity to prefrontal cortex[27] 5-HT system; may account for gender differences in pain modulation[28]

Stress and Ovarian Hormones	
• F IBS pt show[b] ○ Increased vulnerability to life stress ○ Increased depression and anxiety ○ Increased life trauma ○ Increased IBS symptoms to stress No correlation to date between these features and neuroendocrine response	• Studies show ○ F pt with IBS with stress: HPA system not directly activated, effects may be via limbic system[27,29] ○ F pt with IBS: intestinal barrier may be more vulnerable with stress[30]
Ovarian Hormones and Gut Permeability	
• Humans: ERβ preferentially expressed on colon epithelial cells[31] • Rats: E2R modulates intestinal permeability[32,33] F rat: variations in permeability with estrus cycle	• Humans: increased intestinal permeability seen in IBS and correlated with IBS severity ○ Studies suggest E2-dependent maladaptive epithelial response to stress[8,30]

(continued on next page)

Table 2 (continued)	
Known Effects of Ovarian Hormones	**Influences of Hormones in Pathophysiology of IBS**
Hormones and Immune Activation (Limited Data)	

• Gene expression of immune activation and inflammation in F>M[8]
 • Immune cells express E2 and P4
 • E2 increases mast cell activity and T-cell function; P4 has opposite effect
	• GI mucosal mast cell infiltrates increased in IBS[34]
	   ○ F pt with IBS have greater mast cell numbers
	   ○ E2: promotes mast cell activation
	 • Associations between immune activation and IBS postulated to exist (more research needed on effect of menstrual cycle and menopause)

Abbreviations: 5-HT, serotonin; C, constipation; CRD, colorectal distention; D, diarrhea; DRG, dorsal root ganglion; E2, estradiol; ER, estrogen receptor; F, female; fMRI, functional MRI; HPA, hypothalamic-pituitary-adrenal axis; M, male; NO, nitrous oxide; NT, neurotransmitter; P4, progesterone; pt, patients.

[a] Not all data on menstrual cycle consistent.

[b] Methodological problems with menstrual cycle not always considered; stress hormones measured in blood/plasma not tissue.

General Principles

The diagnosis of IBS is made when the patient shows classic symptoms and commonly occurring organic GI diseases have been ruled out. Rome III criteria outline the major diagnostic features of IBS[39] (**Box 1**). The cardinal feature of IBS is abdominal pain or discomfort but symptoms are also characterized by a change in bowel habits involving diarrhea, constipation, or a mixed bowel pattern. It is usual in the diagnostic work-up to identify a predominant bowel type. **Table 3** suggests an approach to the diagnostic work-up using the predominant bowel habit. The Rome III criteria also

---

Box 1
Rome III Criteria for IBS

IBS is defined as recurrent abdominal pain/discomfort[a] occurring at least 3 d/mo for the last 3 months that is associated with 2 or more of the following features:
1. Improvement with defecation
2. Associated with a change in stool frequency
3. Associated with a change in stool form

Criteria should be documented for the last 3 months with symptom onset for at least 6 months before diagnosis.

IBS subtypes
1. IBS-D: loose or watery stools greater than or equal to 25% and hard or lumpy less than 25% of the time.
2. IBS-C: hard or lumpy stools greater than or equal to 25% of the time and liquid stools less than or equal to 25% of the time.
3. IBS-M: hard or lumpy stools greater than or equal to 25% or the time and loose or watery stools greater than or equal to 25% of the time.
4. IBS-U: unable to subtype bowel habit.

Abbreviations: IBS-C, IBS-constipation; IBS-D, IBS-diarrhea; IBS-M, IBS-mixed.

[a] Discomfort; uncomfortable feeling not defined as pain.

Data from Longstreth GF, Thompson WG, Chey WD, et al. Functional bowel disorders. Gastroenterology 2006;130:1480–91.

Table 3
Suggested diagnostic work-up based on IBS bowel subtype (no alarm[a] features)

IBS-C	IBS-D	IBS-M	All IBS

Refractory cases: consider GI referral for work-up of pelvic floor dysfunction or slow-transit constipation	• Celiac disease
	    IgA tTG +
	        quantitative IgA
	• IBD
	    Fecal calprotectin
	        or CRP
	• Bile salt diarrhea
	    SeHCAT, fecal bile
	    acids, or serum C_4
	    where available
	• Microscopic colitis
	    Consider colonoscopy
	    with random
	    biopsies
		• Celiac disease
		    IgA tTG +
		        quantitative IgA
		• IBD
		    Fecal calprotectin
		        or CRP
		• IBS-C
		    ○ Stool diary
		    ○ Consider
		        abdominal
		        radiograph
		        to determine
		        stool burden
			• CBC
			• Age-appropriate
			  CRC
			  Screening (average
			    risk; slight male
			    predominance)
			    white/Asian
			    age ≥ 50 y,
			    African American
			    age ≥ 45 y

Abbreviations: C_4, carbon 4; CBC, complete blood count; CRC, colorectal cancer screening; CRP, C-reactive protein; IBS-C, IBS-constipation; IBS-D, IBS-diarrhea; IBS-M, IBS-mixed; IgA, immunoglobulin A; SeHCAT, selenium homocholic acid taurine; tTG, tissue transglutaminase.

[a] **ALARM FEATURES** include age greater than or equal to 50 years, unintentional weight loss, blood in stools, nocturnal symptoms, change in symptoms, recent antibiotic and family history of organic GI disease (colorectal cancer, celiac disease, and IBD).

rely on stool consistency to help define the predominant bowel habit because this has been shown to better correlate with bowel subtype and transit.[40] The Bristol Stool Form Scale is a validated scale that can be easily referenced at the time of the office visit for clinicians to evaluate the predominant stool type.[41] Other symptoms, such as belching, abdominal distention, or bloating, may be present but are also seen in patients with other functional disorders.[42,43]

Irritable Bowel Syndrome-Constipation

In patients with IBS-constipation (IBS-C), pelvic floor dyssynergia is a particular concern, especially in female patients.[44] Dyssynergia refers to an inability to coordinate the movement of pelvic floor muscles with the anal sphincter and abdominal wall muscles. Patients often present with similar symptoms of abdominal pain/discomfort and bloating, but may also experience feelings of incomplete evacuation and need for digital maneuvers to remove stool. Symptoms may not accurately identify all patients so, if treatment response seems refractory, referral to a motility specialist who can perform anal manometry with balloon expulsion and defecography may be warranted.[45] Referral often facilitates performance of biofeedback, which preliminary data suggests ameliorates both bowel and abdominal symptoms to a significant degree.[46]

Another concern, particularly in patients with IBS-C is colorectal cancer (CRC). The prospective literature, although limited, suggests that the risk of CRC in patients with IBS without alarm features is less than 1%. Although there has been a slight increase in the incidence of CRC in younger patients, this is probably of less concern for younger female patients with IBS because CRC occurs 25% more commonly in men and 20% more commonly in African Americans.[47,48] A recent meta-analysis comparing constipated with nonconstipated individuals supports doing age-appropriate colon cancer screening, particularly in female patients with IBS.[49]

Irritable Bowel Syndrome-Diarrhea

In patients with diarrhea, special consideration should be given to excluding several common disorders: celiac sprue, microscopic colitis, IBD, and bile salt diarrhea. The prevalence of celiac disease in the Western world in the white population is estimated to be about 1% with a slightly higher prevalence in female patients.[50] Decision analysis supports screening for this disorder when the prevalence is at this level, and American College of Gastroenterology (ACG) guidelines have also supported having a low threshold for screening, particularly in patients with IBS-diarrhea (IBS-D) or IBS-mixed (IBS-M)[51,52] Recommended screening consists of a tissue transglutaminase immunglobulin A (tTG-IgA) level as well as an IgA level.[51] Two percent of the celiac population is IgA deficient so obtaining the IgA level helps to determine whether the tTG assay result is valid.[50] For patients with IgA deficiency the recommended test is the deamidated antigliadin IgG antibody with the tTG IgG (less sensitive than tTG-IgA).[53]

Microscopic colitis should be considered in the differential of patients with IBS-D. Certain symptoms, such as age more than 50 years, shorter duration of symptoms, presence of autoimmune disorders, introduction of new medications (nonsteroidal antiinflammatory drugs, proton-pump inhibitors, olmesartan, selective serotonin reuptake inhibitors [SSRIs]), nocturnal symptoms, and weight loss should increase the concern for this disorder.[54] In these cases the literature supports colonoscopy with random biopsies.[51,55]

Concern for Crohn disease and ulcerative colitis (IBD) also enters into the IBS diagnostic picture and patients may have overlapping symptoms. The practical question is how often IBD occurs in patients being screened for IBS. A prospective study of patients with IBS and control patients undergoing colonoscopy revealed that IBD was found in less than 1% of patients with IBS and none of the control patients.[55] Unless there are alarm features, colonoscopy is not the place to start to distinguish these two disorders. Instead, 2 biomarkers, fecal calprotectin and C-reactive protein (CRP), have been assessed in systematic reviews with meta-analyses and have shown utility. Both are measures of inflammation. A fecal calprotectin level less than 40 μg/g or CRP level less than .5 mg/dL were associated with a less than 1% risk of IBD in patients with IBS with usual symptoms.[56] Fecal calprotectin was also found to be a cost-effective screening test.[57]

Bile salt diarrhea should be considered in patients who have undergone cholecystectomy.[58] The presumed mechanism is that unabsorbed bile acids in the colon stimulate water and electrolyte secretion, thereby increasing transit. Usually a trial of a bile salt sequestrant agent (eg, cholestyramine) is tried. Although several assays are available to detect bile salt diarrhea, they have not been widely available. These tests include SeHCAT (tauroselcholic [selenium 75] acid) retention test, serum C4 measurement, and fecal bile acid measurement.[7] Increased availability of these tests would help identify those individuals who would be most likely to respond to treatment with a bile salt sequestrant.

Although IBS-C has been reported to occur after infectious gastroenteritis, IBS-D is more common. This entity, postinfectious IBS (PI-IBS), is thought to occur because of changes in the intestinal flora, which happens in about 10% of patients who develop bacterial gastroenteritis.[14] Some patients remember the precipitating event but others do not. Reliable biomarkers exist for celiac disease but not for IBS to date. However, a recently developed assay holds promise to help in distinguishing IBS-D from IBD. Antivinculin and anti–cytolethal distending toxin B (anti-CdtB) antibodies were recently isolated in an animal model of campylobacter-induced PI-IBS.[59] Vinculin is a cytoplasmic actin-binding protein that is essential to the adhesional system between epithelial cells, and CdtB is a bacterial toxin that develops when cells are infected. Antivinculin and anti-CdtB levels were tested in 2375 patients from the Target 3 study for rifaximin and compared with patients with IBD (N = 142; 73 = Crohn's, 69 = ulcerative colitis), patients with celiac (N = 121), and healthy controls (HC = 43).[59] This assay, which recently became commercially available, had a specificity of 91.6% for anti-CdtB and 83.8% for antivinculin. The levels of these antibodies were statistically significantly higher in patients with IBS-D compared with patients with IBD. It did not perform as well in patients with celiac but a biomarker (tTG) already exists for this disorder.

Irritable Bowel Syndrome-Mixed

Patients with IBS-M may be the most challenging patients to diagnose because, without clinical detective work, it may be more difficult to ascertain whether they have mixed bowel habits or IBS-C that is responding to laxative agents. A careful history is helpful and may reveal that the patient has constipation followed by periods in which they have stools of variable consistency that are interpreted by the patient as diarrhea. A stool diary that records laxative use may also be enlightening. An abdominal radiograph can be used to show stool burden on the right or left side, which is suggestive of stool accumulation.

Overlap Syndromes in Female Patents

Overlap syndromes are more common in women. **Table 4** presents a summary of the overlap conditions that most commonly occur in IBS. The most common conditions include migraine headache, temporomandibular joint syndrome, fibromyalgia, joint hypermobility syndrome, interstitial cystitis, and anxiety and depression.[8] Other functional GI disorders, such as gastroesophageal disease and dyspepsia, are often reported in all patients with IBS. In addition, there are gynecologic conditions that commonly overlap, including endometriosis, dysmenorrhea, chronic pelvic pain, and vulvodynia.[8]

Table 4 Overlap conditions associated with IBS	
Neurologic	Migraine headaches
Musculoskeletal	Fibromyalgia Joint hypermobility syndrome Temporomandibular joint syndrome
GI	GERD Dyspepsia Pelvic floor dysfunction
Genitourinary	Bladder pain/interstitial cystitis Chronic cyclic pelvic pain Dyspareunia Dysmenorrhea Endometriosis Adenomyosis Vulvodynia
Psychological	Anxiety Depression
Other	Chronic fatigue syndrome

Abbreviation: GERD, gastroesophageal reflux disease.

A common pathogenesis for these disorders has not been elucidated but is similar to those suggested in IBS.[8]

The presence of these disorders has implications for diagnosis and treatment and may strengthen the clinical suspicion that a patient has IBS. Lackner and colleagues[60] showed that some patients with IBS have as many as 5 comorbid conditions. These patients usually have more severe symptoms and require a more comprehensive approach to treatment.

Between 12% and 23% of menstruating women have endometriosis. However, there is no good noninvasive screening tests so clinical suspicion is necessary to make this diagnosis.[61] The signs and symptoms of this disorder (abdominal pain and altered bowel function) meet the clinical criteria for IBS. One study showed that women with endometriosis are 6 times more likely to be diagnosed with IBS.[62] Symptoms that correlated with endometriosis in women who had IBS and also had laparoscopically proven endometriosis were worsening of symptoms premenstrually and having intermenstrual bleeding.[62] On physical examination, patients more commonly had vaginal forniceal tenderness. The gold standard for diagnosis is laparoscopic examination with biopsies histologically confirming the presence of endometriosis.

Other gynecologic conditions are also seen in patients with IBS, such as chronic pelvic pain, vulvodynia, and dysmenorrhea.

CLINICAL MANAGEMENT
General Principles

The variable severity of IBS must be taken into account when developing a treatment approach to patients. Although no global consensus definition of severity exists, IBS can be classified as mild, moderate, or severe depending on multiple measures, including symptoms (particularly abdominal pain), health-related quality of life (QOL), presence of comorbid health conditions and psychological distress, and health care costs. In addition, the health care setting may also influence the severity of disease that clinicians encounter; for example, there is a predominance of milder disease in the primary care setting. Although previous studies estimated that 5% of the patients seen had severe disease,[63] newer studies have shown a prevalence as high as 19% to 34%.[64,65] Women have also been described as having more severe disease.[66] Increasingly, evidence supports that patients' perceptions of severity are linked to their health-related QOL as well as their abdominal symptoms.[67] The cornerstone of therapy is developing a therapeutic clinician-patient relation. Drossman[68] outlined the core concepts of optimizing communication skills in patients with functional GI disorders. Drossman[68] detailed many important concepts, such as active listening, empathy, setting realistic goals, educating and reassuring patients, as well as setting boundaries and dealing with time constraints. A video link showing these concepts can be found on http://www.youtube.com/watch?v=IDaG0rlR.[68]

Successful treatment also depends on a global view. The Rome Foundation has developed an invaluable tool called the multidimensional clinical profile to assess and integrate information about the illness of a patient with IBS into a meaningful treatment plan. This profile takes into account and defines the following features: categorical diagnosis (meeting Rome Criteria of diagnosis), clinical modifiers (subtype; eg, IBS-C, PI-IBS), psychosocial factors, the impact of symptoms on daily activities, and the presence of physiologic modifiers on function and biomarkers (eg, a positive lactose breath test).[69]

Dietary Strategies for Management of Irritable Bowel Syndrome Symptoms

Diet and irritable bowel syndrome

Exacerbation of symptoms among patients with IBS has been described to occur most commonly in relation to food ingestion, stress, and the menstrual cycle.[70–72] Up to 90% of patients with IBS restrict their diets to prevent or improve their symptoms.[73] Only recently have food-related symptoms received more attention and emerging evidence supports dietary management for patients with IBS.[74] Ingestion of food, especially fat, stimulates the gastro-colonic motor response, which in those with IBS leads to an exaggerated physiologic response causing postprandial pain and rectal urgency. It has been suggested that tryptophan, histamine, and related compounds may modulate mood and provide an initial stimulus for persistent visceral hypersensitivity.[75,76]

True food allergies are uncommon in IBS, but sensitivities are frequently reported.[73] Only 11% to 27% of patients with IBS correctly identify the offending agent stimulating symptoms in formal, blinded food challenge studies.[77] Immune-mediated responses to food components may play a role. Subtle structural changes were seen in the duodenal mucosa using confocal endomicroscopy when the small intestines of patients with IBS were directly exposed to certain food antigens.[78] This finding suggests that some patients with IBS mount an immunologic response to dietary components leading to a microenteropathy related to primary or acquired food sensitivity such as can be seen PI-IBS.[79] Patients report some food constituents as more problematic, such as wheat, fruit, and vegetables, which has led to substantial focus on the role of 2 dietary triggers: gluten and fermentable oligosaccharides, disaccharides, monosaccharides, and polyols (FODMAPs).[73,80]

Gluten and irritable bowel syndrome

Several studies have shown that a gluten-free diet can improve IBS symptoms in a subset of patients.[81,82] A 4-week, randomized controlled trial evaluating the efficacy of a gluten-free diet in patients with IBS-D and without celiac disease reported increased stool frequency, as well as altered intestinal permeability (measured by urine lactulose/rhamnose ratio) and immune activation, in the presence of gluten. Bowel movement frequency was reduced in patients randomized to a gluten-free diet compared with patients consuming gluten, and this effect was more significant in patients with either of the celiac-associated genes HLA-DQ2 or HLA-DQ8.[81] These genes are seen in virtually all patients with celiac disease but are present in approximately 30% of the general population.[83] In another study, the effect of gluten was assessed by a randomized, double-blind, placebo-controlled, rechallenge trial in 34 patients with IBS with a history of nonceliac gluten sensitivity (NCGS).[82] During 6 weeks, overall IBS symptoms were not adequately controlled in 68% of patients receiving gluten versus 40% receiving a gluten-free diet. Reintroduction of gluten to these patients with IBS was associated with worsened pain, bloating, stool consistency, and notably fatigue.

These patients may have NCGS, which is 1 or more IBS-type symptoms precipitated by ingestion of gluten-containing foods. These individuals do not satisfy the diagnostic criteria for celiac disease and have been ruled out for wheat allergy.[84,85] Mechanisms that have been proposed include an effect of gluten on mucosal integrity or cellular adherence[86] or that another component of wheat, the amylase trypsin inhibitor enzymatic family, triggers the innate immune system stimulating the release of proinflammatory cytokines in cells.[87] In addition, it may be that fructans, a nonabsorbable carbohydrate component of wheat, may cause of symptoms. At present there are no diagnostic criteria or serologic testing available for NCGS.

Fermentable oligosaccharides, disaccharides, monosaccharides, and polyols diet and irritable bowel syndrome

As suggested earlier, it may be fructans that cause IBS symptoms,[88,89] as shown in a double-blind crossover trial of 37 patients with IBS with self-reported NCGS who were randomly assigned to a diet of reduced low-fermentable, poorly absorbed, short-chain carbohydrates and then placed on either a gluten or whey protein challenge. In all participants, GI complaints consistently improved during reduced FODMAP intake, but significantly worsened to a similar degree when their diets included gluten or whey proteins.[88] FODMAPs are found in such foods as wheat, onions, some fruits and vegetables, sorbitol, and some dairy products (**Table 5**). These foods are not efficiently absorbed in the small intestine and therefore arrive in the colon where they produce hydrogen, methane, and hydrogen sulfide gases, which leads to increased colonic water secretion, motility, and sensation.[90] Aside from increased flatulence, FODMAPs do not cause GI symptoms in healthy adults but may be an important trigger of meal-related symptoms in patients with IBS, possibly as a consequence of underlying

Table 5
FODMAP food groups and exemplars

Fermentable Oligosaccharides		Disaccharides	Monosaccharides	Polyols
Fructans	**Galacto-oligosaccharides**	**Lactose**	**Fructose**	**Polyols**
Fruits	Legumes	Condensed milk	Fruits	Fruits
Apples	Chickpeas	Custard	Boysenberry	Apricots
Nectarines	Dry beans	Evaporated milk	Cherries	Avocado
Persimmon		Ice cream	Figs	Blackberries
Pomegranate		Milk	Mangoes	Plums
Watermelon		Soft unripened	Pears	Prunes
White peaches		cheeses	Sweeteners	Vegetables
Cereals/grains/		Yoghurt	Fructose	Cauliflower
starches			High-fructose	Mushrooms
Wheat			corn syrup	Sweet potato
Rye			Honey	Additives/
Barley				sweeteners
Nuts				Isomaltose
Cashews				Maltitol
Pistachios				Mannitol
Additives				Sorbitol
Inulin				Xylitol
Vegetables				
Artichoke				
Asparagus				
Beetroot				
Broccoli				
Brussels sprouts				
Fennel				
Garlic				
Green peas				
Leek				
Onion				
Corn				
Drinks				
Chicory-based				
coffee				
substitutes				

abnormalities in gut physiology and visceral sensation.[91] These theoretical concepts have been evaluated in recent clinical trials that have shown significant beneficial clinical effects on IBS symptoms through the adoption of a low-FODMAP diet.[91,92]

A randomized clinical trial in 30 patients with IBS found lower overall symptom scores on the low-FODMAP diet versus a typical Australian diet.[91] Seventy percent of patients with IBS felt better while receiving the low-FODMAP diet regardless of IBS subtype.

Limiting FODMAPs sounds like a tempting treatment option but the diet is complex, requiring supervision by a qualified dietitian. Also, the diet may suppress the growth of bacterial species such as bifidobacteria that are commonly regarded as important components of a healthy microbiome.[91,93] It is recommended that even responders to full FODMAP exclusion should gradually reintroduce FODMAP foods to identify the level of dietary restriction needed to maintain symptom benefit.

Fiber and irritable bowel syndrome

Fiber and fiber-based supplements accelerate colon transit, increase stool bulk, and facilitate passage, resulting in an increase in stool frequency. This increase can translate into clinically meaningful benefits for patients with chronic constipation and IBS-C. Fiber is often used as a first-line therapy but it should be started at a low dose and gradually titrated up to a total daily intake of 20 to 30 g. A recent meta-analysis reported modest benefits with fiber for global IBS symptoms.[94] In a subgroup analysis, soluble fiber (psyllium and ispaghula husk) but not insoluble fiber (wheat bran) was associated with improved IBS symptoms. **Table 6** outlines different types of fiber and their sources.

Exercise and Sleep

Physically active individuals have more frequent bowel movements and more rapid colon transit than sedentary individuals.[95] A randomized clinical trial of patients with IBS found significant reduction in IBS symptoms in those randomized to physical activity (20–60 minutes of moderate to vigorous exertion 3 times a week for 12 weeks) compared with patients randomized to usual care.[96] Therefore, patients with IBS, regardless of subtype, should be encouraged to increase their physical activity not only for their general well-being but to improve IBS symptoms.

The association between sleep and next-day pain has been shown in patients with chronic pain with nightly sleep disturbance predictive of next-day pain.[97] Self-reported sleep disturbances are associated with next-day symptoms in women with IBS.[98] A recent small study of 24 women found that subjects with poorer

Table 6
Sources of soluble and insoluble fiber (not all inclusive)

Soluble Fiber	Insoluble Fiber
Oatmeal/oat bran	Whole-wheat breads
Nuts and seeds	Barley
Dried peas	Couscous
Beans	Brown rice
Lentils	Wheat bran
Apples	Carrots
Pears	Zucchini
Strawberries	Celery
Blueberries	Whole-grain cereals

self-reported sleep quality predicted higher next-day abdominal pain, anxiety, and fatigue, but not GI symptom scores or depressed mood.[99]

Pharmacotherapy

It should be recognized that patients use many over-the-counter (OTC) medications to obtain symptomatic relief, such as digestive enzymes (lactase, β-galactosidase, and pancreatic enzymes), probiotics, simethicone, antidiarrheal agents, and stimulant and osmotic laxatives. Not all drugs are discussed in detail here but **Table 7** presents data on mechanism of action, dose (where applicable), quality of data and summary recommendations by ACG, and number needed to treat (NNT) for the IBS drugs/therapies discussed later.[77] Women predominate in almost all drug trials.

Complementary Medications

Enteric-coated peppermint oil and STW5 (Iberogast) are complementary medications that have been studied in patients with IBS.[13] STW5 (Iberogast) is an OTC standardized mixture of herbs (angelica root, bitter candy tuft, caraway fruit, celandine, chamomile flowers, lemon balm leaves, liquorice root, peppermint leaves, and St Mary's thistle). This medication has been used to treat other functional disorders, has a good side effect profile, and is thought to work on muscarinic and serotonergic receptors to affect GI muscle tone and secretion.[100] It is used to help bloating, gas, and dyspepsia. There is only 1 randomized placebo-controlled trial in 208 patients. In that small study, it did achieve statistical significance in improving its primary end points of improvement in abdominal pain ($P = .0009$) and global IBS symptoms ($P = .001$) after 4 weeks of treatment.[101]

Peppermint oil (Colpermin, IBGard) has been used for hundreds of years and is reputed to have antibacterial, antiinflammatory, and antispasmodic effects.[102] Peppermint oil has also shown benefit in IBS-D via its antispasmodic properties and also seems to alleviate bloating. Small clinical trials suggest benefit at a dose of 187 to 225 mg 3 times daily.[103] The most recent ACG guidelines on IBS gave peppermint oil a weak recommendation as a therapy but found it superior to placebo in improving IBS symptoms.[77] Two recent formulations (Colpermin, IBGard) are enteric coated to reduce the major side effect of reflux and to ensure that the medication gets to the small intestine, which is the presumed site of action. Both products have been evaluated in small, randomized, placebo-controlled trials and improved global IBS symptoms.[104,105] There is some evidence that peppermint oil may target the microbiome.[106]

DRUGS TARGETING THE MICROBIOME
Probiotics

Because intestinal flora, particularly SIBO, has been implicated in the pathogenesis of IBS, there has been growing interest in treatments targeting bacteria in the gut. Both probiotics and antibiotics have been used in this way. Probiotics are live bacteria that result in a health benefit to the host when taken in sufficient quantities. Probiotics improve global IBS symptoms, including abdominal pain, bloating, and flatulence, according to a recent meta-analysis.[107] However, data supporting the use of particular strains of bacteria are inconsistent and the trials heterogeneous. There have been some data to support use of *Bifidobacterium infantis* as well as *Lactobacillus acidophilus*, although sample sizes were small.[108,109] Overall the recommendation for use of probiotics is still weak.

Antibiotics

Antibiotics, particularly rifaximin, a poorly absorbed broad-spectrum agent, are also used to treat IBS-D and to some extent IBS-M. Patients who clearly have P-IBS

Table 7
Gut-directed pharmacotherapy for IBS

Medication	Mechanism of Action	Dose	ACG Level of Evidence/Recommendation	NNT
Complementary Medications				
Iberogast	Possibly muscarinic Possible serotonergic effects	20 drops in glass of water TID	NA	5
Peppermint oil	Antispasmodic Possibly antibacterial Possibly antiinflammatory	180–225 mg TID	Moderate/weak	3 (2–4)
Drugs Affecting the Microbiome				
Probiotics	Likely multiple	Varies	Weak/low	4
Antibiotics Rifaximin (IBS-D or IBS-M)	Altering gut flora Possibly reducing number of colonic bacteria	550 mg TID for 14 d	Weak/moderate	7–11
Drugs Targeting Diarrhea				
Loperamide	Mu-opioid agonist	Up to 16 mg/d	Very low	NA
Antispasmodics • Hyoscyamine • Dicyclomine	Anticholinergic effects	0.125 mg QID 10–20 mg QID	Low/weak	NA
Bile acid–binding agents • Colesevelam • Obeticholic acid • Colestipol • Cholestyramine	Bind bile acids	Dose varies according to agent	NA	NA

	Mechanism	Dose	Quality/recommendation	NNT
5-HT$_3$ antagonists				
• Alosetron (United States only)	5-HT$_3$ antagonist	0.5–1 mg BID	Moderate/weak recommendation	7–8
• Ondansetron		4–8 mg TID	NA	NA
Opioid receptor modulator				
• Eluxadoline	Mu and kappa opioid agonist, delta opioid antagonist	75–100 mg BID	NA	NA
Drugs Targeting Constipation				
Osmotic laxative				
• PEG-3350	Osmotic effect	17 g daily	Very low/weak	NA
Prosecretory agents				
• Linaclotide	Guanylate cyclase-C agonist	290 µg QD (145 µg QD for CIC)	High/strong	5
• Lubiprostone	Chloride channel (ClC-2 activator)	8 µg BID (24 µg BID for CIC)	Moderate/strong	12
5-HT$_4$ agonist				
• Prucalopride	5-HT$_4$ agonist	2 mg daily	NA	NA

Abbreviations: ACG, American College of Gastroenterology; BID, twice daily; CIC, chronic idiopathic constipation; NA, not applicable; NNT, number needed to treat; QD, daily; TID, 3 times daily.

Data from Halland M, Saito Y. Irritable bowel syndrome: new and emerging treatments. BMJ 2015;350:h1622; and Ford AC, Moayyedi P, Lacy BE, et al. American College of Gastroenterology monograph on the management of irritable bowel syndrome and chronic idiopathic constipation. Am J Gastroenterol 2014; 109(Suppl 1):S2–26.

may also benefit because of the purported role of SIBO in these patients. Two large, randomized clinical trials, Target 1 and 2, revealed that rifaximin 550 mg by mouth 3 times a day for 2 weeks offered more relief of global symptoms than placebo (combined results 41% vs 32%; odds ratio [OR], 1.53; $P<.001$).[110,111] It also significantly relieved bloating (combined 40% vs 30%; OR, 1.56; $P<.001$). The Target 3 study assessed retreatment data on rifaximin and suggested that second and third courses of this antibiotic have efficacy similar to the first course.[112] Based on these data, rifaximin was recently approved by the US Food and Drug Administration (FDA) for the treatment of IBS-D. Other medications used to target IBS-D are discussed later.

DRUGS TARGETING DIARRHEA
Antidiarrheals

First-line therapy for IBS-D includes antidiarrheals, both OTC, such as loperamide, or prescription, such as diphenoxylate atropine. These antidiarrheals work by inhibiting peristalsis, prolonging transit time and reducing fecal volume. Loperamide is preferred to diphenoxylate atropine because it does not cross the blood-brain barrier.[113] It does not improve global symptoms of IBS and was given a very low recommendation by the most recent ACG guidelines.[77]

Antispasmodics

Antispasmodics include hyoscyamine, dicyclomine, and tiropramide (available in Europe), which have anticholinergic or calcium channel blocking properties that relax intestinal smooth muscle. They are generally safe except for dose-dependent effects such as constipation, dry mouth, and blurred vision.[114] They have not been shown to relieve global symptoms but they may have utility in symptomatic relief of postprandial diarrhea.

Bile Acid–binding Agents

Bile salt diarrhea, either caused by increased bile acid synthesis or impaired reabsorption, occurs in up to one-third of patients with IBS-D.[115] Bile acid sequestrants include colesevelam, obeticholic acid, colestipol, and cholestyramine. These medications increase intraluminal binding of bile acids and improve the frequency and form of bowel movements. Many physicians use them empirically to treat IBS-D but they have not been evaluated by the ACG. Recent studies have shown improvement in bowel function but have not assessed global IBS symptom improvement.[116,117]

Serotonergic Agents: 5-Hydroxytryptamine-3 Antagonists

Alosetron is a 5-hydroxytryptamine (5-HT)-3 antagonist that has been studied in patients with severe IBS-D. Alosetron is specifically approved in the United States for women with severe IBS-D that have not responded to traditional medical therapies. It has improved not only diarrhea but global IBS symptoms as well.[118] Because of rare severe side effects of ischemic colitis and significant chronic constipation it was put in a restricted use program that requires clinicians and patients to sign a form acknowledging these side effects. Ondansetron, which is a weaker 5-HT_3 antagonist approved for the treatment of nausea, was recently evaluated for the treatment of IBS-D. In doses of 4 to 8 mg, 1 to 3 times a day, it improved global symptoms as well as stool consistency, urgency, and bloating ($P<.002$ for all symptoms).[119] It did not improve pain.

Opioid Receptor Modulators

Eluxadoline, a mu and kappa opioid receptor agonist, delta receptor antagonist, was approved in 2015 for the treatment of IBS-D and is now available. It can improve abdominal pain and decrease transit time without inducing tolerance.[120] The most common side effects were nausea and abdominal pain with only mild constipation. In clinical trials it was noted to cause spasm of the sphincter of Oddi, resulting in pancreatitis, thus patients predisposed to this problem are discouraged from using this medication. Also, patients with history of constipation, pancreatitis, and obstruction of bile ducts, and those consuming more than 3 alcoholic drinks per day, are urged to avoid taking this medication.

Drugs Targeting Constipation: Osmotic and Stimulant Agents

Clinicians often recommend the osmotic agent polyethylene glycol-3350 as first-line therapy. To date, only 2 randomized placebo-controlled trials have been done. They did not show any improvement in pain and only 1 showed an improvement in bowel movements.[121,122] Hence ACG guidelines indicate that the level of evidence was too low to support its use.[77] Stimulant laxatives, like bisacodyl, are also often tried by providers to improve bowel movement frequency but there are no clinical trials in IBS for these agents. They are not recommended in the treatment of IBS-C.

Prosecretory Agents

The prosecretory agents linaclotide and lubiprostone both improve stool frequency and reduce abdominal pain. Linaclotide is a guanylate cyclase-C agonist that increases luminal chloride and fluid secretion. The approved dose for IBS-C is 290 µg daily. The chief side effect is diarrhea and the lower 145 µg dose approved for chronic idiopathic constipation (CIC) can be used off label for IBS. Taking the medication 30 to 60 minutes before meals can minimize the diarrhea. In October of 2015 results of a study in constipation comparing 72 µg versus 145 µg were presented to the FDA. The lower dose showed efficacy and is likely to yield another dose that can be used off label to treat IBS-C.[123] The higher dose of linaclotide approved in clinical trials showed a positive effect on colonic nociceptors in reducing abdominal pain.[124] Patients need to be encouraged to persevere in treatment because the nociceptive effect can take up 9 weeks to be apparent.[125]

Lubiprostone is a chloride channel activator that stimulates intestinal fluid secretion. The dose approved for IBS-C is 8 µg twice daily.[126] A 24-µg dose is approved for CIC, which allows titration to a higher dose in patients with more refractory symptoms. Nausea and diarrhea are the primary side effects of lubiprostone and nausea is a frequent cause for medication discontinuation. It is recommended that the drug be given with food in an effort to prevent nausea.

5-Hydroxytryptamine-4 Agonists

Prucalopride, a 5-HT$_4$ agonist currently approved in Europe and Canada, works by accelerating colonic transit. It is approved for women with CIC but could be used off label in IBS. It was shown to improve the number of spontaneous bowel movements in a recent meta-analysis.[127] Adverse reactions were minor, with headache being the most common side effect. The cardiac side effects have been extensively studied and it has been found to be safe.[128]

CENTRALLY ACTING MEDICATIONS AND THERAPIES

Tricyclic antidepressants (TCAs), SSRIs, and to a lesser extent selective norepinephrine reuptake inhibitors (SNRIs) have all been evaluated in the treatment of IBS (**Table 8**).[129] The medications are used for their effects on mood, motility, and pain perception. These medications are often used based on their side effect profile; for

Table 8
Centrally acting therapies/lifestyle changes for IBS

Drug/Therapy	IBS Symptom Treated	Dosing	ACG Quality of Evidence/ ACG Recommendation	AGA Level of Evidence	NNT
Centrally Acting Medications					
Tricyclic Antidepressants • Amitriptyline • Desipramine • Trimipramine • Imipramine • Doxepin	Used to treat primarily IBS-D and pain	10–150 mg/d depending on drug; average around 50 mg	High/weak	Low	4
SSRIs • Fluoxetine • Paroxetine • Citalopram	Used to treat global IBS symptoms	20 mg daily 10–50 mg/d 20–40 mg/d	High/weak	Low	4
SNRIs • Duloxetine • Venlafaxine • Desvenlafaxine	Can target pain; not yet adequately studied	30–120 mg/d 75–225 mg/d 50 mg/d	NA	NA	?
Centrally Acting Therapies					
Hypnotherapy/CBT	Global	6–12 sessions	High/weak	NA	2–4
Lifestyle					
Diet	Global	Varies with diet	Very low/weak	NA	NA
Exercise	Global	20–60 min vigorous activity 3–5 times/wk	NA	NA	6

Abbreviation: CBT, cognitive behavior therapy.

Data from Ford AC, Moayyedi P, Lacy BE, et al. American College of Gastroenterology monograph on the management of irritable bowel syndrome and chronic idiopathic constipation. Am J Gastroenterol 2014;109(Suppl 1):S2; and Castro J, Harrington AM, Hughes PA, et al. Linaclotide inhibits colonic nociceptors and relieves abdominal pain via guanylate cyclase-C and extracellular cyclic guanosine 3′,5′-monophosphate. Gastroenterology 2015;145:1334–46.

example, TCAs can cause constipation so are most often used to treat IBS-D. Usually, lower doses (10–25 mg) are used at bedtime to take advantage of their anticholinergic effects to cause drowsiness. SSRIs can have prokinetic effects and may be a better choice for patients with IBS-C or those patients with significant anxiety. SSRIs are also used in lower doses.[130] SNRIs (venlafaxine and duloxetine) potentially can be used in IBS, especially for treatment of abdominal pain, but have not been well studied.

PSYCHOLOGICAL THERAPIES

Psychological therapies are also centrally acting therapies, and are designed to improve anxiety and help manage symptoms (see **Table 8**). In a large meta-analysis of 2000 patients, 4 modalities showed efficacy compared with other therapies: cognitive behavior therapy (CBT), gut-directed hypnosis, multicomponent psychotherapy, and dynamic psychotherapy.[129] The NNT was calculated to be 4 (95% CI, 3–5). Although treatment is effective, lack of available therapists, poor insurance coverage, and social stigma have limited their use. It is hoped that the development of online therapies, particularly for CBT, may help bridge these gaps.

SUMMARY

IBS is a disorder that occurs primarily in women, causing significant morbidity and decreased QOL. It is a heterogeneous disorder whose pathophysiology is currently multifactorial and includes evolving concepts of motility, autonomic nervous system dysregulation, central and peripheral processing, and changes in gut permeability and the microbiome, which clearly are influenced by estrogen and progesterone. However, the full significance of why there is a female predominance in this disorder and the effects of the menstrual cycle and menopause also need to be more fully understood.

A confident diagnosis of IBS can be made based on considering the differential of the predominant bowel habit and excluding alarm features. In female patients, special consideration of overlap syndromes and gynecologic disorders should be made. Successful management of female patients with IBS also needs to include an understanding of female gender roles as well as establishing a caring, positive clinician-patient relationship. Treatment approach should encompass a healthy lifestyle that includes diet, adequate sleep, and physical activity. From there clinicians can use gut symptom–directed pharmacotherapy and psychological therapies as indicated by the severity of the disease. Further understanding of female hormones may eventually help develop therapies that work better in female patients.

REFERENCES

1. Chial HJ, Camilleri M. Gender differences in irritable bowel syndrome. J Gend Specif Med 2002;5:37–45.
2. Lovell RM, Ford AC. Global prevalence of and risk factors for irritable bowel syndrome: a meta-analysis. Clin Gastroenterol Hepatol 2012;10:712–21.
3. Lovell RM, Ford AC. Effect of gender on the prevalence of irritable bowel syndrome in the community: systematic review and meta-analysis. Am J Gastroenterol 2012;107(7):991–1000.
4. Maguen S, Madden E, Cohen B, et al. Association of mental health problems with gastrointestinal disorders in Iraq and Afghanistan veterans. Depress Anxiety 2014;31:160–5.

5. Adeyemo MA, Spiegel B, Chang L. Meta-analysis: do irritable bowel syndrome symptoms vary between men and women? Aliment Pharmacol Ther 2010;32: 738–55.

6. Herman J, Pokkunuri V, Braham L, et al. Gender distribution in irritable bowel syndrome is proportional to the severity of constipation relative to diarrhea. Gend Med 2010;7:240–6.

7. Chey WD, Kurlander J, Eswaran S. Irritable bowel syndrome – A clinical review. JAMA 2015;109:949–57.

8. Meleine M, Matricon J. Gender-related differences in irritable bowel syndrome: potential mechanisms of sex hormones. World J Gastroenterol 2014;20: 6725–43.

9. Eswaran W, Goel A, Chey WD. What role does wheat play in the symptoms of irritable bowel syndrome? Gastroenterol Hepatol 2013;9:85–91.

10. Posserud I, Ageforz P, Ekman R, et al. Altered visceral perceptual and neuroendocrine response in patients with irritable bowel syndrome during mental stress. Gut 2004;53:1102–8.

11. Quigley EM. Bacterial flora in irritable bowel syndrome: role in pathophysiology; implications for management. J Dig Dis 2007;8:2–7.

12. Crowell MD, Harris L, Jones MP, et al. New insights into the pathophysiology of irritable bowel syndrome: implications for future treatments. Curr Gastroenterol Rep 2005;7:272–9.

13. Halland M, Saito Y. Irritable bowel syndrome; new and emerging treatments. BMJ 2015;350:h1622.

14. Spiller R, Lam C. An update on post-infectious irritable bowel syndrome: role of genetics, immune activation, serotonin and altered microbiome. J Neurogastroenterol Motil 2012;3:258–68.

15. Wald A, VanThiel DH, Hoechsttetter L, et al. Gastrointestinal transit: the effect of the menstrual cycle. Gastroenterology 1981;80:1498–500.

16. Shah S, Nathan L, Singh R, et al. E2 and not P4 increases NO release from NANC nerves of the gastrointestinal tract: implications in pregnancy. Am J Physiol Regul Integr Comp Physiol 2001;280:R1546–54.

17. Unruh AM. Gender variations in clinical pain experience. Pain 1996;65:123–67.

18. Papka RE, Storey-Workley M. Estrogen receptor-alpha and -beta coexist in a subpopulation of sensory neurons of female rat dorsal root ganglia. Neurosci Lett 2002;319:71–4.

19. Myers B, Schulkin J, Greenwood-Van Meerveld B. Sex steroids localized to the amygdala increase pain responses to visceral stimulation in rats. J Pain 2011; 12:486–94.

20. Chieng BC, Christie MJ, Osborne PB. Characterization of neurons in the rat central nucleus of the amygdala: cellular physiology, morphology and opioid sensitivity. J Comp Neurol 2006;497:910–27.

21. Chang L, Mayer EA, Labus JS, et al. Effect of sex on perception of rectosigmoid stimuli in irritable bowel syndrome. Am J Physiol Regul Integr Comp Physiol 2006;291:R277–84.

22. Whitehead W, Cheskin LJ, Heller BR, et al. Evidence of exacerbation of irritable bowel syndrome during menses. Gastroenterology 1990;98:1485–9.

23. Houghton L, Jackson NA, Whorwell PJ, et al. Do male sex hormones protect from irritable bowel syndrome? Am J Gastroenterol 2000;95:2296–300.

24. Berman SM, Naliboff BD, Chang L, et al. Enhanced preattentive central nervous system reactivity in irritable bowel syndrome. Am J Gastroenterol 2002;97: 2791–7.

25. Berkley KJ. Sex differences in pain. Behav Brain Sci 1997;20:371–80 [discussion: 435–513].
26. Fillingim RM, Maixner W, Kincaid S, et al. Sex differences in temporal summation but not sensory-discriminative processing of thermal pain. Pain 1998;75:121–7.
27. Naliboff BD, Berman S, Chang L, et al. Sex-related differences in IBS patients: central processing of visceral stimuli. Gastroenterology 2003;124:1738–47.
28. Fukudo S, Kanazawa M, Mizuno T, et al. Impact of serotonin transporter-gene polymorphism on brain activation by colorectal distention. Neuroimage 2009; 47:946–51.
29. Labus J, Gupta A, Coveleskie K, et al. Sex differences in emotion-related cognitive processes in irritable bowel syndrome and healthy control subjects. Pain 2013;154:2088–99.
30. Alonso C, Guilarte M, Vicario M, et al. Maladaptive intestinal epithelial responses to life stress may predispose healthy women to gut mucosal inflammation. Gastroenterology 2008;135:163–72.e1.
31. Enmark E, Pelto-Huikko M, Grandien K, et al. Human estrogen receptor beta-gene structure, chromosomal localization, and expression pattern. J Clin Endocrinol Metab 1997;82:4258–65.
32. Homma H, Hu E, Xu DZ, et al. The female intestine is more resistant than the male intestine to gut injury and inflammation when subjected to conditions associated with shock states. Am J Physiol Gastrointest Liver Physiol 2005;288: G466–72.
33. Looijer-van Langen M, Hotte N, Dieleman LA, et al. Estrogen receptor-β signaling modulates epithelial barrier function. Am J Physiol Gastrointest Liver Physiol 2011;300:G621–6.
34. Cremon C, Gargano L, Morselli-Labate AM, et al. Mucosal immune activation in irritable bowel syndrome: gender-dependence and association with digestive symptoms. Am J Gastroenterol 2009;104:392–400.
35. Toner QB, Akman D. Gender role and irritable bowel syndrome: literature review and hypothesis. Am J Gastroenterol 2000;95:11–6.
36. Cheney AM. "Most girls want to be skinny": body (dis)satisfaction among ethnically diverse women. Qual Health Res 2011;21:1347–59.
37. Jack DC. Silencing the self: women and depression. Cambridge (MA): Harvard University Press; 1991.
38. Ali A, Toner BB, Stuckless N, et al. Emotional abuse, self-blame, and self-silencing in women with irritable bowel syndrome. Psychosom Med 2000;62: 76–82.
39. Longstreth GF, Thompson WG, Chey WD, et al. Functional bowel disorders. Gastroenterology 2006;130:1480–91.
40. Saad RJ, Rao SS, Koch KL, et al. Do stool form and frequency correlate with whole-gut and colonic transit? Results from a multicenter study in constipated individuals and healthy controls. Am J Gastroenterol 2010;105(2):403–11.
41. Lewis SJ, Heaton KW. Stool form scale as a useful guide to intestinal transit time. Scand J Gastroenterol 1997;32:920–4.
42. Ringel Y, Williams RE, Kalilani L, et al. Prevalence, characteristics, and impact of bloating symptoms in patients with irritable bowel syndrome. Clin Gastroenterol Hepatol 2009;7:68–72.
43. Tuteja AK, Talley NJ, Joos SK, et al. Abdominal bloating in employed adults: prevalence, risk factors, and association with other bowel disorders. Am J Gastroenterol 2008;103:1241–8.

44. Ratuapli SK, Bharucha AE, Noelting J, et al. Phenotypic identification and classification of functional defecatory disorders using high-resolution anorectal manometry. Gastroenterology 2013;144(2):314–22.e2.

45. Wald A, Bharucha AE, Cosman BC, et al. ACG clinical guidelines: management of benign anorectal disorders. Am J Gastroenterol 2014;109:1141–57.

46. Chey WD, Baker JRB, Shifferd J. Assessment of abdominal symptoms before and after biofeedback therapy in patients with dyssynergic defecation. Am J Gastroenterol 2012;107(Suppl 1):S718.

47. Davis DM, Marcet JE, Frattini JC, et al. Is it time to lower the recommended screening age for colorectal cancer? J Am Coll Surg 2011;213:352.

48. Torre LA, Bray F, Siegel RL, et al. Global cancer statistics. CA Cancer J Clin 2012;2015(65):87.

49. Power AM, Talley NJ, Ford AC. Association between constipation and colorectal cancer: systematic review and meta-analysis of observational studies. Am J Gastroenterol 2013;108(6):894–903.

50. Rönnblom A, Holmström T, Tanghöj H, et al. Celiac disease, collagenous sprue and microscopic colitis in IBD. Observations from a population-based cohort of IBD (ICURE). Scand J Gastroenterol 2015;50:1234–40.

51. Brandt LJ, Chey WD, Foxx-Orenstein AE, et al, American College of Gastroenterology Task Force on Irritable Bowel Syndrome. An evidence-based position statement on the management of irritable bowel syndrome. Am J Gastroenterol 2009;104(Suppl 1):S1–35.

52. Chow MA, Lebwohl B, Reilly NR, et al. Immunoglobulin A deficiency in celiac disease. J Clin Gastroenterol 2012;46(10):850–4.

53. Oxentenko AS, Murray JA. Ten things every gastroenterologist should know. Clin Gastroenterol Hepatol 2015;13:1396–404.

54. Macaigne G, Lahmek P, Locher C, et al. Microscopic colitis or functional bowel disease with diarrhea: a French prospective multicenter study. Am J Gastroenterol 2014;109:1461–70.

55. Chey WD, Nojkov B, Rubenstein JH, et al. The yield of colonoscopy in patients with non-constipated irritable bowel syndrome: results from a prospective, controlled US trial. Am J Gastroenterol 2010;105:859–65.

56. Menees SB, Kurlander J, Goel A, et al. Meta-analysis of the utility of common serum and fecal biomarkers in adults with IBS. Gastroenterology 2014;146:S194.

57. Yang Z, Clark N, Park KT. Effectiveness and cost-effectiveness of measuring fecal calprotectin in diagnosis of inflammatory bowel disease in adults and children. Clin Gastroenterol Hepatol 2014;12:253–62.

58. Wedlake L, A'Hern R, Russell D, et al. Systematic review: the prevalence of idiopathic bile acid malabsorption as diagnosed by SeHCAT scanning in patients with diarrhoea-predominant irritable bowel syndrome. Aliment Pharmacol Ther 2009;30:707–17.

59. Pimentel M, Morales W, Rezaie A, et al. Development and validation of a biomarker for diarrhea-predominant irritable bowel syndrome in human subjects. PLoS One 2015;10(5):e0126438, eCollection 2015.

60. Lackner JM, Ma CX, Keefer L, et al. Type, rather than number, of mental and physical comorbidities increases the severity of symptoms in patients with irritable bowel syndrome. Clin Gastroenterol Hepatol 2013;11(9):1147–57.

61. Brown J, Farquhar C. Endometriosis: an overview of Cochrane Reviews. Cochrane Database Syst Rev 2014;(3):Cd009590.

62. Seaman HE, Ballard KD, Wright JT, et al. Endometriosis and its coexistence with irritable bowel syndrome and pelvic inflammatory disease: findings from a national case-control study–Part 2. BJOG 2008;115:1392–6.
63. Drossman DA, Thompson WG. The irritable bowel syndrome: review and a graduated multicomponent treatment approach. Ann Intern Med 1992;116:1009–16.
64. Ricci J, Jhingran P, Harris W, et al. Impact of differences in severity of irritable bowel syndrome (IBS) on patient's well-being and resource use. Gastroenterology 2001;120:A406.
65. Luttecke KA. A three-part controlled study of trimebutine in the treatment of irritable colon syndrome. Curr Med Res Opin 1980;6:437–43.
66. Coffin B, Dapoigny M, Cloarec D, et al. Relationship between severity of symptoms and quality of life in 858 patients with irritable bowel syndrome. Gastroenterol Clin Biol 2004;28:11–5.
67. Lembo A, Ameen VZ, Drossman D. Irritable bowel syndrome: toward an understanding of severity. Clin Gastroenterol Hepatol 2005;3:717–25.
68. Drossman DA. 2012 David Sun lecture: helping your patient by helping yourself – how to improve the patient-physician relationship by optimizing communication skills. Am J Gastroenterol 2013;108:521–8.
69. Drossman DA. In: Multi-dimensional clinical profile (MDCP) for the functional gastrointestinal disorders. Raleigh (NC): The Rome Foundations; 2015. p. 3–14.
70. Cuomo R, Andreozzi P, Zito FP, et al. Irritable bowel syndrome and food interaction. World J Gastroenterol 2014;20:8837–45.
71. Posserud I, Strid H, Störsrud S, et al. Symptom pattern following a meal challenge test in patients with irritable bowel syndrome and healthy controls. United European Gastroenterol J 2013;1:358–67.
72. Shekhar PJ, Monaghan C, Morris J, et al. Rome III functional constipation and irritable bowel syndrome with constipation are similar disorders within a spectrum of sensitization regulated by serotonin. Gastroenterology 2013;145:749–57.
73. Hayes P, Corish C, O'Mahony E, et al. A dietary survey of patients with irritable bowel syndrome. J Hum Nutr Diet 2014;27(Suppl 2):36–47.
74. Heizer WD, Southern S, McGovern S. The role of diet in symptoms of irritable bowel syndrome in adults: a narrative review. J Am Diet Assoc 2009;109:1204–14.
75. Wouters MM. Histamine antagonism and postinflammatory visceral hypersensitivity. Gut 2014;63:1836–7.
76. Kelly JR, Kennedy PJ, Cryan JF, et al. Breaking down the barriers: the gut microbiome, intestinal permeability and stress-related psychiatric disorders. Front Cell Neurosci 2015;9:392.
77. Ford AC, Moayyedi P, Lacy BE, et al. American College of Gastroenterology monograph on the management of irritable bowel syndrome and chronic idiopathic constipation. Am J Gastroenterol 2014;109(Suppl 1):S2–26.
78. Fritscher-Ravens A, Schuppan D, Ellrichmann M, et al. Confocal endomicroscopy shows food-associated changes in the intestinal mucosa of patients with irritable bowel syndrome. Gastroenterology 2014;147:1012–20.e1014.
79. Rostami K. From microenteropathy to villous atrophy: what is treatable? Dig Liver Dis 2003;35:758–9.
80. Guo YB, Khuang K-M, Kuang L, et al. Association between diet and lifestyle habits and irritable bowel syndrome: a case-control study. Gut Liver 2015;9:649–56.

81. Vazquez-Roque MI, Camilleri M, Smyrk T, et al. A controlled trial of gluten-free diet in patients with irritable bowel syndrome-diarrhea: effects on bowel frequency and intestinal function. Gastroenterology 2013;144:903–11.e3.

82. Biesiekierski JR, Newnham ED, Irving PM, et al. Gluten causes gastrointestinal symptoms in subjects without celiac disease: a double-blind randomized placebo-controlled trial. Am J Gastroenterol 2011;106:508–14.

83. Sollid LM, Markussen G, Ek J, et al. Evidence for a primary association of celiac disease to a particular HLA-DQ alpha/beta heterodimer. J Exp Med 1989;169: 345–50.

84. Bizzaro N, Tozzoli R, Villalta D, et al. Cutting-edge issues in celiac disease and in gluten intolerance. Clin Rev Allergy Immunol 2012;42:279–87.

85. Ludvigsson JF, Leffler DA, Bai J, et al. The Oslo definitions for coeliac disease and related terms. Gut 2013;62:43–52.

86. Di Sabatino A, Corazza GR. Nonceliac gluten sensitivity: sense or sensibility? Ann Intern Med 2012;156:309–11.

87. Junker Y, Zeissig S, Kim SJ, et al. Wheat amylase trypsin inhibitors drive intestinal inflammation via activation of toll-like receptor 4. J Exp Med 2012;209:2395–408.

88. Biesiekierski JR, Peters SL, Newnham ED, et al. No effects of gluten in patients with self-reported non-celiac gluten sensitivity after dietary reduction of fermentable, poorly absorbed, short-chain carbohydrates. Gastroenterology 2013;145: 320–8.e1-3.

89. Rodrigo L, Blanco I, Bobes J, et al. Effect of one year of a gluten-free diet on the clinical evolution of irritable bowel syndrome plus fibromyalgia in patients with associated lymphocytic enteritis: a case-control study. Arthritis Res Ther 2014; 16:421103.

90. Murray K, Wilkinson-Smith V, Hoad C, et al. Differential effects of FODMAPs (fermentable oligo-, di-, mono-saccharides and polyols) on small and large intestinal contents in healthy subjects shown by MRI. Am J Gastroenterol 2014; 109:110–9.

91. Halmos EP, Power VA, Shepherd SJ, et al. A diet low in FODMAPs reduces symptoms of irritable bowel syndrome. Gastroenterology 2014;146:67–75.e5.

92. Ong DK, Mitchell SB, Barrett JS, et al. Manipulation of dietary short chain carbohydrates alters the pattern of gas production and genesis of symptoms in irritable bowel syndrome. J Gastroenterol Hepatol 2010;25:1366–73.

93. Staudacher HM, Lomer MCE, Anderson JL, et al. Fermentable carbohydrate restriction reduces luminal bifidobacteria and gastrointestinal symptoms in patients with irritable bowel syndrome. J Nutr 2012;142:1510–8.

94. Moayyedi P, Quigley EM, Lacy BE, et al. The effect of fiber supplementation on irritable bowel syndrome: a systematic review and meta-analysis. Am J Gastroenterol 2014;109:1367–74.

95. Song BK, Cho KO, Jo Y, et al. Colon transit time according to physical activity level in adults. J Neurogastroenterol Motil 2012;18:64–9.

96. Johannesson E, Simren M, Strid H, et al. Physical activity improves symptoms in irritable bowel syndrome: a randomized controlled trial. Am J Gastroenterol 2011;106:915–22.

97. Palermo TM, Law E, Churchill SS, et al. Longitudinal course and impact of insomnia symptoms in adolescents with and without chronic pain. J Pain 2012;13:1099–106.

98. Jarrett M, Heitkemper M, Cain KC, et al. Sleep disturbance influences gastrointestinal symptoms in women with irritable bowel syndrome. Dig Dis Sci 2000;45: 952–9.

99. Buchanan DT, Cain K, Heitkemper M, et al. Sleep measures predict next-day symptoms in women with irritable bowel syndrome. J Clin Sleep Med 2014; 10:1003–9.

100. Ottillinger B, Storr M, Malfertheiner P, et al. STW 5 (Iberogast®)—a safe and effective standard in the treatment of functional gastrointestinal disorders. Wien Med Wochenschr 2013;163:65–72.

101. Madisch A, Holtmann G, Plein K, et al. Treatment of irritable bowel syndrome with herbal preparations: results of a double-blind, randomized, placebo-controlled, multi-centre trial. Aliment Pharmacol Ther 2004;19:271–9.

102. Rozza AL, Meira de Faria F, Souza Brito AR, et al. The gastroprotective effect of menthol: involvement of anti-apoptotic, antioxidant and anti-inflammatory activities. PLoS One 2014;9:1–6.

103. Khanna R, MacDonald J, Levesque B. Peppermint oil for the treatment of irritable bowel syndrome: a systematic review and meta-analysis. J Clin Gastroenterol 2014;48:505–12.

104. Merat S, Khalili S, Mostajabi P, et al. The effect of enteric-coated, delayed-release peppermint oil on irritable bowel syndrome. Dig Dis Sci 2010;55: 1385–90.

105. Cash BD, Epstein MS, Shah SM. A novel delivery system of peppermint oil is an effective therapy for irritable bowel syndrome symptoms. Dig Dis Sci 2015; 61(2):560–71.

106. Imai H, Osawa K, Yasuda H, et al. Inhibition by the essential oils of peppermint and spearmint of the growth of pathogenic bacteria. Microbios 2001;106(Suppl 1):31–9.

107. Ford AC, Quigley EM, Lacy BE, et al. Efficacy of prebiotics, probiotics and synbiotics in irritable bowel syndrome and chronic idiopathic constipation systematic review and meta-analysis. Am J Gastroenterol 2014;109:1547–61.

108. Whorwell PJ, Altringer L, Morel J, et al. Efficacy of an encapsulated probiotic Bifidobacterium infantis 35624 in women with irritable bowel syndrome. Am J Gastroenterol 2006;101:1581–90.

109. Sinn DH, Song JH, Kim HJ, et al. Therapeutic effect of Lactobacillus acidophilus-SDC 2012, 2013 in patients with irritable bowel syndrome. Dig Dis Sci 2008; 53:2714–8.

110. Menees S, Maneerattannaporn M, Kim HM, et al. Efficacy of rifaximin in patients with irritable bowel syndrome: a meta-analysis. Am J Gastroenterol 2012;107: 28–35.

111. Pimentel M, Lembo A, Chey WD, et al. Rifaximin therapy for patients with irritable bowel syndrome without constipation. N Engl J Med 2011;364:22–32.

112. FDA approves 2 therapies to treat IBS-D. Available at: http://www.fda. gov/NewsEvents/Newsroom/PressAnnouncements/ucm448328.htm. Accessed February 11, 2015.

113. Jailwala J, Imperiale TF, Kroenke K, et al. Pharmacologic treatment of the irritable bowel syndrome: a systematic review of randomized, controlled trials. Ann Intern Med 2000;133:136–47.

114. Ford AC, Talley NJ, Spiegel BM, et al. Effect of fibre, antispasmodics, and peppermint oil in the treatment of irritable bowel syndrome: systematic review and meta-analysis. BMJ 2008;337:a2313.

115. Bajor A, Tomblom H, Rudling M, et al. Increased colonic bile acid exposure: a relevant factor for symptoms and treatment in IBS. Gut 2015;6:84–92.

116. Camilleri M, Acosta A, Busciglio I, et al. Effect of colesevelam on faecal bile acids and bowel functions in diarrhoea-predominant irritable bowel syndrome. Aliment Pharmacol Ther 2015;41(5):438–48.

117. Walters JR, Johnston IM, Nolan JD, et al. The response of patients with bile acid diarrhoea to the farnesoid X receptor agonist obeticholic acid. Aliment Pharmacol Ther 2015;41(1):54–64.

118. Camilleri M, Mayer EA, Drossman DA, et al. Improvement in pain and bowel function in female irritable bowel patients with alosetron, a 5-HT3 receptor antagonist. Aliment Pharmacol Ther 1999;13:1149–59.

119. Garsed K, Chernova J, Hastings M, et al. A randomised trial of ondansetron for the treatment of irritable bowel syndrome with diarrhoea. Gut 2014;63:1617–25.

120. Dove LS, Lembo A, Randall CW, et al. Eluxadoline benefits patients with irritable bowel syndrome with diarrhea in a phase 2 study. Gastroenterology 2013; 145(2):329–38.

121. Awad RA, Camacho S. A randomized, double-blind, placebo-controlled trial of polyethylene glycol effects on fasting and postprandial rectal sensitivity and symptoms in hypersensitive constipation-predominant irritable bowel syndrome. Colorectal Dis 2010;12:1131–8.

122. Chapman RW, Stanghellini V, Geraint M, et al. Randomized clinical trial: macrogol/PEG 3350 plus electrolytes for treatment of patients with constipation associated with irritable bowel syndrome. Am J Gastroenterol 2013;108:1508–15.

123. Ironwood reports positive top-line results from phase III trial of 72 mcg linaclotide in adults with chronic idiopathic constipation. Available at: http://investor. ironwoodpharma.com/releasedetail.cfm?ReleaseID=936437. Accessed May 11, 2015.

124. Castro J, Harrington AM, Hughes PA, et al. Linaclotide inhibits colonic nociceptors and relieves abdominal pain via guanylate cyclase-C and extracellular cyclic guanosine 3',5'-monophosphate. Gastroenterology 2015;145:1334–46.

125. Rao S, Lembo AJ, Shiff SJ, et al. A 12-week, randomized, controlled trial with a 4-week randomized withdrawal period to evaluate the efficacy and safety of linaclotide in irritable bowel syndrome with constipation. Am J Gastroenterol 2012;11:1714–24.

126. Drossman DA, Chey WD, Johanson JF, et al. Clinical trial: lubiprostone in patients with constipation-associated irritable bowel syndrome-results of two randomized, placebo-controlled studies. Aliment Pharmacol Ther 2009;29: 329–41.

127. Shin A, Camilleri M, Kolar G, et al. Systematic review with meta-analysis: highly selective 5-HT4 agonists (prucalopride, velusetrag or naronapride) in chronic constipation. Aliment Pharmacol Ther 2014;39:239–53.

128. Mendzelevski B, Ausma J, Chanter DO, et al. Assessment of the cardiac safety of prucalopride in healthy volunteers: a randomized, double-blind, placebo- and positive-controlled thorough QT study. Br J Clin Pharmacol 2012;73:203–9.

129. Ford AC, Quigley EM, Lacy BE, et al. Effect of antidepressants and psychological therapies, including hypnotherapy, in irritable bowel syndrome: systematic review and meta-analysis. Am J Gastroenterol 2014;109:1350–65.

130. Drossman DA. Beyond tricyclics: new ideas for treating patients with painful and refractory functional gastrointestinal symptoms. Am J Gastroenterol 2009;104: 2897–902.

Chronic Constipation

Darren M. Brenner, MD, AGAF[a],*, Marmy Shah, MD[b]

KEYWORDS

- Constipation • Pathophysiology • Motility • Diagnostic testing
- Anorectal manometry • Laxatives • Secretagogues

KEY POINTS

- Chronic constipation is a disabling disorder affecting approximately 20% of the world's population. In outpatient clinics in the United States it is 1 of the 5 most commonly diagnosed gastrointestinal disorders.
- There are many etiologies for constipation and these can overlap. Constipation may be due to a combination of normal or slow transit, an evacuation disorder, or secondary to an underlying medical condition.
- Old and newer diagnostics are available to differentiate the causes of chronic constipation. Those most commonly used include radiopaque marker testing, anorectal manometry, balloon expulsion testing, defecography, and wireless motility capsule.
- Regularly used therapeutic classes include stool softeners, emollients, bulking substances, stimulant and osmotic agents, and the newest category of agents: the secretagogues.

CHRONIC CONSTIPATION
Introduction

Chronic idiopathic constipation (CIC) is one of the most common digestive complaints in the general population. This disorder affects approximately 20% of individuals, and is 1 of the 5 most common issues assessed by practicing gastroenterologists in the United States.[1,2] Data recently collected from the National Ambulatory Medical Care Survey and National Hospital Ambulatory Medical Care Survey recently identified CIC as the fourth most common gastrointestinal (GI) diagnosis made in emergency departments (EDs) between 2006 and 2012. This study found 800,000 visits representing

Disclosures: Nothing to disclose (M. Shah). Consultant/Advisor for the following: Astra Zeneca, Ironwood, Actavis, Salix, P&G, QoL Medical, Commonwealth Laboratories, GI Health Foundation. Speaker: Astra Zeneca, Ironwood, Actavis, Salix, P&G, GI Health Foundation Pending Grants: AstraZeneca (D.M. Brenner).
[a] Division of Gastroenterology, Northwestern University Feinberg School of Medicine, 675 North Saint Clair Avenue, Suite 17-250, Chicago, IL 60611, USA; [b] Division of Gastroenterology and Nutrition, Loyola University Medical Center, 2160 South First Avenue, Building 54-Room 167, Maywood, IL 60153, USA
* Corresponding author.
E-mail address: darren-brenner@northwestern.edu

Gastroenterol Clin N Am 45 (2016) 205–216
http://dx.doi.org/10.1016/j.gtc.2016.02.013
0889-8553/16/$ – see front matter © 2016 Elsevier Inc. All rights reserved.

a 60% increase over this time period. Combining ED, office, and hospital outpatient visits in 2010, CIC represented 3.7 million evaluations, ranking as the fourth most commonly diagnosed GI disorder in the United States.[3]

Although considered benign in most cases, CIC can result in chronic illness with potentially serious complications including fecal impaction, incontinence, hemorrhoids, anal fissures, bleeding, and in the most extreme cases colon perforation. These aside, the disorder alone is associated with significantly impaired quality of life.[4] Chronic constipation is most commonly associated with increasing age. There is also increased prevalence among women (median female-to-male ratio of 1:5:1) with women more likely to use laxatives and seek health care for their constipation. Although the exact etiologic mechanisms have yet to be elucidated, anatomic and hormonal differences (ie, elevations in serum progesterone) appear to play a role. This may also explain why some women experience increased rates or exacerbations of their symptoms with pregnancy and/or during hormonal fluctuations within their menstrual cycles. Other risk factors correlated with the development of CIC include decreased daily physical activity and/or low fiber intake, low socioeconomic status, and reduced education.[1]

Currently, CIC is defined via the Rome III criteria as documented later in this article.[5] However, updates to these are expected with the publication of the Rome IV criteria in 2016 (**Box 1**).

Etiology/Pathophysiology

The pathogenesis of CIC is complex; it has the potential to be derived from a singular entity or multiple overlapping etiologies (**Fig. 1**). Based on current schemata, chronic constipation is usually classified into 2 categories: idiopathic (or primary) and secondary constipation. The distinctions between the 2 types are important, as identification of etiology can help guide therapy.[6]

Secondary Constipation

Multiple biological, environmental, and pharmaceutical precipitants exist with the potential to cause CIC (**Fig. 2**). Pharmaceuticals are one of the most common contributors to the development of constipation. Major categories of secondary systemic

---

Box 1
Rome III diagnostic criteria for functional constipation

Infrequent loose stools

Insufficient criteria for a diagnosis of irritable bowel syndrome (IBS)

≥ 2 of the following symptoms present for ≥ 6 months

<3 bowel movements (BMs) per week

Lumpy or hard stools $\geq 25\%$ BM

Straining $\geq 25\%$ of BM

Sensation of incomplete evacuation $\geq 25\%$ BM

Sensation of anorectal blockage $\geq 25\%$ BM

Use of manual maneuvers to facilitate defecation $\geq 25\%$ BM

Data from Longstreth GF, Thompson WG, Chey WD, et al. Functional bowel disorders. Gastroenterology 2006;130:1480

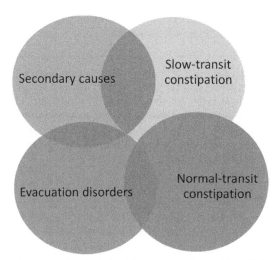

Fig. 1. Potential etiologies of CIC. (*Adapted from* Brenner DM, Chey WD. An evidence-based review of novel and emerging therapies for constipation in patients taking opioid analgesics. Am J Gastroenterol Suppl 2014;2:40; with permission.)

disorders include endocrinopathies (eg, diabetes, hypothyroidism), metabolic abnormalities (eg, hypercalcemia or hypocalcemia, hypokalemia), neuropathic or myopathic disorders (eg, scleroderma, multiple sclerosis, Parkinson disorder, amyotrophic lateral sclerosis), and mechanical or pseudo-obstructions.[6] An extensive list of potential causal factors is well described elsewhere in the clinical literature.[7]

Idiopathic Constipation

Normal transit
Normal transit constipation is usually defined as a subtype of CIC in which adults have adequate colonic transit rates. Individuals often complain of difficult evacuation,

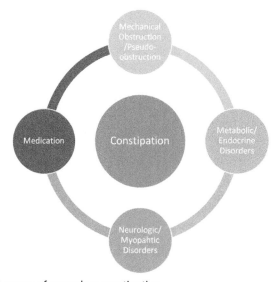

Fig. 2. Potential causes of secondary constipation.

straining, the passage of hard stools, and abdominal discomfort. Most are subsequently diagnosed with irritable bowel syndrome.[8]

Slow transit

Slow transit constipation (STC) is most commonly characterized by infrequent defecation and blunted urge to defecate due to delayed transit of fecal material through the colon. These changes have been associated with impaired colonic propulsive motor activity, delayed emptying of the proximal colon, and an attenuated gastrocolic reflex. Immunohistochemical studies have revealed a paucity of interstitial cells of Cajal. Whether this a secondary consequence of CIC or the driving factor for the development of CIC has yet to be elucidated.[9]

Evacuation Disorders

This refers to difficulty or an inability to expel stool and is usually due to anatomic (ie, rectocele, enterocele, anal stenosis, excessive perineal descent, intussusception, rectal prolapse) or functional disorders of the anorectum. The most frequently identified of such disorders is dyssynergic defecation, which is known by many pseudonyms including pelvic floor dyssynergia, anismus, or obstructive defecation. All indicate a failure to coordinate abdominopelvic musculature leading to inadequate rectal propulsive forces, paradoxic anal sphincter and/or puborectalis muscle contraction, inadequate anal sphincter relaxation, or a combination thereof.[7]

CLINICAL EVALUATION

A meticulous history and physical examination are the most important elements of initial evaluation of patient with chronic constipation. Laboratory tests, endoscopic evaluation, and radiographic studies are not routinely recommended. These procedures should, however, be considered in patients with alarm features, such as hematochezia, weight loss, a family history of colon cancer or inflammatory bowel disease, anemia, positive fecal occult blood, or acute constipation in elderly. Further diagnostic workup is recommended for patients who fail conservative treatment and the etiology of their constipation remains unknown.[9]

History

A careful history focuses on the onset/duration of symptoms, bowel movement frequency, stool texture and caliber, straining, sensations of incomplete evacuation or mechanical obstruction, and the need for manual maneuvers to facilitate evacuation. However, no subjective symptom is sine qua none for a particular constipation subtype. The Bristol Stool Form Scale and symptoms diaries are useful adjunctive tools for defining fecal transit and overall bowel patterns.[10] A complete medical, surgical, dietary, and medication history are key to identifying secondary causes of constipation. Prior laxative use, doses, frequency, and response are important to help guide therapy.

Physical Examination

The most valuable components of a physical examination for chronic constipation include careful inspection of the perineum and the digital rectal examination. Inspection of the perineum is performed to identify fissures, hemorrhoids, excoriations, a gaping or patulous anus, or evidence of stool leakage. An assessment for appropriate perineal descent while a patient strains also should be observed. Identification of rectal prolapse may require the patient to strain in a squatting position. Palpation of the anal canal and rectum can identify rectal masses, strictures, hemorrhoids, rectoceles, and rectal tenderness. If stool is palpated in the rectal vault, the consistency and any evidence of blood should be noted. Sphincter tone at rest, with squeeze, and bear down are defined as normal, weak, or increased. During bear down or simulating defecation, the examiner may assess abdominal push effort by placing the other hand on patient's abdomen. A lack of anal sphincter and puborectalis relaxation, paradoxic contraction of these muscles, or poor abdominal push efforts may suggest dyssynergia.[11]

Diagnostic Testing

Routine bloodwork, including a complete blood count, chemistry panel, and thyroid function test, are often routinely performed to evaluate for metabolic diseases. Colonoscopy is recommended in those who meet age-appropriate guidelines for colon cancer screening or in those with alarming symptoms, as previously mentioned. Routine radiographic evaluation by x-ray or barium enema has little utility when routinely obtained and should be discouraged. However, patients who have medication-refractory symptoms should be further evaluated and updated algorithms for the assessment of these individuals have been recently published by both the American Gastroenterological Association (AGA) and the American College of Gastroenterology (ACG).[12,13]

Physiologic Testing

Anorectal manometry

Anorectal manometry (ARM) in association with balloon expulsion testing (BET) is considered a first-line diagnostic in patients with medication-refractory CIC.[12,13] It is used to evaluate the functional performance of the pelvic floor musculature. A probe (usually high-resolution or high-definition) with circumferential pressure sensors along its length and a balloon at the tip is placed across the anal canal of a patient who is positioned in left later decubitus position. This probe can then be used to measure puborectalis and anal sphincter pressures at rest, with squeeze, during a cough maneuver, and attempted defecation, rectal sensation and compliance, the presence of the rectoanal inhibitory reflex, which is typically absent in patients with Hirschsprung and scleroderma.[14]

Rectal balloon expulsion test

The BET is another first-line diagnostic in the evaluation for dyssynergic defecation. The test is usually performed using a balloon filled with 50 mL water or air. However, some experts are advocating using a volume threshold consistent with a patient's desired urge to defecate. Although there are discrepancies and a lack of standardization regarding the amount of time considered appropriate for a positive study, most physicians agree that more than 5 minutes is abnormal, with many advocating a threshold of more than 1 minute.[7] This study is usually performed in conjunction with an ARM.

Radiopaque marker study

The radiopaque marker study (ROM) attempts to assess the rate of transit of stool through the colon to determine whether the etiology of constipation is transit related. Although many techniques are available, the simplest, the Hinton technique, uses a single capsule of 24 radiopaque markers. This is ingested on day 1 by the patient. An abdominal radiograph is obtained 120 hours later (day 6) and STC is indicated if there is retention of greater than 20% of markers. As up to 50% or patients with dyssynergic defecation may have comorbid slow transit, it is recommended to exclude dyssynergia before performing ROM testing.[14]

Defecography

Defecography is performed by injecting contrast material into the rectum and monitoring of defecation parameters via fluoroscopy. The study is useful for evaluating potential anatomic abnormalities causing CIC. Although not recommended as an initial diagnostic maneuver, it has benefits including testing in the natural-seated position. Findings suggestive of pelvic floor dysfunction, ineffective stool evacuation, and structural abnormalities (ie, rectoceles, rectal prolapse, or intussusception) can be identified on defecography. Patients with impaired mobility and embarrassment often find this examination difficult to tolerate. In addition, there is variation in quality of the test depending on operator and intraobserver bias. Recently, functional MRI has emerged as a tool to evaluate the anatomy and dynamics of the pelvic floor but this is performed in the left lateral decubitus position similar to ARM.[7]

Wireless motility capsule

Wireless motility capsule (WMC) is a newer technology used to assess regional and whole-gut transit times. Patients who have failed or become refractory to laxative therapy and other conservative measures are candidates for WMC testing. Given the high cost and similar clinical benefit as ROM, this test is not extensively performed, but saved in many instances for use in individuals with potential global dysmotility syndromes or to evaluate for concurrent upper gastrointestinal dysmotility in patients when a colectomy for isolated STC is being considered.[15]

Colonic manometry

Colonic manometry (CM) measures intraluminal colonic and rectal pressures to quantify colonic motor activity. In addition, CM attempts to identify complex contractile patterns in the colon at rest, during sleep, and with meals or other propagating stimuli. CM is predominately used when necessary to differentiate neuropathic from myopathic disorders. Currently, this diagnostic is relegated to large academic centers and used primarily for research purposes.[16]

Treatment

Multiple classes of agents are currently available for treating CIC: bulking agents, stimulant and osmotic laxatives, stool softeners, emollients, secretagogues, and serotonergic agents (**Table 1**). Each works via a specific mechanism of action. Given the array of currently available therapies and the availability of many of these agents as over-the-counter (OTC) therapeutics, it can be difficult for patients and physicians alike to choose first-line and second-line agents. In a recent survey of US gastroenterologists, 97% endorsed using an OTC therapy as a first-line agent, specifically recommending fiber (52%) and osmotic laxatives (40%) as their initial treatments of choice. Interestingly, if these failed, osmotic laxatives were used as the most common second-line intervention (46%), but there was a sharp decline in the use of fiber (6%) in favor of prescription secretagogues (24%).[17] Recent guidelines, including the ACG monograph on the treatment of CIC[18] and the AGA technical review on constipation,[7] have been congruous in their recommendations and appear to echo these general practice principles.

Bulking Agents

Dietary fiber supplements are carbohydrate polymers that are poorly digested in the small intestine; consequently, they are delivered almost unchanged to the colon where they bulk stool by drawing fluid into the intestinal lumen, and accelerate colon transit time. However, these agents can also undergo fermentation by colonic flora,

Table 1
Common chronic idiopathic constipation therapies

Medications	Important Information
Bulk laxatives	
Soluble: Psyllium Insoluble: Bran, methylcellulose, calcium polycarbophil	Increase stool bulk stimulating peristalsis
Stimulant laxatives	
Anthraquinones: (Senna/Casacara)	Stimulate intestinal secretion and motility. These may cause melanosis coli → No direct association to colon cancer or myenteric nerve damage proven
Diphenylmethane derivatives	
Bisacodyl	Hydrolyzed to active form by small intestine and colon enzymes
Sodium picosulfate	Hydrolyzed to active form by colon bacteria
Saline laxatives	
Mg hydroxide/Mg citrate	Hypermagnesemia can occur in renal failure and children
Sodium phosphate	Acute phosphate nephropathy can occur; black box warning
Osmotic laxatives	
Lactulose	Synthetic disaccharide consisting of galactose/fructose and resistant to degradation by disaccharidases but not bacteria. Gas/bloating common
Polyethylene glycol 3350	Organic polymer poorly absorbed and not metabolized by colonic bacteria; may cause less gas/bloating
Secretagogues	
Lubiprostone	Chloride ClC_2 agonist promoting luminal secretion and accelerated transit. May cause nausea (25%–33%)
Linaclotide	Guanylate Cyclase-C agonist promoting luminal secretion and accelerated transit. May cause diarrhea
Plecanatide	Guanylate Cyclase-C agonist currently completing Phase III clinical trials
Serotonergic agents	
Tegaserod	Withdrawn from US market due to small but significant increased risk of cardiovascular events
Prucalopride	Highly selective 5-HT_4 agonist approved for the treatment of chronic idiopathic constipation in Canada and Europe
Stool softeners	
Docusate sodium	Ionic detergent softens stool by lowering surface tension resulting in increased stool H_2O retention
Lubricants	
Mineral oil	Provides lubrication for the passage of stool.

generating hydrogen, methane, and carbon dioxide, which can increase gas and bloating. Fiber supplements can be soluble or insoluble in nature depending on their interactions with water. The most commonly used and tested fiber is the soluble fiber psyllium (ispaghula) derived from the seeds of the *Plantago ovata* plant. Insoluble fibers include the natural supplement bran and the semisynthetic agents: methylcellulose and calcium polycarbophil.

Although high-quality studies on the overall effectiveness of fiber are sparse, data from a recent meta-analysis of 3 trials comparing psyllium with placebo (PBO) suggested beneficial effects from its use (number needed to treat [NNT] = 2; 95% confidence interval 1.6–3.0).[18] Furthermore, a recent systematic review identified 7 studies published over the past decade with 5 of 7 yielding beneficial effects in favor of fiber supplementation. However, these studies were small (enrolling 30–80 individuals), used variable fiber supplements and dosages, assessed different endpoints, and evaluated these findings over short durations.[19] Thus, longer more rigorously standardized trials are warranted. Currently, the ACG strongly endorses the use of fiber, particularly soluble fiber, for increasing stool frequency, but admits that this recommendation is based on low-quality evidence.[18]

Stimulant Laxatives

Stimulant laxatives exert their effect on the GI tract via induction of colonic peristalsis and/or fluid and electrolyte secretion. Although many are available, the data for the effectiveness of these therapeutics are sparse. To date, only 2 randomized, PBO-controlled trials have been completed: one using bisacodyl and the other liquid sodium picosulfate (SPS). Although different prodrugs, these molecules are activated in the small intestine to the same active molecule: bis-(p-hydroxyphenyl)-pyridyl-2-methane. In the first study, 267 individuals meeting Rome III criteria for CIC were randomized to receive 10 mg (18 gtts) of SPS or PBO in a 2:1 ratio for 4 weeks. At trial completion those receiving SPS experienced a significant increase in complete spontaneous bowel movements (CSBMs) compared with PBO (3.4 vs 1.7; $P<.0001$).[20] In the second study, 247 patients also meeting Rome III criteria were randomized to consume 10 mg bisacodyl or PBO. Four weeks later, patients receiving the bisacodyl also experienced a significant improvement in CSBMs compared with PBO (5.2 vs 1.9; $P<.0001$).[21] Unfortunately, their use can be limited by side effects including diarrhea and cramping with a recent meta-analysis yielding a number needed to harm of 3, which was equivalent to overall NNT of 3.[22] Stimulant laxatives are strongly recommended for the treatment of CIC with this recommendation based on moderate levels of evidence.[18]

Osmotic Laxatives

A mainstay of daily therapy, these agents function by retaining water in the intestinal lumen. Four major classes of osmotic agents current exist: polyethylene glycol (PEG)-based solutions, nonabsorbable carbohydrates, magnesium-containing solutions, and sodium phosphate–based products (see **Table 1**). Of these, PEG and lactulose have been most extensively studied. In the largest and longest laxative trial to date, 304 patients were randomized to receive PEG (n = 204) or PBO (n = 100) for 6 months. At completion of the study, individuals in the PEG cohort experienced a significant increase in bowel movements per week compared with PBO (7.9 vs 5.6; $P<.001$) and the percentage of individuals achieving a goal of 3 or more bowel movements per week was also significantly greater in favor of PEG (52% vs 11%; $P<.001$).[23] Multiple meta-analyses have also consistently yielded positive results favoring the use of osmotic agents. Ford and Suarez[22] recently pooled 5 studies comparing PEG and lactulose with PBO and identified a nonresponder rate of 37.2% compared with 68.9% of PBO (NNT = 3). Belsey and colleagues[24] analyzed 10 studies and found that PEG was superior to PBO and lactulose for increasing stool frequency. Furthermore, a recent Cochrane analysis of 10 clinical trials comparing PEG and lactulose revealed PEG to be superior for improving stool frequency, stool texture, relieving abdominal pain, and reducing the need for additional laxative use.[25] Both PEG and lactulose are strongly recommended by the ACG for the treatment of CIC; however, the quality of evidence supporting the use of PEG is high, whereas for lactulose it is low.[18]

Secretagogues

Secretagogues, the newest class of agents, exert their effects by enhancing intestinal fluid secretion and accelerating small bowel and colonic transit. There are currently 2 commercially available agents in the class: the chloride channel activist lubiprostone and the guanylyl cyclase-C (GC-C) agonist linaclotide. Both are approved by the Food and Drug Administration (FDA) for the treatment of CIC. A second GC-C agonist, plecanatide, just completed phase III evaluation and a new drug application is currently being drafted to the FDA. The benefits of lubiprostone have been shown in 2 double-blind PBO-controlled trials randomizing 479 individuals with CIC. Patients received 24 µg lubiprostone twice daily or PBO for 4 weeks. In both studies a significantly higher percentage of subjects receiving lubiprostone experienced an increase in spontaneous bowel movements at the end of the first week of treatment (5.69 and 5.89 vs 3.46 and 3.99 in trials 1 and 2, respectively; $P<.05$), and these effects were maintained throughout all subsequent weeks of the study. Nausea was the most common adverse event affecting 21% to 32% of individuals.[26,27] Linaclotide has also been evaluated in 2 phase III trials enrolling 1272 individuals to either 145 mg or PBO for 12 weeks. The primary endpoint, the percentage of individuals experiencing 3 or more CSBMs per week plus an increase of at least 1 CSBM per week for 9 of 12 weeks of the study, was achieved by 18% of patients receiving linaclotide compared with 4.5% in the PBO arm. The most common adverse event was diarrhea, affecting 16% of those receiving linaclotide.[28] Both received strong recommendations from the ACG for treating CIC based on high levels of evidence[18] with NNT of 4 and 6 for lubiprostone and linaclotide, respectively.[22] Plecanatide is the first agent to be tested under the FDA's new guidance endpoint for CIC trials. To be considered an overall responder, individuals must have 3 or more CSBMs per week and an increase of at least 1 CSBM per week from baseline for 9 of 12 study weeks; however, now both endpoints must be met for at least 3 of the last 4 weeks of the trial. In these studies, 2683 individuals were enrolled to consume 3 or 6 mg of plecanatide or PBO once daily. At the end of 12 weeks, 20.5% and 19.75% of all test subjects in the 3-mg and 6-mg cohorts, respectively, achieved this endpoint compared with 11.5% in the PBO group ($P<.001$ for both comparisons to PBO). The most common adverse event was diarrhea, occurring in 4.55%, 5.00%, and 1.30% of those consuming 3 or 6 mg of the test drug and PBO, respectively.[29,30]

Serotonin Agonists

Serotonin (5-HT) plays a major role in the GI tract, influencing motility, secretion, and sensory functions, and although there are 7 major 5-HT receptor subtypes, the 5-HT$_4$ subtype has been most frequently targeted in this class. Tegaserod, a partial 5-HT$_4$ agonist, was the first in this class to be approved for the treatment of CIC but was withdrawn from the US market in March 2007, as postmarketing trials revealed the potential for increased cardiovascular events.[31] Currently, none of the drugs in this class are approved for the treatment of CIC in the United States; however, prucalopride, a highly selective 5-HT$_4$ agonist is approved for the treatment of CIC in Canada and Europe. A recent meta-analysis of 6 international trials compared the likelihood of response to prucalopride characterized as the percentage of individuals experiencing an average of 3 or more CSBMs over a period of 12 weeks. Twenty-eight percent of patients receiving prucalopride compared with 13% of patients receiving PBO achieved this endpoint ($P<.001$; NNT = 6.8). The most common adverse events included headaches, nausea, and diarrhea.[32] Prucalopride has received a strong recommendation for improving CIC symptoms based on moderate levels of evidence.[18]

Miscellaneous Agents

Multiple therapeutics are currently being used to treat clinically refractive patients based on their mechanisms of action or anecdotal/case reports documenting their benefits. These include the anti-inflammatory agent colchicine and the synthetic prostaglandin E_1 molecule misoprostol. Both are known to induce diarrhea as a side effect, and thus may be beneficial in rare cases. Other common agents, such as the macrolide antibiotic erythromycin, which stimulates motilin receptors throughout the GI tract, are also under investigation. Early data suggested that erythromycin may be an effective intervention[33]; however, subsequent motility testing has revealed a lack of prokinetic effects in children and adolescents[34] and also a paucity of colokinetic activity in adults.[35] Each of these interventions is also associated with severe side-effect profiles including abortifacient properties (misoprostol) and an ability to prolong cardiac QT(c) intervals (erythromycin). Consequently, these drugs should be considered only in rare instances when other laxatives have failed and other causes for CIC (eg, dyssynergia) have been ruled out.

SUMMARY

Constipation is a common chronic disorder that can significantly impact an individual's quality of life. Despite advances in our therapeutic armamentarium, the rates of CIC in this country continue to rise. Much of this can be explained by currently identified precipitants. The diagnosis of CIC can be made using standard criteria and, once made, a determination of the underlying etiology/etiologies should be undertaken. In many instances, these will be gleaned from the history and physical examination with routine diagnostic studies unnecessary in the absence of alarming clinical signs or symptoms. Specialized diagnostic testing may be warranted after the failure of initial laxative trials.

REFERENCES

1. Higgins PD, Johansen JF. Epidemiology of constipation in North America: a systemic review. Am J Gastroenterol 2004;99:750.
2. Shaheen NJ, Hansen RA, Morgan DR, et al. The burden of gastrointestinal and liver diseases, 2006. Am J Gastroenterol 2006;101:2128–38.
3. Peery AF, Crockett SD, Barritt AS, et al. Burden of gastrointestinal, liver, and pancreatic diseases in the United States. Gastroenterology 2015;149:1731–41.
4. Belsey J, Greenfield S, Candy D, et al. Systematic Review: impact of constipation on quality of life in adults and children. Aliment Pharmacol Ther 2010;31:938–49.
5. Longstreth GF, Thompson WG, Chey WD, et al. Functional bowel disorders. Gastroenterology 2006;130:1480.
6. Brenner DM, Chey WD. An evidence-based review of novel and emerging therapies for constipation in patients taking opioid analgesics. Am J Gastroenterol Suppl 2014;2:38–48.
7. Bharucha AE, Pemberton JH, Locke GR III, et al. American Gastroenterological Association technical review on constipation. Gastroenterology 2013;144:218–38.

8. Brenner DM. Chronic constipation: where we have been and where we are going. Gastroenterol Rep 2006;1:4–11.

9. Lembo A, Camilleri M. Chronic constipation. N Engl J Med 2003;349(14):1360–8.

10. Saad RJ, Rao SSC, Koch KL, et al. Do stool form and frequency correlate which whole-gut and colonic transit? Results from a multicenter study in constipated individuals and healthy controls. Am J Gastroenterol 2010;195:403–11.

11. Talley NJ. How do I do and interpret a rectal exam in gastroenterology. Am J Gastroenterol 2008;103:820–2.

12. Bharucha AE, Pemberton JH, Locke GR. American Gastroenterological Association Medical Position Statement on Constipation. Gastroenterology 2013;144: 211–7.

13. Wald A, Bharucha AE, Cosman BC, et al. ACG clinical guideline: management of benign anorectal disorders. Am J Gastroenterol 2014;109:1141–57.

14. Rao SS, Ozturk R, Laine L. Clinical utility of diagnostic tests for constipation in adults: a systematic review. Am J Gastroenterol 2005;100:1605.

15. Agency for Healthcare Research and Quality (AHRQ). Wireless motility capsule versus other diagnostic technologies for evaluating gastroparesis and constipation: a comparative effectiveness review (No. 110). Available at: http://effectivehealthcare. ahrq.gov/ehc/products/392/1498/Constipation-gastroparesis-wireless-capsule-report-130520.pdf. Accessed October 27, 2015.

16. Rao S, Singh S. Clinical utility of colonic and anorectal manometry in chronic constipation. J Clin Gastroenterol 2010;44(9):597–609.

17. Menees SB, Guentner A, Chey SW, et al. How do US gastroenterologists use over-the-counter and prescription medications in patients with gastroesophageal reflux and chronic constipation? Am J Gastroenterol 2015;110(11):1516–25.

18. Ford AD, Moayyedi P, Lacy BE, et al. American College of Gastroenterology monograph on the management of irritable bowel syndrome and chronic idiopathic constipation. Am J Gastroenterol 2014;109:S2–26.

19. Rao SSC, Yu S, Fedewa A. Systematic review: dietary fibre and FODMAP-restricted diet in the management of constipation and irritable bowel syndrome. Aliment Pharmacol Ther 2015;41:1256–70.

20. Muller-Lissner S, Kamm MA, Wald M, et al. Multicenter, 4-week, double-blind, randomized, placebo-controlled trial of sodium picosulfate in patients with chronic constipation. Am J Gastroenterol 2010;105:897–903.

21. Kamm MA, Mueller-Lissner S, Wald A, et al. Oral bisacodyl is effective and well-tolerated in patients with chronic constipation. Clin Gastroenterol Hepatol 2011;9: 577–83.

22. Ford AC, Suarez NC. Effect of laxatives and pharmacological therapies in chronic idiopathic constipation: Systematic review and meta-analysis. Gut 2011;60: 209–18.

23. DiPalma JA, Cleveland MV, McGowan J, et al. A randomized, multicenter, placebo-controlled trial of polyethylene glycol laxative for the chronic treatment of chronic constipation. Am J Gastroenterol 2007;102:1436–41.

24. Belsey JD, Geraint M, Dixon TA. Systematic review and meta-analysis: polyethylene glycol in adults with non-organic constipation. Int J Clin Pract 2010;64: 944–55.

25. Lee-Robichaud H, Thomas K, Morgan J, et al. Lactulose versus polyethylene glycol for chronic constipation. Cochrane Database Syst Rev 2010;(7):CD007570.

26. Johanson J, Morton D, Geenen J, et al. Multicenter, 4-week double-blind, randomized, placebo-controlled trial of lubiprostone, a locally-active type-2 chloride

channel activator in patients with chronic constipation. Am J Gastroenterol 2008; 103:170–7.

27. Barish C, Drossman D, Johanson J, et al. Efficacy and safety of lubiprostone in patients with chronic constipation. Dig Dis Sci 2010;55:1090–7.

28. Lembo AJ, Schneier HA, Shiff SJ, et al. Two randomized trials of linaclotide for chronic constipation. N Engl J Med 2011;365:527–36.

29. Available at: http://www.businesswire.com/news/home/20150617005307/en/ Synergy-Pharmaceuticals-Announces-Positive-Results-Phase-3. Accessed October 26, 2015.

30. Available at: http://finance.yahoo.com/news/synergy-pharmaceuticals-announces-positive-results-100000891.html. Accessed October 26, 2015.

31. Available at: http://www.fda.gov/Drugs/DrugSafety/DrugSafetyPodcasts/ucm 078972.html. Accessed October 29, 2015.

32. Piessevaux H, Camilleri M, Yiannakou Y, et al. Efficacy and safety of prucalopride in chronic constipation. Gastroenterology 2015;148(4 Suppl 1):S-311.

33. Sharma SS, Bhargava N, Mathur SC. Effect of oral erythromycin on colon transit in patients with idiopathic constipation: A pilot study. Dig Dis Sci 1995;40(11): 2446–9.

34. Dranove J, Horn D, Reddy SN, et al. Effect of intravenous erythromycin on the colonic motility of children and young adults during colonic manometry. J Pediatr Surg 2010;45(4):777–83.

35. Bassotti G, Chiarioni G, Vantini I, et al. Effect of different doses of erythromycin on colonic motility in patients with slow transit constipation. Z Gastroenterol 1998; 36(3):209–13.

Fecal Incontinence and Pelvic Floor Dysfunction in Women: A Review

 CrossMark

Alison Freeman, MD, MPH, Stacy Menees, MD, MS*

KEYWORDS

- Pelvic floor dysfunction • Fecal incontinence • Accidental bowel leakage
- Anal sphincter • Women's health • Sphincter injury

KEY POINTS

- Pelvic floor dysfunction, which includes pelvic organ prolapse, urinary incontinence, and fecal incontinence (FI), is very common among parous women.
- FI is also common, particularly among older women, can be socially isolating, and often goes under-reported to their health care providers. Physicians should actively ask their patients about these symptoms.
- FI is commonly associated with older age, change in bowel habits (typically loose and/or frequent stools, fecal urgency), and debility. FI is common in institutionalized patients.
- Treatment of FI initially involves a combination of dietary and lifestyle modifications, medications, and biofeedback training. If conservative methods fail to improve FI symptoms, then other interventions can be considered, including nerve stimulation, anal sphincter augmentation, and surgical options.

INTRODUCTION/EPIDEMIOLOGY

Pelvic floor dysfunction, which includes urinary incontinence, fecal incontinence (FI), and pelvic organ prolapse (POP),[1] affects 25% or more of women.[2,3] These disorders will become more prevalent with an aging population. In 2008, there were 38.6 million and 5.4 million Americans aged 65 years and 85 years and older, respectively. In 2050, the 65-year-old and 85-year-old and older segments of the population will more than double to 88.5 million and 19 million, respectively. With increasing age, women comprise a higher percentage of the population among all older age groups: 54% in those aged 65 to 69 years, 69% of those aged 85 to 89 years, and 80% of those

Disclosures: The authors have no conflicts of interest and nothing to disclose.
Division of Gastroenterology, Department of Internal Medicine, University of Michigan Health System, 3912 Taubman Center, 1500 East Medical Center Drive, SPC 5362, Ann Arbor, MI 48109, USA
* Corresponding author.
E-mail address: sbartnik@med.umich.edu

Gastroenterol Clin N Am 45 (2016) 217–237
http://dx.doi.org/10.1016/j.gtc.2016.02.002
0889-8553/16/$ – see front matter © 2016 Elsevier Inc. All rights reserved.

gastro.theclinics.com

aged 95 to 99 years.[4] Wu and colleagues[5] estimated the future prevalence of pelvic floor disorders in women using the US Census Bureau population projections from 2010 to 2050. FI is expected to have the largest increase at 59% (10.6 million to 16.8 million affected women). They estimated that the number of women with urinary incontinence will increase 55% from 18.3 million in 2010 to 28.4 million in 2050, whereas POP will increase 46% from 3.3 million to 4.9 million from 2010 to 2050.[5] This article focuses largely on fecal incontinence, but discusses these other pelvic floor disorders because they are pertinent in the evaluation and work-up of FI.

FI, sometimes referred to as accidental bowel leakage,[6] is defined as the involuntary loss or passage of solid or liquid stool in patients with a developmental age greater than 4 years.[7] However, the definition can vary based on consistency of stools and frequency or duration of symptoms. FI does not include flatal incontinence or fecal soilage. Anal incontinence comprises both liquid and stool incontinence along with gas incontinence. Fecal soilage is the staining or streaking of underwear with fecal material or mucus.

The prevalence of FI in women ranges from 2% to 25%,[6,8–11] but this varies based on definition used, age, and living situation (independently living vs nursing home). The prevalence of FI increases from 2.6% in young women (aged 20–29 years) to 15.3% by age 70 years or older.[10,12] In addition, 88% of women with FI develop their symptoms after age 40 years.[13] Women living in nursing homes or other institutionalized settings are at high risk for FI, with a prevalence among this population between 14% and 47%.[14,15]

The reported prevalence of FI likely underestimates the true prevalence because FI is significantly under-reported to physicians.[16,17] Patients are often reluctant to discuss their symptoms because it is embarrassing.[18,19] In the recent Mature Women's Health Study, Brown and colleagues[16] found that two-thirds of women with FI do not seek care for their symptoms even though 40% of them had symptoms severe enough to affect their quality of life.[20] However, physicians also bear the burden for the underdiagnosis of FI. Dunivan and colleagues[21] showed that practitioners routinely fail to inquire about FI during patient visits.

Quality of life can be significantly affected in patients with FI, resulting in patient embarrassment, psychological stress, social isolation, and job loss,[20,22] and it is the second leading cause of placement in a skilled nursing facility[23] (**Box 1**).

Box 1
Reflections on the anal sphincter as presented at the International Academy of Proctology, April 1959

They say man has succeeded where the animals fail because of the clever use of his hands, yet when compared to the hands, the sphincter ani is far superior. If you place into your cupped hands a mixture of fluid, solid, and gas and then through an opening at the bottom, try to let only the gas escape, you will fail. Yet the sphincter can do it. The sphincter apparently can differentiate between solid, fluid, and gas. It apparently can tell whether its owner is alone or with someone, whether standing up or sitting down, whether its owner has his pants on or off. No other muscle of the body is such a protector of the dignity of man, yet so ready to come to his relief.[24]

—Walter C. Borneimeier, General Surgeon and former president of the American Medical Association, Chicago, IL.

PATHOPHYSIOLOGY

Continence is a complex process involving the internal and external anal sphincters, compliant rectum, puborectalis muscle, neurologically intact anal sphincter complex, and functional pelvic floor muscles. FI can develop when bowel motility is altered (either diarrhea or constipation), or from weakening of the anal sphincter muscles, rectal inflammation or other causes of poor rectal compliance, rectal sensory abnormalities, or dysfunction of the pelvic floor musculature.[25,26] In 80% of patients there is more than 1 pathophysiologic factor that causes FI.[27] There are multiple physiologic factors associated with aging. Both sphincters can be affected with fibrosis and thickening leading to decreased resting tone, with thinning of the external anal sphincter producing a weak squeeze pressure. In addition, decreased rectal sensation, rectal compliance, and rectal capacity all cause impairment of the colorectal sensorimotor function and impaired rectal reservoir function.[26,28,29]

RISK FACTORS

Multiple studies have described risk factors for FI.[8–11,13,22,30–33] These risk factors are listed in **Box 2**. Although the impact of most of these risk factors is debatable, the major risk factors for FI in women seem to be advanced age, alterations in bowel movements, and institutionalization. The major gastrointestinal symptom strongly associated with FI is diarrhea, and any disease that can cause loose/watery stools or frequent bowel movements (more than 21 stools per week) can lead to FI.[10,13,30] However, a portion of these cases may be caused by underlying constipation with or without fecal impaction, causing overflow diarrhea.[14] The mechanism of incontinence with diarrhea is likely multifactorial, but it may be caused by increased difficulty retaining loose or watery stool, overwhelming the anal sphincter with high volumes delivered to the rectum in a short interval of time, reflex inhibition of the internal anal sphincter (IAS), and/or interactions between the consistency of the stool and sphincter defects. Other major risk factors include concurrent stress urinary incontinence, prior vaginal delivery with forceps or stitches, rectal urgency, and multiple chronic comorbidities.[8,10,13,22,30–33]

EVALUATION

An algorithm for the evaluation and management of FI is shown in **Fig. 1**. The first step in this process involves obtaining a detailed history and examination, including digital rectal examination to assess for sphincter defects, rectal tone, and fecal impaction. If fecal impaction is present, then treatment should focus on the management of constipation. The clinicians must determine whether the patient has symptoms of fecal soilage or of true incontinence. If incontinent, is it solid or liquid stool? Current medications should be reviewed to identify anything that may exacerbate FI (**Table 1**). Also consider constipating medications as a cause for overflow diarrhea/overflow incontinence.

Fecal Soilage

The initial work-up for women with fecal soilage only should include anorectal manometry (ARM) to evaluate for dyssynergic defecation. If present, then the patient should be referred to physical therapy (PT) for biofeedback training (BFT) and consideration of the nonpharmacologic treatment options described later (see **Fig. 1**).

Box 2
Risk factors for fecal incontinence

Patient characteristics

Increased age
Female gender
Current smoking
Obesity
Institutionalization

Gastrointestinal factors

Loose or watery stools
Frequent bowel movements (>21/wk)
Rectal urgency
Functional bowel disorders
Inflammatory bowel disease
Fecal impaction/severe constipation with overflow incontinence
Rectocele

Obstetric history factors

Multiparity
Sphincter laceration/episiotomy
Prolonged second stage of labor
Vacuum extraction
Vaginal delivery with forceps

Other medical comorbidities

Urinary incontinence
Multiple chronic illnesses
Debility
Dementia
Dietary intolerances/dietary factors
Enteral tube feeding
Medication side effects
Anxiety/depression
Diabetes
Neurologic disease/prior stroke
History of pelvic radiation

Effects of prior surgery

Hysterectomy
Cholecystectomy
Anal sphincterotomy
Hemorrhoidectomy
Colectomy with ileoanal pouch anastomosis

Postvoid enemas can be considered to remove residual stool in the rectum and anal canal.

Liquid Stool Incontinence

If incontinent of liquid stool only, then evaluation for causes of diarrhea should be pursued, including possible colonoscopy, and treatment tailored to the cause. Common causes of diarrhea include medication side effects, diet, carbohydrate intolerance,

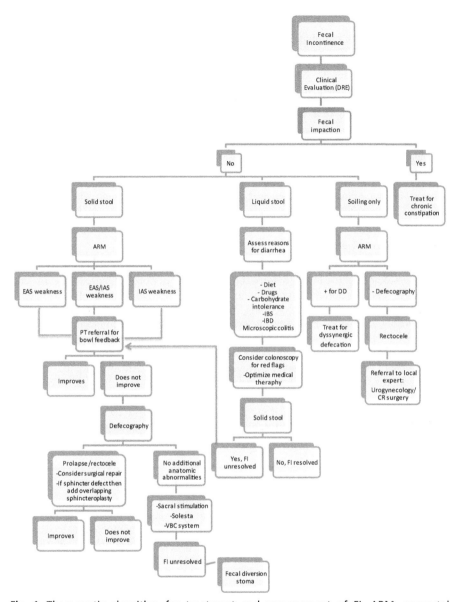

Fig. 1. Therapeutic algorithm for treatment and management of FI. ARM, anorectal manometry; CR, colorectal; DD, dyssynergic defecation; DRE, digital rectal examination; EAS, external anal sphincter; IBD, inflammatory bowel disease; IBS, irritable bowel syndrome; FI, fecal incontinence; PT, physical therapy; VBC, vaginal bowel control.

small intestinal bacterial overgrowth, microscopic colitis, bile acid malabsorption, irritable bowel syndrome (IBS), inflammatory bowel disease, and autonomic dysfunction. Management generally focuses on dietary and lifestyle interventions as well as the antidiarrheal pharmacologic options described later (see **Fig. 1**), but varies based on the cause.

Table 1 Medications that can contribute to or worsen FI	
Drugs	**Mechanism**
Nitrates, CCB, BB, sildenafil, SSRI	Reduce sphincter tone
Glyceryl trinitrate ointment, diltiazem gel, bethanechol cream, botulinum toxin A injection	Reduce sphincter tone via application of topical medications to the anus
Antibiotics, laxatives, metformin, orlistat, SSRI, magnesium-containing antacids, digoxin, PPI	Cause loose stools or diarrhea
Benzodiazepines, SSRI, antipsychotics	Relaxant, hypnotic

Abbreviations: BB, β-blockers; CCB, calcium channel blockers; PPI, proton pump inhibitors; SSRI, selective serotonin reuptake inhibitors.

Solid Stool Incontinence

The approach for patients with solid stool incontinence should begin with ARM to evaluate for weakness in the IAS or external anal sphincter or both. If present, then referral to PT for BFT is appropriate. If incontinence does not improve, then functional imaging with either fluoroscopic defecography, dynamic cystocolpoproctography, or MRI defecography should be performed to evaluate for concomitant anatomic abnormalities.[34,35] If POP or rectocele is identified, then referral for surgical intervention should be considered, with or without sphincter repair as indicated. If no anatomic abnormalities are identified, then minimally invasive approaches, such as injectable bulking agents, sacral nerve stimulator, or vaginal bowel control system, can be attempted. If these methods fail, then definitive surgical intervention, including fecal diversion, can be considered (see **Fig. 1**). If surgical options are being considered, then first perform endoscopic ultrasonography or transanal ultrasonography to assess sphincter integrity.

TREATMENT OF FECAL INCONTINENCE

Treatment options for FI vary from noninvasive strategies such as dietary and lifestyle changes, PT with BFT, and pharmacologic agents, to minimally invasive options such as nerve stimulation, sphincter augmentation methods with injectable bulking agents or radiofrequency energy, and bowel control systems, to more invasive surgical interventions of sphincteroplasty, sphincter repair, and fecal diversion surgery. These options are listed in **Table 2**.

Dietary and Lifestyle Modification

Potentially modifiable risk factors, such as obesity, inactivity, and smoking, should be addressed.[36] Weight loss has been shown to improve FI in obese women.[37] Behavioral techniques for FI can be implemented, including bowel-retraining techniques such as pausing to perform Kegel exercises rather than rushing to the bathroom, which increases abdominal wall strength and reduces the focus on the pelvic floor, aiding in continence. Toileting strategies such as performing a few Kegel exercises between wiping can also help improve episodes of incontinence.[9]

Some patients may also benefit from vaginal splinting and/or techniques such as anal wicking with a cotton ball or rectal enemas to prevent fecal soilage or mild

Table 2
Treatment options for FI

Noninvasive Interventions	Minimally Invasive Procedures	Surgical
Dietary modification (increase dietary fiber intake; avoid common trigger foods such as caffeine, dairy, high-fat foods)	Sphincter augmentation with injectable bulking agents or radiofrequency energy	Sphincteroplasty
Modifiable behavioral risks (weight loss, smoking cessation, increased exercise)	Sacral nerve stimulation	Artificial anal sphincter[a]
Pharmacologic therapies	Percutaneous tibial nerve stimulation	Muscle transposition
Anal wicking	Eclipse System[b]	Diversion surgery
Increased fiber/bulking agents	Magnetic anal sphincter[b]	
Bowel regimen (if constipated)	TOPAS system[b]	
PT with BFT		

[a] Technique largely abandoned because of severe adverse events, including sphincter erosion.
[b] Technique still investigational or not yet widely available.

incontinence.[38] Anal wicking is the technique of placing a long piece of cotton or a cotton ball shaped into a wick between the buttocks, resting directly on the anus so that mild seepage of fecal material is contained. Vaginal splinting is discussed in further detail later.

Dietary interventions can focus on foods that are known to cause loose stools or urgency. Avoidance of common triggers such as caffeine, dairy products, or high-fat foods can be helpful. Dietary fiber and/or stool bulking agents, such as psyllium, can improve symptoms of FI. A cross-sectional survey of elderly Korean women showed that those with the lowest weekly intake of dietary fiber had a 2.66-fold increased likelihood of having FI (overall prevalence of FI in this population, 15.5%).[39] Bliss and colleagues,[40] in a randomized, double-blind, placebo-controlled trial, showed a significant decrease in reported symptoms of FI in patients receiving 1 month of daily fiber supplementation with either psyllium (with 49% of stools at baseline associated with FI to 17% with psyllium) or gum arabic (with 66% of stools at baseline associated with FI to 18% with gum arabic) compared with placebo. Only 1 study has assessed the efficacy of a fiber supplement compared with a medication in a randomized fashion.[41] Markland and colleagues[41] recently conducted a randomized, double-blind, placebo-controlled, crossover study that compared daily loperamide versus psyllium in the treatment of FI. Eighty adults (68% male) were given either daily loperamide (with a concurrent placebo powder) or psyllium powder (with a concurrent placebo pill) for 4 weeks, followed by a 2-week wash-out period, then another 4 weeks of the opposite treatment in the crossover arm. Both groups showed improvement in number of FI episodes per week and quality of life, but there was no difference between loperamide and psyllium among these end points. Loperamide was associated with higher rates of constipation than psyllium, but no other adverse effects were noted.

Pharmacologic Therapy

Medications that target causes of diarrhea should be considered. Common medications that can be effective for loose stools and FI are listed in **Table 3**.[42] They include

| Table 3 |
| Medications for treatment of FI |

Mechanism of Action	Medications
Stool bulking agents	Psyllium, methylcellulose, gum arabic
Antidiarrheal/antimotility	Loperamide, diphenoxylate/atropine, codeine
Bile acid resins	Cholestyramine, colestipol, colesevelam
Bacterial overgrowth	Various antibiotics
Tricyclic antidepressants	Nortriptyline, amitriptyline
Enhancement of anal sphincter tone	Phenylepinephrine gel, sodium valproate, zinc-aluminum ointment, L-erythro methoxamine gel
Barrier creams	Zinc oxide, Calmoseptine ointment, Alkagin powder, Aquaphor ointment

antidiarrheal/antimotility agents, stool bulking agents, bile acid resins, tricyclic antidepressants, and others that can enhance the anal sphincter tone.

In a recent Cochrane Review, Omar and Alexander[42] identified only 16 trials evaluating the efficacy of various medications for the treatment of FI. This review included 7 antidiarrheal medication trials, 6 trials for medications that enhance the anal sphincter tone (phenylephrine gel or sodium valproate), 1 trial of zinc-aluminum ointment, and 2 trials of laxatives in patients with FI caused by constipation and overflow diarrhea. There were no included studies of medications compared with other treatment modalities. Overall, although these data are limited, all of these studies showed improvement in FI but most reported side effects (only zinc-aluminum ointment had no reported adverse effects). There were insufficient data to recommend one type of medication rather than another.[42]

Some patients may also benefit from perianal barrier creams to prevent skin excoriation and incontinence-associated dermatitis, or from techniques such as anal wicking with a cotton ball, or the routine use of rectal enemas to prevent fecal soilage or mild incontinence.[38] The incidence of incontinence-associated perianal dermatitis is 41% among community-dwelling adults with FI. This rate is mildly associated with severity of FI, but not with age, gender, or concurrent urinary incontinence.[43]

Biofeedback Therapy

Pelvic floor muscle training (PFMT) alone has been shown to be effective for the treatment of urinary incontinence,[44] but outcomes for FI seem to be improved with the addition of BFT in uncontrolled studies.[45] However, a randomized trial of biofeedback compared with either PFMT or advice alone showed no additional benefit from BFT.[46] BFT is a form of PT that uses electronic instrumentation to monitor specific, often unconscious, physiologic activities, and then uses a visual or auditory signal to provide the information as feedback to the patient. Although biofeedback techniques vary, the methods, which may be used independently or in combination, include rectal sensory training and compliance, strength and endurance training of the pelvic floor and anal sphincter, and coordination training of the anal sphincter. In addition to pelvic floor exercises, biofeedback instrument modalities include electrical stimulation, rectal distention balloons, surface and/or intra-anal electromyography (EMG), manometric pressures, and transanal ultrasonography.[45,47] The success of BFT is variable, from 0% to 80%.[47] A multicenter study found that success is best achieved if biofeedback uses a combination of

EMG, electrical stimulation, and a long duration of treatment (>3 months).[48] In a recent Cochrane Review, Norton and Cody[45] did not find any evidence that specific types of biofeedback or exercise were more beneficial than others, but that BFT or electrical stimulation is more efficacious than PFMT alone in patients who have failed to respond to other conservative measures.

Anal Sphincter Augmentation

Two minimally invasive options exist that augment the native anal sphincter, including injectable bulking agents and radiofrequency energy. These methods can be considered in patients with mild to moderate FI, no anatomic anal sphincter abnormalities, and who have failed the conservative medical therapies described earlier.

Injectable bulking agents

The current most common injectable medication is dextranomer with hyaluronic acid (NASHA/Dx; Solesta, Salix Pharmaceuticals, Raleigh, NC), although other injectable materials can be used (collagen, silicone, autologous fat, glutaraldehyde, and carbon-coated beads, among others[47,49]). NASHA/Dx is a biocompatible injectable gel consisting of dextranomer microspheres stabilized in hyaluronic acid that is injected submucosally in all 4 quadrants of the anal sphincter just proximally to the dentate line. This procedure is performed via anoscope, and can be performed with only local anesthesia. A multicenter, randomized, sham-controlled study found that approximately half of their patients receiving NASHA/Dx had a greater than 50% reduction in the number of FI events compared with 30% of patients with the sham injections (odds ratio, 2.36; confidence interval, 1.24–4.27; $P = .0089$).[50] An earlier trial showed similar efficacy results that lasted at least 12 months after treatment.[51] Frequent adverse events have been reported with the use of NASHA/Dx, including serious rare complications of rectal and prostate abscesses.[50]

Radiofrequency energy

The SECCA procedure (Curon Medical, Inc, Fremont, CA) delivers radiofrequency energy[52,53] to the IAS in order to stimulate increased collagen deposition in the IAS and improve continence and sphincter tone.[54] Through the use of a commercially available device, temperature-controlled radiofrequency energy (RFE) is applied multiple times to all 4 quadrants of the anal sphincter. This procedure is typically performed under conscious sedation in an endoscopy suite or operating room. A recent review of the SECCA procedure found only 11 studies for a total of 220 patients, but did find that SECCA may be useful for well-selected patients (those with adequate muscle mass and collagen in the sphincter at baseline) to reduce the number of incontinence episodes and improve quality of life.[55] However, the results of SECCA have been variable, including a recent small prospective cohort trial that failed to show any significant clinical response or durability up to 3 years following the procedure in most of their patients.[56] In addition, Lam and colleagues[56] failed to show any changes in anorectal pressures or rectal compliance, as measured by rectal endoscopic ultrasonography and anorectal manometry. One advantage is that RFE may lead to fewer adverse events compared with other types of procedures, such as injectable bulking medications, nerve stimulation, and surgery.

Nerve Stimulation

In patients with moderate to severe FI who have failed to respond to more conservative measures, nerve stimulation can be considered. Sacral nerve stimulation (SNS) has been used for the last 20 years, whereas percutaneous tibial nerve stimulation (PTNS) for the treatment of FI was developed more recently.

Sacral nerve stimulation

SNS (Interstim, Medtronic, Minneapolis, MN) is thought to improve FI by chronically stimulating the sacral nerves, and therefore the corresponding muscles, by applying a low-voltage electrical current via an implanted electrode through the corresponding sacral foramen.[57] Most commonly, SNS placement is performed in a 2-stage process. During the first stage, a tined electrode lead is placed parallel to the sacral nerve through the S3 sacral foramen and stimulated with a percutaneous nerve stimulator for a 1-week to 2-week trial period. If a reduction in FI symptoms is seen, then a permanent implanted nerve stimulator is implanted in the buttock and connected to the tined lead. The implanted device is then programmed to the individual's response pattern.[47]

A recent Cochrane Review found that SNS can be effective for improving FI.[57] In multiple small crossover studies, when the SNS device is turned on, episodes of FI can improve from 59% to 88% compared with conventional medical therapy.[58–60] One study failed to show any improvement in episodes of FI when the device was on versus off.[61] The improvement in FI symptoms seems to be durable, with Hull and colleagues[62] reporting 89% of patients reporting continued significant reduction in weekly episodes of FI at 5 years postimplantation compared with baseline (mean 9.1 episodes of FI per week at baseline compared with 1.7 per week at 5 years), and about a third of patients had complete resolution of symptoms. Multiple studies have shown impressive results with SNS even in patients with known sphincter defects,[63–67] and that the degree of defect does not affect results.[66]

Percutaneous tibial nerve stimulation

The tibial nerve shares nerve fibers with the sacral nerve. PTNS is a technique whereby the posterior tibial nerve is stimulated with a needle. PTNS is performed weekly in the outpatient setting for 12 weeks, for about 30 minutes per session.[68] The major advantage compared with SNS is that it is much less invasive and does not require the placement of an implantable device. Stimulation of the tibial nerve is comparable with SNS in the treatment of urinary incontinence,[69–72] and initial studies for the treatment of FI have been promising.[68] Thin and colleagues[73] showed that PTNS and SNS had comparable results in the treatment of FI, at least in the short term. However, when PTNS was compared with a sham electrical stimulation procedure, no difference was seen in FI clinical outcomes between the two groups.[74] Further confirmatory studies will determine its utility in FI treatment.

Surgical Options

Options for surgical intervention are considered when more conservative therapies have failed. Surgical options include sphincteroplasty, muscle transposition, antegrade continence enema, and fecal diversion.

Sphincteroplasty

Sphincteroplasty, or repair of the anal sphincter, commonly using an anterior overlapping technique, has long been used to treat FI caused by external anal sphincter injury when conservative therapies have failed.[47,52,75,76] Most women with FI caused by anal sphincter injury have a history of vaginal delivery, and the most common risk factors include multiple vaginal deliveries, need for vaginal instrumentation during labor, third-degree or fourth-degree tear, pudendal nerve injury, and failed prior sphincteroplasty.[77,78] Short-term outcomes for sphincteroplasty are generally much better than long-term outcomes. In the short term, the median rate of either good or excellent fecal continence with sphincteroplasty is 70%,[79] ranging from 30% to 83%.[52] However, numerous recent long-term studies have shown less promising results for the durability of the procedure. Long-term continence decreases to 0% to 60% in most studies.[76,79–86] Although many of these studies concluded that advanced age at the time of the surgery was a risk factor for long-term failure,[76,79,83] a recent systematic review did not find any consistent factors, including age, that were predictive for failure.[85] In addition, a recent large retrospective review of 321 women did not show any significant difference in long-term severity of FI, quality of life, or postoperative satisfaction between younger versus older women.[87]

Muscle transposition

Muscle transposition is another surgical technique that was used more commonly in the past for medically refractory FI, but is rarely used now because of the high rate of adverse events associated with this procedure and the availability of other less invasive but equally effective treatment options.[52] This technique, which is now typically only performed at highly specialized surgical centers, involves the surgical harvesting of functional skeletal muscle with either the gluteus maximus or gracilis muscle, and wrapping around the nonfunctional anal sphincter complex to create a new sphincter in vivo. Graciloplasty can be either unstimulated (adynamic) or stimulated (dynamic). The unstimulated technique relies on patients to learn how to voluntarily contract the muscle to aid in continence, whereas the stimulated technique has the addition of an implanted neuromodulator to help keep the skeletal muscles tonically contracted, allowing superior results.[52] Outcomes are good with muscle transposition, with a reported success of 60% to 75%,[47] but postsurgical complications are common. These complications include surgical site infection, rectal pain, rectal injury, stimulator malfunction, and device erosion,[47,52] and the prevalence of postsurgical obstructive constipation symptoms can be as high as 50%.[88]

Antegrade continence enema

Use of antegrade continence enemas (ACE) for the treatment of FI has long been described and used in the pediatric population with good success.[89] However, it is rarely used in the adult population. This procedure involves the creation of a stoma from the appendix, terminal ileum, or cecum, or other type of proximal access point (such as gastrostomy tube placement into cecum), instilling water or enema solution via this access point, and allowing fecal material to be flushed from the colon in an antegrade manner, alleviating symptoms of both FI and constipation. A recent systematic review found that most adults (47%–100%) were still performing ACE at 6 to 55 months' follow-up, and at least a third of patients achieved full continence.[90]

Fecal diversion

Creation of an end colostomy or ileostomy for fecal diversion can be considered when all other modalities of treatment have failed, or with specific rare indications such as severe neurogenic incontinence, complete pelvic floor denervation, severe perianal trauma, severe radiation-induced incontinence, or significant physical or mental incapacitation.[91,92] This surgical approach is aggressive, but for some patients can dramatically improve quality of life compared with those dealing with fecal incontinence.[93] Norton and colleagues[94] found that 83% of patients who had undergone colostomy placement for their FI had little or no restriction in their life caused by their ostomy, and that 84% would choose to have the stoma placement again.

Potential Future Treatments

Future FI treatment strategies that may soon (or not so soon) become available include a vaginal bowel control system called the Eclipse system, magnetic anal sphincter, Trans-obturator Post-Anal Sling (TOPAS) pelvic floor repair system, and autologous cell or stem cell transplant.

The eclipse system

The Eclipse System (Pelvalon Inc, Sunnyvale, CA) is a vaginally placed device for the treatment of FI that was approved by the US Food and Drug Administration in early 2015. It is fitted like a vaginal pessary, and has a posteriorly directed inflatable balloon.[95] When the balloon is inflated, it occludes the rectal vault and prevents incontinence. However, for defecation, the patient is then able to temporarily deflate the system. The major advantages of this device are that it is easily reversible, dynamically controlled by the patient, and low risk. In a study of 61 women, Richter and colleagues[95] reported that 86% of women, in a per-protocol analysis considered bowel symptoms to be very much better or much better after 1 month of use, which was still stable at 3 months, and quality of life was significantly improved. In that study, there were no serious adverse events. The most common side effect was cramping or discomfort, typically during fitting.

Magnetic anal sphincter

An investigational device called the Magnetic Anal Sphincter (MAS; Fenix, Torax Medical Inc, Shoreline, MN) is a small, flexible band of interlinked titanium beads with magnetic cores. It is surgically implanted around the external anal sphincter and functions to reinforce and improve competence of the sphincter.[96,97] The magnets separate with Valsalva maneuver, allowing defecation.

Lehur and colleagues[96] first described their experiences with, and results of, MAS in 2010. Fourteen women, all of whom had previously failed other treatments, were implanted with MAS. Only 5 of 14 were followed for at least 6 months, but, among this group, they reported a 91% mean reduction in average weekly FI episodes and had significant improvement in quality of life. Two of the 14 patients had the device explanted because of infection, and 1 had spontaneous passage of the device. Other observed adverse events included bleeding, pain, and obstructed defecation.

Another study by Pakravan and colleagues[98] described the results of 18 patients implanted with MAS for FI, followed up to 2 years (mean follow-up, 607 days). One of the 18 patients had an intraoperative rectal perforation, and the procedure was aborted. Of the 17 remaining, 76% of patients showed at least a 50% reduction in number of weekly FI events. None of the patients required explantation, but 29% had pain and/or swelling.

In the short term, MAS performs comparably with artificial bowel sphincters.[99] However, in a 10-year follow-up study, artificial bowel sphincters had high complication rates, typically caused by risk for infection. Fifty percent of the patients with artificial bowel sphincters have required explantation or revision because of device malfunction or infection.[100]

TOPAS pelvic floor repair system

The TOPAS pelvic floor repair system (American Medical Systems, Minnetonka, MN) is an investigational device consisting of a single-use, self-affixing polypropylene mesh sling.[101] It is intended to reinforce soft tissues in the pelvic floor where there are areas of weakness in the gastrointestinal and gynecologic anatomic structures. The center point of the mesh is surgically placed posterior to the anorectum and is brought out through both obturator foramen, similar to a transobturator urinary sling.[97,101]

Initial data by Rosenblatt and colleagues[101] describe the results of 29 women with FI that had failed at least 1 prior therapy, followed up to 2 years postplacement. Fifty-five percent of the women reported treatment success, which was defined as at least a 50% reduction in the number of FI episodes per week. Improvements in continence (as measured by the Cleveland Clinic Incontinence Score) and quality of life (as measured by the Fecal Incontinence Quality of Life) were sustainable through the 2-year follow-up period.[101] The most common adverse events were de novo urinary incontinence (n = 6 of 29), worsening FI (n = 2 of 29), and constipation (n = 2 of 29). No device erosions or extrusions were reported. A larger, multicenter trial by Fenner and colleagues[102] involving 152 women with similar end points showed efficacy in 69.1% and complete continence in 19% of women. The TOPAS system is not yet commercially available, but is currently under investigation.

Cell transplant
Injection of autologous skeletal muscle cells into the external anal sphincter to stimulate muscle growth and regeneration in humans has been described, and mesenteric stem cell transplant has been described in animal models.[103,104] Pathi and colleagues[105] showed that direct injection of mesenteric stem cells into injured rat anal sphincters stimulated increased contractility. Frudinger and colleagues[106] followed 10 women with obstetric-related anal sphincter injury over a 5-year follow-up period. They harvested autologous skeletal muscle–derived cells from each patient's pectoralis muscle and directly injected these cells into the external anal sphincter defect. Improvement in continence and quality of life was seen, which was sustainable for the duration of the follow-up period.[106] Although there may be promise for this method in the future, more research into the utility of autologous or stem cell transplant must be undertaken before it becomes more widely used.

Pyloric valve transplant
In 2011, Goldsmith and Chandra[107] described a novel surgical technique in humans whereby a poorly functional anal sphincter complex is recreated by transplantation of an autologous pyloric valve. This procedure is described in patients with end-stage FI as an alternative to permanent end colostomy. Chandra and colleagues[108] showed better continence outcomes when the pyloric valve was used to augment the native anal sphincter rather than replace it, although there was improvement in both groups.

OTHER CONSIDERATIONS FOR PELVIC ORGAN PROLAPSE

It is common for gastroenterologists to encounter symptoms or complications of pelvic floor dysfunction, including POP. POP is defined as the descent of pelvic organs into or out of the vagina or anus, and includes rectoceles, enteroceles, cystoceles, urethroceles, uterine prolapse, and vaginal vault prolapse (**Fig. 2**). Vaginal delivery and its associated complications can damage the pelvic floor muscles, nerves, and/or connective tissues,[109] which can then result in POP, urinary incontinence, and/or FI. Risk factors for the development of pelvic floor dysfunction include vaginal delivery, prolonged second stage of labor, vacuum-assisted delivery, and third-degree and fourth-degree perineal lacerations or episiotomies.[109,110] Patients with POP, including rectoceles, may report symptoms of incomplete emptying following a bowel movement, bulging sensation, pelvic pressure, and/or need for digital manipulation or splinting in order to complete a bowel movement.[111] However, several studies have shown that there is no correlation between these bowel symptoms and the severity

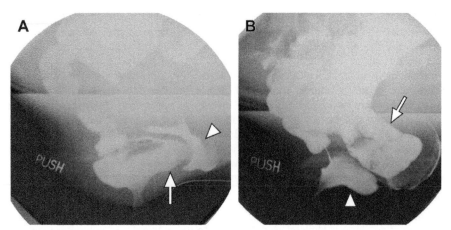

Fig. 2. (A) Rectocele, as seen on defecography. Arrow points to rectocele and arrowhead points to vagina. (B) Enterocele, as seen on defecography. Arrow points to the enterocele and arrowhead points to rectum.

of prolapse.[112–114] Experts agree that the only "consistent symptom with posterior vaginal wall prolapse is its inconsistency."[115] In addition, the symptoms for enteroceles are just as nonspecific, and are compounded by the fact that experts cannot agree on a single definition.[115]

Managing patients with multiple factors, such as those with FI plus POP (rectocele, enterocele, and so forth) plus urinary incontinence, can be challenging. Diagnosis of POP can be made with dynamic imaging as discussed earlier. However, multiple studies have shown that the degree of bowel symptoms does not correlate with severity of prolapse (and therefore response to surgical intervention).[112–114] Furthermore, when physiologic tests (ARM, pudendal nerve latency testing, surface EMG, transanal ultrasonography, or defecography) were added to the work-up, there was still no correlation between degree of bowel symptoms and severity of posterior vaginal wall prolapse.[116]

Patients with rectoceles should be counseled on the use of vaginal splinting during bowel movements. Splinting often refers to manually pressing on the posterior vaginal wall in order to reduce the rectocele bulge such that stool can pass more easily through the anal canal. If conservative measures fail, then a referral to surgical colleagues can be considered. Gustilo-Ashby and collegues[117] followed 106 women who had undergone rectocele repair (technique of repair was variable) for 1 year postoperatively. At 1 year after surgery, there were significant improvements in the individual symptoms of splinting to defecate (baseline, 51% [52 of 102]; 1-year visit, 16% [15 of 94]; $P = .0001$), hard straining (baseline, 71% [72 of 102]; 1-year visit, 40% [37 of 93]; $P = .0001$), and incomplete emptying (baseline, 71% [73 of 99]; 1-year visit, 42% [32 of 92]; $P = .0001$).[117]

SUMMARY

FI with pelvic organ prolapse is a common and debilitating condition in women, particularly as women age, and often goes under-reported to health care providers. As a provider, it is important to ask patients about possible symptoms and the characteristics of those symptoms. Although there have been many possible risk factors associated with pelvic floor dysfunction and FI, the most significant seem to be advanced age, history of vaginal delivery and its associated complications, stool consistency (loose or frequent bowel movements), fecal urgency, and institutionalization or generalized debility.

A therapeutic algorithm is presented in **Fig. 1**. Evaluation and management can be tailored to the specific symptoms and characteristics of the incontinence. Work-up often begins with anorectal manometry plus any other procedures as needed based on symptoms (colonoscopy, dynamic pelvic floor imaging, and so forth), followed by conservative therapies. Typically, initial therapies involve a combination of dietary and lifestyle modifications, pharmacologic agents, and PT with BFT. If these methods fail to improve FI symptoms, then other interventions can be considered. In general, less invasive options should be tried first, such as nerve stimulation and anal sphincter augmentation, before surgical options are explored.

However, in some women, the symptoms may be more suggestive of POP. In these cases, conservative measures, including vaginal splinting, can be tried before surgical options are considered.

REFERENCES

1. Nygaard I, Barber MD, Burgio KL, et al. Prevalence of symptomatic pelvic floor disorders in US women. JAMA 2008;300(11):1311–6.
2. Sung VW, Hampton BS. Epidemiology of pelvic floor dysfunction. Obstet Gynecol Clin North Am 2009;36(3):421–43.
3. DeLancey JO. The hidden epidemic of pelvic floor dysfunction: achievable goals for improved prevention and treatment. Am J Obstet Gynecol 2005; 192(5):1488–95.
4. He W, Sengupta M, Velkoff VA, et al. Current population reports P23-209, 65+ in the United States: 2005. Washington, DC: US Government Printing Office; 2005. p. 23–209.
5. Wu JM, Hundley AF, Fulton RG, et al. Forecasting the prevalence of pelvic floor disorders in U.S. women: 2010 to 2050. Obstet Gynecol 2009;114(6):1278–83.
6. Brown HW, Wexner SD, Segall MM. Accidental bowel leakage in the Mature Women's Health Study: prevalence and predictors. Int J Clin Pract 2012; 66(11):1101–8.
7. Bharucha AE, Wald A, Enck P, et al. Functional anorectal disorders. Gastroenterology 2006;130(5):1510–8.
8. Nelson R, Norton N, Cautley E, et al. Community-based prevalence of anal incontinence. JAMA 1995;274(7):559–61.
9. Norton C, Whitehead WE, Bliss DZ, et al, Conservative management of fecal incontinence in adults Committee of the International Consultation on Incontinence. Management of fecal incontinence in adults. Neurourol Urodyn 2010; 29(1):199–206.
10. Whitehead WE, Borrud L, Goode PS, et al. Fecal incontinence in US adults: epidemiology and risk factors. Gastroenterology 2009;137(2):512–7, 517.e1–2.
11. Goode PS, Burgio KL, Halli AD, et al. Prevalence and correlates of fecal incontinence in community-dwelling older adults. J Am Geriatr Soc 2005;53(4): 629–35.
12. Melville JL, Fan M-Y, Newton K, et al. Fecal incontinence in US women: a population-based study. Am J Obstet Gynecol 2005;193(6):2071–6.
13. Bharucha AE, Zinsmeister AR, Schleck CD, et al. Bowel disturbances are the most important risk factors for late onset fecal incontinence: a population-based case-control study in women. Gastroenterology 2010;139(5):1559–66.

14. Nelson R, Furner S, Jesudason V. Fecal incontinence in Wisconsin nursing homes. Dis Colon Rectum 1998;41(10):1226–9.
15. Aslan E, Beji NK, Erkan HA, et al. The prevalence of and the related factors for urinary and fecal incontinence among older residing in nursing homes. J Clin Nurs 2009;18(23):3290–8.
16. Brown HW, Wexner SD, Lukacz ES. Factors associated with care seeking among women with accidental bowel leakage. Female Pelvic Med Reconstr Surg 2013;19(2):66–71.
17. Whitehead WE. Diagnosing and managing fecal incontinence: if you don't ask, they won't tell. Gastroenterology 2005;129(1):6.
18. Bharucha AE, Zinsmeister AR, Locke GR, et al. Symptoms and quality of life in community women with fecal incontinence. Clin Gastroenterol Hepatol 2006; 4(8):1004–9.
19. Norton C. Nurses, bowel continence, stigma, and taboos. J Wound Ostomy Continence Nurs 2004;31(2):85–94.
20. Brown HW, Wexner SD, Segall MM, et al. Quality of life impact in women with accidental bowel leakage. Int J Clin Pract 2012;66(11):1109–16.
21. Dunivan GC, Heymen S, Palsson OS, et al. Fecal incontinence in primary care: prevalence, diagnosis, and health care utilization. Am J Obstet Gynecol 2010; 202(5):493.e1–6.
22. Smith TM, Menees SB, Xu X, et al. Factors associated with quality of life among women with fecal incontinence. Int Urogynecol J 2013;24(3):493–9.
23. Szurszewski DJH, Holt PR, Schuster M. Proceedings of a workshop entitled "Neuromuscular function and dysfunction of the gastrointestinal tract in aging". Dig Dis Sci 1989;34(7):1135–46.
24. Bornemeier WC. Sphincter protecting hemorrhoidectomy. Am J Proctol 1960; 11(1):48–52.
25. Jorge JM, Wexner SD. Etiology and management of fecal incontinence. Dis Colon Rectum 1993;36(1):77–97.
26. Yu SWB, Rao SSC. Anorectal physiology and pathophysiology in the elderly. Clin Geriatr Med 2014;30(1):95–106.
27. Rao SSC. Fecal incontinence in a 56-year-old female executive. Clin Gastroenterol Hepatol 2007;5(4):422–6.
28. Lewicky-Gaupp C, Hamilton Q, Ashton-Miller J, et al. Anal sphincter structure and function relationships in aging and fecal incontinence. Am J Obstet Gynecol 2009;200(5):559.e1–5.
29. Lewicky-Gaupp C, Brincat C, Yousuf A, et al. Fecal incontinence in older women: are levator ani defects a factor? Am J Obstet Gynecol 2010;202(5): 491.e1–6.
30. Markland AD, Goode PS, Burgio KL, et al. Incidence and risk factors for fecal incontinence in black and white older adults: a population-based study. J Am Geriatr Soc 2010;58(7):1341–6.
31. Bharucha AE, Zinsmeister AR, Locke GR, et al. Risk factors for fecal incontinence: a population-based study in women. Am J Gastroenterol 2006;101(6): 1305–12.
32. Quander CR, Morris MC, Melson J, et al. Prevalence of and factors associated with fecal incontinence in a large community study of older individuals. Am J Gastroenterol 2005;100(4):905–9.
33. Altman D, Zetterström J, López A, et al. Effect of hysterectomy on bowel function. Dis Colon Rectum 2004;47(4):502–9.

34. Maglinte DDT, Hale DS, Sandrasegaran K. Comparison between dynamic cystocolpoproctography and dynamic pelvic floor MRI: pros and cons: which is the "functional" examination for anorectal and pelvic floor dysfunction? Abdom Imaging 2013;38(5):952–73.
35. Silva ACA, Maglinte DDT. Pelvic floor disorders: what's the best test? Abdom Imaging 2013;38(6):1391–408.
36. Townsend MK, Matthews CA, Whitehead WE, et al. Risk factors for fecal incontinence in older women. Am J Gastroenterol 2013;108(1):113–9.
37. Markland AD, Richter HE, Burgio KL, et al. Weight loss improves fecal incontinence severity in overweight and obese women with urinary incontinence. Int Urogynecol J 2011;22(9):1151–7.
38. Madoff RD, Parker SC, Varma MG, et al. Faecal incontinence in adults. Lancet 2004;364:621–32.
39. Joh H-K, Seong M-K, Oh S-W. Fecal incontinence in elderly Koreans. J Am Geriatr Soc 2010;58(1):116–21.
40. Bliss DZ, Jung HJ, Savik K, et al. Supplementation with dietary fiber improves fecal incontinence. Nurs Res 2001;50(4):203–13.
41. Markland AD, Burgio KL, Whitehead WE, et al. Loperamide versus psyllium fiber for treatment of fecal incontinence: the fecal incontinence prescription (Rx) management (FIRM) randomized clinical trial. Dis Colon Rectum 2015;58(10):983–93.
42. Omar MI, Alexander CE. Drug treatment for faecal incontinence in adults. Cochrane Database Syst Rev 2013;(6):CD002116.
43. Bliss DZ, Funk T, Jacobson M, et al. Incidence and characteristics of incontinence-associated dermatitis in community-dwelling persons with fecal incontinence. J Wound Ostomy Continence Nurs 2015;42(5):525–30.
44. Dumoulin C, Hay-Smith J. Pelvic floor muscle training versus no treatment, or inactive control treatments, for urinary incontinence in women. Cochrane Database Syst Rev 2010;(1):CD005646.
45. Norton C, Cody JD. Biofeedback and/or sphincter exercises for the treatment of faecal incontinence in adults. Cochrane Database Syst Rev 2012;(7):CD002111.
46. Norton C, Chelvanayagam S, Wilson-Barnett J, et al. Randomized controlled trial of biofeedback for fecal incontinence. Gastroenterology 2003;125(5):1320–9.
47. Van Koughnett JA, Wexner SD. Current management of fecal incontinence: choosing amongst treatment options to optimize outcomes. World J Gastroenterol 2013;19(48):9216–30.
48. Schwandner T, König IR, Heimerl T, et al. Triple target treatment (3T) is more effective than biofeedback alone for anal incontinence: the 3T-AI study. Dis Colon Rectum 2010;53(7):1007–16.
49. Watson NFS, Koshy A, Sagar PM. Anal bulking agents for faecal incontinence. Colorectal Dis 2012;14(Suppl 3):29–33.
50. Graf W, Mellgren A, Matzel KE, et al. Efficacy of dextranomer in stabilised hyaluronic acid for treatment of faecal incontinence: a randomised, sham-controlled trial. Lancet 2011;377(9770):997–1003.
51. Dodi G, Jongen J, de la Portilla F, et al. An open-label, noncomparative, multicenter study to evaluate efficacy and safety of NASHA/Dx Gel as a bulking agent for the treatment of fecal incontinence. Gastroenterol Res Pract 2010;2010:467136.
52. Wexner SD, Bleier J. Current surgical strategies to treat fecal incontinence. Expert Rev Gastroenterol Hepatol 2015;9(12):1577–89.

53. Efron JE. The SECCA procedure: a new therapy for treatment of fecal incontinence. Surg Technol Int 2004;13:107–10.
54. Herman RM, Berho M, Murawski M, et al. Defining the histopathological changes induced by nonablative radiofrequency treatment of faecal incontinence–a blinded assessment in an animal model. Colorectal Dis 2015;17(5):433–40.
55. Frascio M, Mandolfino F, Imperatore M, et al. The SECCA procedure for faecal incontinence: a review. Colorectal Dis 2014;16(3):167–72.
56. Lam TJ, Visscher AP, Meurs-Szojda MM, et al. Clinical response and sustainability of treatment with temperature-controlled radiofrequency energy (SECCA) in patients with faecal incontinence: 3 years follow-up. Int J Colorectal Dis 2014; 29(6):755–61.
57. Thaha MA, Abukar AA, Thin NN, et al. Sacral nerve stimulation for faecal incontinence and constipation in adults. Cochrane Database Syst Rev 2015;(8):CD004464.
58. Leroi AM, Parc Y, Lehur PA, et al. Efficacy of sacral nerve stimulation for fecal incontinence: results of a multicenter double-blind crossover study. Ann Surg 2005;242(5):662–9.
59. Vaizey CJ, Kamm MA, Roy AJ, et al. Double-blind crossover study of sacral nerve stimulation for fecal incontinence. Dis Colon Rectum 2000;43(3):298–302.
60. Kahlke V, Topic H, Peleikis HG, et al. Sacral nerve modulation for fecal incontinence: results of a prospective single-center randomized crossover study. Dis Colon Rectum 2015;58(2):235–40.
61. Sorensen M, Thomsen F. Sacral nerve stimulation increased rectal sensitivity in patients with faecal incontinence: results of randomized, double-blinded crossover study. In: Proceedings of the Joint Meeting of the International Continence Society and the International Urogynecologic Association. Toronto, Canada, Aug 23–27, 2010. p. 437.
62. Hull T, Giese C, Wexner SD, et al. Long-term durability of sacral nerve stimulation therapy for chronic fecal incontinence. Dis Colon Rectum 2013;56(2):234–45.
63. Ratto C, Litta F, Parello A, et al. Sacral nerve stimulation is a valid approach in fecal incontinence due to sphincter lesions when compared to sphincter repair. Dis Colon Rectum 2010;53(3):264–72.
64. Ratto C, Litta F, Parello A, et al. Sacral nerve stimulation in faecal incontinence associated with an anal sphincter lesion: a systematic review. Colorectal Dis 2012;14(6):e297–304.
65. Brouwer R, Duthie G. Sacral nerve neuromodulation is effective treatment for fecal incontinence in the presence of a sphincter defect, pudendal neuropathy, or previous sphincter repair. Dis Colon Rectum 2010;53(3):273–8.
66. Boyle DJ, Knowles CH, Lunniss PJ, et al. Efficacy of sacral nerve stimulation for fecal incontinence in patients with anal sphincter defects. Dis Colon Rectum 2009;52(7):1234–9.
67. Iachetta RP, Cola A, Villani RD. Sacral nerve stimulation in the treatment of fecal incontinence - the experience of a pelvic floor center: short term results. J Interv Gastroenterol 2012;2(4):189–92.
68. Horrocks EJ, Thin N, Thaha MA, et al. Systematic review of tibial nerve stimulation to treat faecal incontinence. Br J Surg 2014;101(5):457–68.
69. Bosch JL, Groen J. Sacral (S3) segmental nerve stimulation as a treatment for urge incontinence in patients with detrusor instability: results of chronic electrical stimulation using an implantable neural prosthesis. J Urol 1995;154:504–7.
70. Shaker HS, Hassouna M. Sacral nerve root neuromodulation: an effective treatment for refractory urge incontinence. J Urol 1998;159(5):1516–9.

71. Vandoninck V, van Balken MR, Finazzi Agró E, et al. Posterior tibial nerve stimulation in the treatment of urge incontinence. Neurourol Urodyn 2003;22(1): 17–23.
72. MacDiarmid SA, Siegel SW. Posterior tibial nerve stimulation before a trial of sacral nerve stimulation for refractory urge incontinence. J Urol 2014;191(6): 1652–4.
73. Thin NN, Taylor SJC, Bremner SA, et al. Randomized clinical trial of sacral versus percutaneous tibial nerve stimulation in patients with faecal incontinence. Br J Surg 2015;102(4):349–58.
74. Knowles CH, Horrocks EJ, Bremner SA, et al. Percutaneous tibial nerve stimulation versus sham electrical stimulation for the treatment of faecal incontinence in adults (CONFIDeNT): a double-blind, multicentre, pragmatic, parallel-group, randomised controlled trial. Lancet 2015;386(10004):1640–8.
75. Parks AG, McPartlin JF. Late repair of injuries of the anal sphincter. Proc R Soc Med 1971;64(12):1187–9.
76. Oom DMJ, Gosselink MP, Schouten WR. Anterior sphincteroplasty for fecal incontinence: a single center experience in the era of sacral neuromodulation. Dis Colon Rectum 2009;52(10):1681–7.
77. Johnson E, Carlsen E, Steen TB, et al. Short- and long-term results of secondary anterior sphincteroplasty in 33 patients with obstetric injury. Acta Obstet Gynecol Scand 2010;89(11):1466–72.
78. Dudding TC, Vaizey CJ, Kamm MA. Obstetric anal sphincter injury: incidence, risk factors, and management. Ann Surg 2008;247(2):224–37.
79. Bravo Gutierrez A, Madoff RD, Lowry AC, et al. Long-term results of anterior sphincteroplasty. Dis Colon Rectum 2004;47(5):727–31 [discussion:731–2].
80. Lehto K, Hyöty M, Collin P, et al. Seven-year follow-up after anterior sphincter reconstruction for faecal incontinence. Int J Colorectal Dis 2013;28(5):653–8.
81. Halverson AL, Hull TL. Long-term outcome of overlapping anal sphincter repair. Dis Colon Rectum 2002;45(3):345–8.
82. Maslekar S, Gardiner AB, Duthie GS. Anterior anal sphincter repair for fecal incontinence: good longterm results are possible. J Am Coll Surg 2007;204(1): 40–6.
83. Zutshi M, Tracey TH, Bast J, et al. Ten-year outcome after anal sphincter repair for fecal incontinence. Dis Colon Rectum 2009;52(6):1089–94.
84. Karoui S, Leroi AM, Koning E, et al. Results of sphincteroplasty in 86 patients with anal incontinence. Dis Colon Rectum 2000;43(6):813–20.
85. Glasgow SC, Lowry AC. Long-term outcomes of anal sphincter repair for fecal incontinence: a systematic review. Dis Colon Rectum 2012;55(4):482–90.
86. Barisic GI, Krivokapic ZV, Markovic VA, et al. Outcome of overlapping anal sphincter repair after 3 months and after a mean of 80 months. Int J Colorectal Dis 2006;21(1):52–6.
87. El-Gazzaz G, Zutshi M, Hannaway C, et al. Overlapping sphincter repair: does age matter? Dis Colon Rectum 2012;55(3):256–61.
88. Thornton MJ, Kennedy ML, Lubowski DZ, et al. Long-term follow-up of dynamic graciloplasty for faecal incontinence. Colorectal Dis 2004;6(6):470–6.
89. Sinha CK, Grewal A, Ward HC. Antegrade continence enema (ACE): current practice. Pediatr Surg Int 2008;24(6):685–8.
90. Patel AS, Saratzis A, Arasaradnam R, et al. Use of antegrade continence enema for the treatment of fecal incontinence and functional constipation in adults: a systematic review. Dis Colon Rectum 2015;58(10):999–1013.

91. Meurette G, Duchalais E, Lehur PA. Surgical approaches to fecal incontinence in the adult. J Visc Surg 2014;151(1):29–39.

92. Hocevar B, Gray M. Intestinal diversion (colostomy or ileostomy) in patients with severe bowel dysfunction following spinal cord injury. J Wound Ostomy Continence Nurs 2008;35(2):159–66.

93. Colquhoun P, Kaiser R, Efron J, et al. Is the quality of life better in patients with colostomy than patients with fecal incontinence? World J Surg 2006;30(10): 1925–8.

94. Norton C, Burch J, Kamm MA. Patients' views of a colostomy for fecal incontinence. Dis Colon Rectum 2005;48(5):1062–9.

95. Richter HE, Matthews CA, Muir T, et al. A vaginal bowel-control system for the treatment of fecal incontinence. Obstet Gynecol 2015;125(3):540–7.

96. Lehur P-A, McNevin S, Buntzen S, et al. Magnetic anal sphincter augmentation for the treatment of fecal incontinence: a preliminary report from a feasibility study. Dis Colon Rectum 2010;53(12):1604–10.

97. Rosenblatt P. New developments in therapies for fecal incontinence. Curr Opin Obstet Gynecol 2015;27(5):353–8.

98. Pakravan F, Helmes C. Magnetic anal sphincter augmentation in patients with severe fecal incontinence. Dis Colon Rectum 2015;58(1):109–14.

99. Wong MTC, Meurette G, Stangherlin P, et al. The magnetic anal sphincter versus the artificial bowel sphincter: a comparison of 2 treatments for fecal incontinence. Dis Colon Rectum 2011;54(7):773–9.

100. Wong MTC, Meurette G, Wyart V, et al. The artificial bowel sphincter: a single institution experience over a decade. Ann Surg 2011;254(6):951–6.

101. Rosenblatt P, Schumacher J, Lucente V, et al. A preliminary evaluation of the TOPAS system for the treatment of fecal incontinence in women. Female Pelvic Med Reconstr Surg 2014;20(3):155–62.

102. Fenner DE, Lucente V, Zutshi M, et al. TOPAS: a new modality for the treatment of fecal incontinence in women. J Minim Invasive Gynecol 2015;22(3):S3–4.

103. Zakhem E, Rego SL, Raghavan S, et al. The appendix as a viable source of neural progenitor cells to functionally innervate bioengineered gastrointestinal smooth muscle tissues. Stem Cells Transl Med 2015;4(6):548–54.

104. Bitar KN, Bohl J, Fortunato JE, et al. 600 In Situ implantation of autologous Biosphincter™ re-instates continence in a large animal model of passive fecal incontinence. Gastroenterology 2015;148(4 Supp 1):S–117.

105. Pathi SD, Acevedo JF, Keller PW, et al. Recovery of the injured external anal sphincter after injection of local or intravenous mesenchymal stem cells. Obstet Gynecol 2012;119(1):134–44.

106. Frudinger A, Pfeifer J, Paede J, et al. Autologous skeletal-muscle-derived cell injection for anal incontinence due to obstetric trauma: a 5-year follow-up of an initial study of 10 patients. Colorectal Dis 2015;17(9):794–801.

107. Goldsmith HS, Chandra A. Pyloric valve transposition as substitute for a colostomy in humans: a preliminary report. Am J Surg 2011;202(4):409–16.

108. Chandra A, Kumar A, Noushif M, et al. Perineal antropylorus transposition for end-stage fecal incontinence in humans: initial outcomes. Dis Colon Rectum 2013;56(3):360–6.

109. Bortolini MAT, Drutz HP, Lovatsis D, et al. Vaginal delivery and pelvic floor dysfunction: current evidence and implications for future research. Int Urogynecol J 2010;21(8):1025–30.

110. Patel DA, Xu X, Thomason AD, et al. Childbirth and pelvic floor dysfunction: an epidemiologic approach to the assessment of prevention opportunities at delivery. Am J Obstet Gynecol 2006;195(1):23–8.
111. Ellerkmann RM, Cundiff GW, Melick CF, et al. Correlation of symptoms with location and severity of pelvic organ prolapse. Am J Obstet Gynecol 2001;185(6): 1332–8.
112. Fialkow MF, Gardella C, Melville J, et al. Posterior vaginal wall defects and their relation to measures of pelvic floor neuromuscular function and posterior compartment symptoms. Am J Obstet Gynecol 2002;187(6):1443–9.
113. Burrows LJ, Meyn LA, Walters MD, et al. Pelvic symptoms in women with pelvic organ prolapse. Obstet Gynecol 2004;104(5 Pt 1):982–8.
114. Bradley CS, Brown MB, Cundiff GW, et al. Bowel symptoms in women planning surgery for pelvic organ prolapse. Am J Obstet Gynecol 2006;195(6):1814–9.
115. Hale DS, Fenner D. Consistently Inconsistent, the posterior vaginal wall. Am J Obstet Gynecol 2015. http://dx.doi.org/10.1016/j.ajog.2015.09.001.
116. da Silva GM, Gurland B, Sleemi A, et al. Posterior vaginal wall prolapse does not correlate with fecal symptoms or objective measures of anorectal function. Am J Obstet Gynecol 2006;195(6):1742–7.
117. Gustilo-Ashby AM, Paraiso MFR, Jelovsek JE, et al. Bowel symptoms 1 year after surgery for prolapse: further analysis of a randomized trial of rectocele repair. Am J Obstet Gynecol 2007;197(1):76.e1–5.

Upper Gastrointestinal Tract Motility Disorders in Women, Gastroparesis, and Gastroesophageal Reflux Disease

CrossMark

Jasmine K. Zia, MD[a],*, Margaret M. Heitkemper, RN, PhD[b]

KEYWORDS

- Sex differences • Women's health • Gastrointestinal dysmotility • GERD
- Gastroparesis • Estrogen • Progesterone

KEY POINTS

- Female ovarian hormones (ie, progesterone, estrogen) are one of the main causes for the observed sex differences in upper gastrointestinal motility.
- Men have increased stomach acid production and more physiologic gastroesophageal reflux (GERD) than women, possibly explaining the increased complication rates of GERD in men.
- Healthy women's stomachs empty out slower than men. Women also perceive fullness and nausea more quickly and for longer periods of time than men.
- Women with gastroparesis tend to be more symptomatic than men. Their symptoms are also less likely to improve over time compared with men.

INTRODUCTION

There are known sex differences in gastrointestinal (GI) motility in both healthy and diseased states, likely due to the effect of female hormones. Both estrogen and progesterone receptors are found throughout the GI tract and likely influence its motility.[1] There are several mechanisms that may account for the influence of these hormones on GI motility. In vitro studies suggest that estrogen is needed to prime and enhance

Disclosures/Conflicts of Interests: None.
[a] Division of Gastroenterology and Hepatology, Department of Medicine, University of Washington, 1959 Northeast Pacific Street, Box 356424, Seattle, WA 98195-6424, USA; [b] Department of Biobehavioral Nursing and Health Systems, University of Washington, 1959 Northeast Pacific Street, Box 357266, Seattle, WA 98195-7266, USA
* Corresponding author. Division of Gastroenterology, Department of Medicine, University of Washington, 1959 Northeast Pacific Street, Box 356424, Seattle, WA 98195-6424.
E-mail address: JZia@medicine.washington.edu

Gastroenterol Clin N Am 45 (2016) 239–251
http://dx.doi.org/10.1016/j.gtc.2016.02.003
0889-8553/16/$ – see front matter © 2016 Elsevier Inc. All rights reserved.

the inhibitory effects of progesterone.[2] These hormones also likely mediate GI motility effects by eliciting changes in nitric oxide–containing neurons in the myenteric plexus and by affecting the number and function of mast cells in GI mucosa.[3,4]

Given the fluctuations of these female hormones during the menstrual cycle, pregnancy, and menopause, including the perimenopausal transition, one may also expect significant differences in GI motility during each of these female hormonal stages. Such differences have in fact been found in some studies and are described in this article. During the menses stage of the menstrual cycle, estrogen and progesterone are at their lowest levels. In the follicular phase that follows, estrogen levels begin to increase. It is this increase that triggers ovulation. Once ovulation has occurred, estrogen levels peak a second time followed by an increase in progesterone levels during the luteal phase to prepare the uterus lining for possible fertilization. If the egg is not fertilized, the corpus luteum degenerates and no longer produces progesterone, followed by a decrease in estrogen levels. The menstrual cycle then repeats itself. Menstruation is considered an inflammatory state characterized by increases in proinflammatory cytokines (eg, tumor necrosis factor-α) and other mediators before menstrual flow. Evidence suggests that the inflammatory response is linked to declining progesterone levels in the late luteal phase.[5,6] During pregnancy, there is a progressive and substantial increase in progesterone and estrogen. After menopause, the opposite occurs: estrogen and progesterone levels drop significantly. The age at which menopause occurs and the pattern of the drop in hormone levels are variable. This transition is referred to as the perimenopause phase.

Despite the growing evidence that sex differences exist, most practitioners continue to diagnose and treat conditions of GI dysmotility without acknowledging them. Providers often generalize associated risk factors and prognoses of GI dysmotility conditions to both men and women. The effect of female hormonal stages (ie, menses, pregnancy, menopause) on GI motility is also not factored into treatment plans. To more accurately and effectively manage conditions of GI dysmotility for both men and women, providers should better understand the sex differences in both healthy and GI dysmotility conditions. More studies need to be conducted to better understand these sex differences.

This article specifically reviews sex differences in esophageal and gastric motility, first for healthy participants and then for the most common dysmotility conditions. For esophageal conditions, it will focus on gastroesophageal reflux disease (GERD) and other esophageal motor disorders. For gastric conditions, it discusses gastroparesis and accelerated gastric emptying. Although limited by the currently available literature, this article describes any known differences in signs and symptoms during each female hormonal stage for each aforementioned healthy and abnormal condition.

THE ESOPHAGUS
Sex Differences in Esophageal Anatomy and Motility in Healthy Participants

Table 1 summarizes the sex differences in esophageal anatomy, motility, sensation, and pH studies. Women may have shorter esophageal sphincter lengths than men.[7,8] In healthy participants undergoing esophageal manometry, women are more likely to have longer esophageal body contractile duration than men.[9–11] Studies investigating sex differences in esophageal mechanical pain thresholds have conflicting results, possibly due to differences in balloon distention methods.[12–15] Although no sex differences in esophageal thermal pain thresholds have been found, women report higher chemical pain thresholds and larger referred pain areas compared with men,

Table 1
Gender differences in esophageal anatomy, motility, sensation, and pH studies in healthy participants

Variable	Healthy Participants (Women vs Men)
Anatomy	
LES length	Slightly shorter vs no difference[7,8]
Motility	
Esophageal body	
% Peristalsis	No difference[9,10]
Amplitude	No difference[10–12]
Contractile duration	Longer[9–11]
Velocity	Conflicting: lower vs no difference[9–12]
LES	
Resting pressures	Conflicting: higher vs no difference[9,11,12]
Duration of relaxation	No difference[10,11]
Sensation	
Mechanical pain	Conflicting: higher, lower vs no difference[12–15]
Chemical pain	Higher[13]
Thermal pain	No difference[13]
Referred pain areas	Larger[13]
pH studies	
% time pH <4	Lower[16]
Total reflux episodes	Lower[16]
Episodes >5min	Lower[16]
Longest reflux episodes	Shorter[16]

possibly reflecting sex differences in central processing of pain to visceral stimuli.[13] In healthy participants undergoing esophageal pH studies, women are found to have decreased physiologic GERD.[16]

The Effect of Female Hormonal Stages on Esophageal Motility

Table 2 summarizes the known effects of specific female hormonal stages (ie, menses, pregnancy, menopause) on esophageal motility. The authors were unable to find any studies directly examining the effects of the menopause transition on esophageal motility.

During the luteal phase of the menstrual cycle, Van Thiel and colleagues[1] observed a small but significant reduction in lower esophageal sphincter pressures (LESP). However, other studies found no LESP differences during the human menstrual cycle.[17,18] The clinical significance of a mildly reduced LESP during normal menstrual cycles is likely unimportant. The frequency of symptomatic heartburn does not differ for women during their menstrual cycle.[1] The menstrual cycle also has no effect on esophageal sensory perception, distal esophageal contraction, or esophageal emptying.[10,14,16,17,19]

LESP are reduced in pseudopregnant women (healthy participants given a potent estrogen followed by progesterone exposure).[20] This finding is discussed further with its clinical implications in the next section. Esophageal dysmotility is rare in pregnancy, although some studies have documented reduced esophageal amplitudes and

Table 2
Effect of female hormonal stages on esophageal motility

Hormonal Stage	Effect on Esophagus
Menstrual cycle	
Sensory perception	None[12,14]
LES pressure	Possibly reduced during the luteal phase of the menstrual cycle[1]
Distal contraction	None[10,17,19]
Esophageal emptying	None[10,17,19]
Pregnancy	
LES pressure	Likely reduced[20]
Distal contraction	Reduced amplitude[16]
% Peristalsis	Reduced % transmitted contractions[16]
Menopause	
—	Unknown

increased nontransmitted contractions during pregnancy.[16] These patterns may be attributed to gestational hormones and/or, at least later in pregnancy, from increased intragastric pressures from an enlarging uterus.

Sex Differences in Gastroesophageal Reflux Disease

The prevalence of GERD is similar among men and nonpregnant women.[21] The following complications of GERD, however, are more common in men: erosive esophagitis, esophageal ulceration, Barrett's esophagus and esophageal adenocarcinoma.[21] Similar to the sex differences found in healthy participants, men with GERD also have more acid reflux than women with GERD. Stomach acid production, both basal and maximum output, is increased in men with GERD compared with women with GERD, possibly because of the increased number of stomach parietal cells.[22] In one study, there seems to be only a weak correlation between gastric acid output and GERD severity in both genders.[21] Estrogen may play a role in attenuating esophageal damage through luminal nitric oxide–related pathways.[23] To date, there are no studies on sex differences in transient lower esophageal sphincter (LES) relaxations.[16] Despite having more sequelae of reflux disease though, men have similar hospitalization rates for GERD complications as women.[24]

GERD-associated factors differ among the sexes based on a study by Murao and colleagues.[25] In women, age and lack of exercise are associated factors with GERD, possibly due to fat accumulation in internal organs as women age, resulting in an increase in intra-abdominal pressure. In men, smoking and fewer hours of sleep are associated factors. In both men and women, a hiatal hernia and higher body mass index (BMI) are associated factors. A stronger association between increasing BMI and reflux symptoms is seen in women than in men.[26]

Table 3 outlines known sex differences in the response to common GERD therapies.

Effect of Female Hormonal Stages on Gastroesophageal Reflux Disease

The authors were unable to find any studies highlighting symptom variation across the menstrual cycle for women with GERD.

During pregnancy, 85% of women report heartburn.[27] The incidence of GERD increases with each trimester: 8%, 40%, and 52% for the first, second, and third

Table 3
Sex differences in the response to common therapies for gastroesophageal reflux disease and gastroparesis

Common Therapies	Known Sex Differences
GERD	
Lifestyle modifications	No available data[56,57]
Medications	
Acid-lowering drugs	
Proton pump inhibitors (PPI)	Controversial: no difference vs poorer response rates in women[58,59]
	Association between long-term PPI therapy and hip fractures is lower in women than men[60]
Histamine$_2$-receptor antagonists	No available data
Surgery	
Nissen fundoplication	Most studies have concluded no significant differences in efficacy[59,61,62]
	In the US, women are more likely to undergo antireflux surgeries[59,63]
Gastroparesis	
Dietary modifications	No available data
Medications	
Promotility agents	
Metoclopramide	Similar response rates to oral, but women may respond better to intranasal formulations[64,65]
Domperidone	No reported differences in efficacy[65,66]
Erythromycin	No available data
	Associated with more cardiac arrhythmias in women than men[67]
Cisapride	No available data
Antiemetics	No reported differences in efficacy[65]
	Women were more likely to have side effects to metoclopramide[68]
Neuromodulators/analgesics	No reported differences (although limited data)[65]
Procedures	
Pyloric botulinum injections	Conflicting: men may have superior responses than women overall, but women may respond to larger doses than men. No differences in durability[69,70]
Nasojejunal tube feeds	No available data
Gastric electrical stimulator	No reported differences in efficacy[71]

trimester, respectively.[16] Following delivery, the incidence of GERD becomes greatly reduced or absent. Increasing maternal age, higher prepregnancy BMI, certain ethnic groups (ie, Caucasian, Native American), tobacco/coffee consumption, and prepregnancy upper GI complaints are associated with higher prevalence of heartburn during pregnancy.[27] Of note, some pregnant women with symptoms of GERD have normal ambulatory esophageal pH testing.[16]

The cause of GERD during pregnancy is likely multifactorial and can vary by trimester. Throughout pregnancy, the progressive increase in progesterone and estrogen can reduce LESPs and effective esophageal body peristalsis to help with the clearance of reflux contents.[17,28] Later in pregnancy, the enlarging uterus compressing the stomach can increase intragastric pressures and cause a mass effect resulting in mechanical alterations of the LES such as loss of the intra-abdominal LES segment and/or shifting of supporting anatomic structures surrounding the LES (eg, diaphragm).

In a survey study by Infantino,[29] postmenopausal women were 2.9 times more likely to have GERD symptoms than premenopausal women. This finding is somewhat inconsistent with 2 prior studies that found only a slight association between age and increased prevalence of GERD symptoms up until the ages of 55 to 69 years old, from which point the trend reversed.[30] If progesterone and estrogen substantially contribute to the cause of GERD in women, one would expect the opposite: a decreased incidence of GERD in postmenopausal women. Other factors associated with aging likely contribute to this increased incidence of GERD with age, such as weight gain, fat redistribution, alcohol, smoking, medications, comorbidities, and so on.[31] In the aforementioned study, women in the postmenopausal group were in fact heavier and consumed more alcohol.

However, the association between BMI and reflux symptoms seems to be stronger in premenopausal than postmenopausal women in the study by Nilsson and colleagues.[26] This study also observed a dose-dependent increase in the risk of reflux symptoms for women on hormone replacement therapy (HRT), which was greater with increasing BMI. These findings support female hormones playing a role in the association between BMI and reflux symptoms.

Sex Differences in Other Esophageal Motor Disorders

In an Australian study by Andrews and colleagues,[32] there was a higher prevalence of ineffective or reflux-related esophageal motility disorder in men than women (34% vs 23%, $P = .01$). In an American study by Tsuboi and colleagues,[33] there was a higher prevalence of nutcracker esophagus in women than men (8.5% vs 4.6%, $P<.001$), while men had a higher prevalence of nonspecific esophageal motility disorders (13.7% vs 10.7%, $P = .003$). Sex otherwise has no effect on other esophageal motor disorder diagnoses: normal, achalasia, or diffuse esophageal spasms.[32,34] In the former Australian study, women were more commonly referred to a specialist for evaluation of esophageal motor disorders.

THE STOMACH
Sex Differences in Stomach Anatomy and Motility in Healthy Participants

Table 4 summarizes the sex differences in stomach anatomy, motility, sensory thresholds, and acid production among healthy participants. Gastric emptying of both solids and liquids are slower in women than men.[35–37] This difference in gastric-emptying time is attributed to a combination of longer proximal gastric relaxation times and decreased postprandial distal stomach contractility (both frequency and amplitude) observed in women. Using dynamic antral scintigraphy to assess postprandial antral contractions, women exhibit more irregular contraction patterns with smaller vertical displacements than men.[35] Using antroduodenal manometry, the frequency of antral contractions drop immediately after meal ingestion in women compared with its temporary increase in men.[35] During gastric-emptying studies, meal retention emptying curves begin to diverge between the sexes at 50 minutes.[35]

Normal gastric-emptying rates can often be described as "biphasic" with a lag phase (thought to allow the stomach time to process food into small enough particles for emptying) followed by a linear phase characterized by a constant rate of emptying.

Table 4
Gender differences in gastric motility, sensation, and acid production in healthy participants

Variable	Healthy Participants (Women vs Men)
Anatomy	
Gastric surface area	Smaller (correlates with body size)[21]
Motility	
Emptying	Slower, both solids and liquids[35–37]
Fundic relaxation	Prolonged[39]
Antral contractility	Decreased with lower amplitudes and frequencies[35]
Sensation	
Satiety perception	Increased, in both intensity and duration[39]
Mechanical pain	No difference[39]
Acid production	
Basal acid output	Lower[16,21]
Maximum acid output	Lower[16,21]
Parietal cells	Less[16]

No sex differences are observed in lag times, but during the linear phase, the slope is less steep in women than men.[35,38]

In healthy participants who participated in barostat studies, there are no sex differences in pain thresholds to balloon distention.[39] However, there are differences in perception. During fasting conditions, the perception of fullness and abdominal pressure increases more rapidly in women than men. During fed states, the perception of nausea is increased, and the perception of fullness remains longer in women than men. This difference can possibly be explained by a delayed return of intragastric volume to basal 30 to 90 minutes postprandial in women compared with men.

Women have lower basal and maximum gastric acid output, likely due to decreased gastric surface areas, which correlates with body size, and thus decreased number of parietal cells.[22]

The Effect of Female Hormonal Stages on Gastric Motility

Table 5 summarizes the known effects of female hormonal stages on gastric motility.

Gastric emptying is significantly delayed in female ovariectomized rats treated with progesterone and estradiol but not testosterone, presumably because of the inhibitory effects of progesterone on stomach smooth muscle.[40] One would therefore expect a delay in gastric emptying during the luteal phase when progesterone is at its highest. Gill and colleagues[41] did observe such delayed gastric emptying of solid-phase markers during the luteal phase in 7 normally menstruating women, which correlated with elevated serum levels of progesterone. Other human studies have not confirmed this finding. Horowitz and colleagues[42] found no significant differences in gastric emptying of solids and liquids in 10 healthy women between the follicular and luteal phases when using a dual isotope scintigraphic technique. Madsen[43] reported the opposite finding: delayed gastric emptying during the follicular phase in 8 women, ages 21 to 27, consuming a meal containing ^{99}m Tc-labeled cellulose fiber and 2- to 3-mm ^{111}In-labeled plastic particles. No differences in manometric antral contractility were found to support the inhibitory effect of progesterone on smooth muscle in this latter study.[43] Perhaps progesterone results in prolonged effects on stomach smooth muscle contractility or even low levels can affect gastric

Table 5
Effect of female hormonal stages on gastric motility

Hormonal Stage	Effect
Menstrual cycle	
Gastric emptying	Conflicting but likely no effect[41–43]
Antral contractility	No effect[43]
Basal gastric pH	No effect[1,20]
Pregnancy	
Intra-abdominal pressure	Increased by enlarging uterus up to twice that of normal[16]
Gastric emptying	Likely no effect[44]
CCK, gastrin levels	No effect[44]
Motilin levels	Decreased[39]
Menopause[a]	
Gastric emptying	Accelerated compared with premenopausal women[47]
Lag phase	Shorter than premenopausal women[47]
Linear phase	Steeper emptying rate than premenopausal women[47]

[a] Not on HRT.

motility. The menstrual cycle, confirmed by changes in progesterone levels, also does not affect fasting gastrin levels (a known stimulant of gastric motility) or basal gastric pH.[1,20]

Most human studies have found that pregnancy has no effect on gastric emptying.[39,44] Although Simpson[45] came to a different conclusion: pregnancy delays liquid gastric emptying, they used the rate of paracetamol absorption, rather than ultrasound examinations, as their primary measure in 28 women undergoing termination of pregnancy. The rate of paracetamol absorption likely involves multiple factors including gastric transit time. Pregnancy does not affect cholecystokinin (CCK) or gastrin levels but does decrease motilin levels.[39,44] In one study, an enlarging uterus was associated with a 2-fold increase in intragastric pressures compared with pre-pregnancy pressures, likely contributing to the increased incidence of GERD during pregnancy.[16]

High levels of progesterone and estrogen can also cause "morning sickness" or nausea during pregnancy. Gastric dysrhythmias, both bradygastria and tachygastria, have been observed from electrogastrography studies in pregnant women and nonpregnant women given progesterone and estrogen doses to mimic pregnancy.[46] Such gastric electrical abnormalities have been linked to nausea and vomiting during pregnancy.

During menopause, there is a trend toward faster gastric emptying similar to men with shorter lag phases and steeper linear emptying rates.[47] If postmenopausal women are taking HRT though, all aforementioned measures are closer to their premenopausal rates.[47] This finding supports the influence of progesterone and estrogen on gastric motility despite the lack of gastric-emptying differences found in women during the menstrual cycle and pregnancy. It may be that the absolute level of progesterone and estrogen is not as important as the rate of change in these female hormones.

Sex Differences in Gastroparesis

Gastroparesis affects women more commonly than men for all main subtypes: idiopathic (80%), diabetic (76%), and possibly postsurgical (89%).[48,49] Like healthy participants, women with gastroparesis have slower gastric-emptying rates and thus higher gastric retention percentages at 4 hours than men.[48]

Women suffering from gastroparesis tend to be more symptomatic than men with gastroparesis. Women with diabetic gastroparesis report significantly more nausea, early satiety, postprandial excessive fullness, and loss of appetite than men.[50] Similarly, women with idiopathic gastroparesis report more nausea, stomach fullness, inability to finish a meal, postprandial excessive fullness, bloating, abdominal distention, and constipation than men.[48] No sex differences in vomiting and retching in either diabetic and idiopathic gastroparesis participants have been reported.[48,50] Although not completely understood, such differences are again attributed to differences in female hormones and baseline gastric function. As outlined in **Table 4**, even healthy women have slower gastric-emptying rates, prolonged fundic relaxation, decreased antral contractility, and increased sensitivity when compared with men. Perhaps this lower reserve of "normal" gastric function makes women more susceptible to the onset and symptoms of gastroparesis.

The prevalence and severity of symptoms of diabetic gastroparesis are higher among women who are obese and who have long-standing, poorly controlled diabetes.[50] Obese/overweight people may be at increased risk of developing gastroparesis due to its proinflammatory effects. Pathologically, myenteric inflammation has been observed in some patients with gastroparesis.[48] The adipose tissue of obese women may also secrete more estrogen.[50] Associated factors for women with idiopathic gastroparesis include smoking, drinking alcohol, and a history of migraine headaches.[48]

Although not extensively studied, there are some known sex differences in the response to certain medications and investigational treatments for gastroparesis, as outlined in **Table 3**. Despite superior responses observed in women for some gastroparesis therapies, symptoms are less likely to improve over time in women compared with men. Male sex is an independent predictor of symptomatic improvement at 48 weeks and is associated with more than a 2-fold improvement over women.[51]

Effect of Female Hormonal Stages on Gastroparesis

In a study by Verrengia and colleagues[52] with 20 premenopausal gastroparesis women not on oral contraceptive agents, nausea and early satiety seem to worsen during the luteal phase of the menstrual cycle. No cyclical differences are otherwise observed for other gastroparesis-related symptoms, such as vomiting, bloating, abdominal pain, fullness, or loss of appetite.

Gastroparesis, especially if severe, is a relative contraindication for pregnancy because of an associated increased risk of maternal morbidity and poor perinatal outcomes.[53] The authors are only able to find one clinical study investigating menopause and gastroparesis. In this study by Parkman and colleagues,[48] 67 of the 214 (31.3%) women with gastroparesis were postmenopausal. Postmenopausal women tend to have less severe gastroparesis symptoms than their counterparts. No significant differences are otherwise found for weight, acute versus insidious onset of symptoms, or gastric retention percentages at 4 hours between premenopausal and postmenopausal women.

Accelerated Gastric Emptying

Accelerated gastric emptying seems to be a more common condition in men than women[54,55]; this can possibly be explained, at least partly, by the uniform cutoff used for both men and women. Overall, healthy women have slower gastric-emptying rates than men. Therefore, this uniform cutoff may not capture what is considered "accelerated gastric emptying" for women. Underlying causes of accelerated gastric emptying (eg, surgery, diabetes, duodenal ulcer, endocrinopathies, hypertension, idiopathic) do not appear to be sex-related. No sex differences are reported for presenting symptoms.

SUMMARY

This article summarizes the known sex differences in both esophageal and gastric motility in healthy participants and those with common upper GI dysmotility conditions. It also discusses the effect of female hormonal stages on the aforementioned states.

More research needs to be conducted to further highlight sex differences in esophageal and gastric motility, for both healthy and disease states. These sex differences may affect diagnostic parameters and treatment strategies of upper GI dysmotility conditions. In some cases, such sex differences have already been taken into account, such as screening guidelines for Barrett's esophagus. A lower LES pressure cutoff could perhaps be considered for women during esophageal manometry. Similarly, different gastric-emptying times could be set for men and women for the diagnosis of gastroparesis. Female patients with either GERD or gastroparesis could be instructed to prepare themselves for feeling more symptomatic during the luteal phase of their menstrual cycle. Clinicians could better guide their therapeutic approach to upper GI dysmotility conditions based on sex as future research expands the knowledge on the sex differences in the response to common therapies (see **Table 3**). Such changes could potentially result in more accurate diagnoses and prognoses, and most importantly, tailored treatment strategies for greater symptom reduction.

REFERENCES

1. Van Thiel D, Gavaler J, Stremple J. Lower esophageal sphincter pressure during the normal menstrual cycle. Am J Obstet Gynecol 1979;134:64–7.
2. Fisher R, Roberts G, Grabowski C, et al. Inhibition of lower esophageal sphincter circular muscle by female sex hormones. Am J Physiol 1978;3:E243–7.
3. Shah S, Nathan L, Singh R, et al. E2 and not P4 increases NO release from NANC nerves of the gastrointestinal tract: implications in pregnancy. Am J Physiol Regul Integr Comp Physiol 2001;280:R1546–54.
4. Bradesi S, Eutamene H, Theodorou V, et al. Effect of ovarian hormones on intestinal mast cell reactivity to substance P. Life Sci 2001;68:1047–56.
5. Evans J, Salamonsen LA. Inflammation, leukocytes and menstruation. Rev Endocr Metab Disord 2012;13:277–88.
6. Whitcomb BW, Mumford SL, Perkins NJ, et al. Urinary cytokine and chemokine profiles across the menstrual cycle in healthy reproductive-aged women. Fertil Steril 2014;101:1383–91.
7. Li Q, Castell J, Castell D. Manometric determination of esophageal length. Am J Gastroenterol 1994;89:722–5.
8. Diamant N. Physiology of the esophagus. Gastrointestinal disease. Philadelphia: WB Saunders Company; 1993.
9. Vega KJ, Palacio C, Langford-Legg T, et al. Gender variation in oesophageal motor function: analysis of 129 healthy individuals. Dig Liver Dis 2010;42:482–4.
10. Dantas R, Ferriolli E, Souza M. Gender effects on esophageal motility. Braz J Med Biol Res 1998;31:539–44.

11. Grande L, Lacima G, Ros E, et al. Deterioration of esophageal motility with age: a manometric study of 79 healthy subjects. Am J Gastroenterol 1999; 94:1795–801.

12. Rao S. Effects of gender and age on esophageal biomechanical properties and sensation. Am J Gastroenterol 2003;98:1688–95.

13. Reddy H, Arendt-Nielsen L, Staahl C, et al. Gender differences in pain and biomechanical responses after acid sensitization of the human esophagus. Dig Dis Sci 2005;50:2050–8.

14. Nguyen P, Lee S, Castell D. Evidence of gender differences in esophagal pain threshold. Am J Gastroenterol 1995;90:901–5.

15. Paterson W, Wang H, Vanner S. Increasing pain sensation to repeated esophageal balloon distention in patients with chest pain of undetermined etiology. Dig Dis Sci 1995;40:1325–31.

16. RB T. Gender differences in gastroesophageal reflux disease. J Gend Specif Med 2000;3:42–4.

17. Nelson J, Richter J, Johns D, et al. Esophageal contraction pressures are not affected by normal menstrual cycles. Gastroenterology 1984;87:867–71.

18. Alvarez-Sanchez A, Rey E, Achem S, et al. Does progesterone fluctuation across the menstrual cycle predispose to gastroesophageal reflux? Am J Gastroenterol 1999;94:1468–71.

19. Hsu J, Kim C, O'Connor M, et al. Effect of menstrual cycle on esophageal emptying of liquid and solid boluses. Mayo Clin Proc 1993;68:753–6.

20. Van Thiel D, Gavaler J, Stremple J. Lower esophageal sphincter pressure in women using sequential oral contraceptives. Gastroenterology 1976;71:232–4.

21. Sonnenberg A. Effects of environment and lifestyle on gastroesophageal reflux disease. Dig Dis 2011;29:229–34.

22. Ter RB, Johnston BT, Castell DO. Influence of age and gender on gastroesophageal reflux in symptomatic patients. Dis Esophagus 1998;11:106–8.

23. Iijima K, Shimosegawa T. Involvement of luminal nitric oxide in the pathogenesis of the gastroesophageal reflux disease spectrum. J Gastroenterol Hepatol 2014; 29:898–905.

24. Sonnenberg A. Time trends of US hospitalization for esophageal disease. J Clin Gastroenterol 2014;48:e71–5.

25. Murao T, Sakurai K, Mihara S, et al. Lifestyle change influences on GERD in Japan: a study of participants in a health examination program. Dig Dis Sci 2011;56:2857–64.

26. Nilsson M, Johnsen R, Ye W, et al. Obesity and estrogen as risk factors for gastroesophageal reflux symptoms. JAMA 2003;290:66–72.

27. Naumann CR, Zelig C, Napolitano PG, et al. Nausea, vomiting, and heartburn in pregnancy: a prospective look at risk, treatment, and outcome. J Matern Fetal Neonatal Med 2012;25:1488–93.

28. Eliakim R, Abulafia O, Sherer D. Estrogen, progesterone and the gastrointestinal tract. J Reprod Med 2000;45:781–8.

29. Infantino M. The prevalence and pattern of gastroesophageal reflux symptoms in perimenopausal and menopausal women. J Am Acad Nurse Pract 2008;20: 266–72.

30. Dent J, El-Serag HB, Wallander MA, et al. Epidemiology of gastro-oesophageal reflux disease: a systematic review. Gut 2005;54:710–7.

31. Greenwald DA. Aging, the gastrointestinal tract, and risk of acid-related disease. Am J Med 2004;117:8–13.

32. Andrews JM, Heddle R, Hebbard GS, et al. Age and gender affect likely mano-metric diagnosis: audit of a tertiary referral hospital clinical esophageal manom-etry service. J Gastroenterol Hepatol 2009;24:125–8.
33. Tsuboi K, Hoshino M, Srinivasan A, et al. Insights gained from symptom evalua-tion of esophageal motility disorders: a review of 4,215 patients. Digestion 2012; 85:236–42.
34. Sonnenberg A. Hospitalization for achalasia in the United States 1997–2006. Dig Dis Sci 2009;54:1680–5.
35. LC K, Parkman HP, Brown K, et al. Delayed gastric emptying and decreased antral contractility in normal premenopausal women compared with men. Am J Gastroenterol 1997;92:968–75.
36. Datz F, Christian P, Moore J. Gender-related differences in gastric emptying. J Nucl Med 1987;28:1204–7.
37. Camilleri M, Iturrino J, Bharucha AE, et al. Performance characteristics of scinti-graphic measurement of gastric emptying of solids in healthy participants. Neu-rogastroenterol Motil 2012;24:1076–1076.e562.
38. Kerrigan D, Mangnall Y, Read N, et al. Influence of acid-pepsin secretion on gastric emptying of solids in humans: studies with cimetidine. Gut 1991;32: 1295–7.
39. Mearadji B, Penning C, Vu MK, et al. Influence of gender on proximal gastric mo-tor and sensory function. Am J Gastroenterol 2001;96:2066–73.
40. Chen T, Doong M, Chang F, et al. Effects of sex steroid hormones on gastric emptying and gastrointestinal transit in rats. Am J Physiol Gastrointest Liver Phys-iol 1995;268:G171–6.
41. Gill R, Murphy P, Hooper H, et al. Effect of the menstrual cycle on gastric emptying. Digestion 1987;36:168–74.
42. Horowitz M, Maddern G, Chatterton B, et al. The normal menstrual cycle has no effect on gastric emptying. Br J Obstet Gynaecol 1985;92:743–6.
43. Madsen J. Effects of gender, age, and body mass index on gastrointestinal transit times. Dig Dis Sci 1992;37:1548–53.
44. Chiloiro M, Darconza G, Piccioli E, et al. Gastric emptying and orocecal transit time in pregnancy. J Gastroenterol 2001;36:538–43.
45. Simpson K. Pregnancy delays paracetamol absorption and gastric emptying in patients undergoing surgery. Br J Anaesth 1988;60:24–7.
46. Walsh J, Hasler WL, Nugent C, et al. Progesterone and estrogen are potential me-diators of gastric slow-wave dysrhythmias in nausea of pregnancy. Am J Physiol 1996;270:G506–14.
47. Hutson W, Roehrkasse R, Wald A. Influence of gender and menopause on gastric emptying and motility. Gastroenterology 1989;96:11–7.
48. Parkman HP, Yates K, Hasler WL, et al. Clinical features of idiopathic gastropare-sis vary with sex, body mass, symptom onset, delay in gastric emptying, and gastroparesis severity. Gastroenterology 2011;140:101–15.
49. Yang D-D, He K, Wu X-L, et al. Risk factors of gastroparesis syndrome after abdominal non-gastroduodenal operation and its prevention. Asian Pac J Trop Med 2013;6:497–9.
50. Dickman R, Wainstein J, Glezerman M, et al. Gender aspects suggestive of gas-troparesis in patients with diabetes mellitus: a cross-sectional survey. BMC Gas-troenterol 2014;14:34–9.
51. Pasricha PJ, Yates KP, Nguyen L, et al. Outcomes and factors associated with reduced symptoms in patients with gastroparesis. Gastroenterology 2015; 149(7):1762–74.e4.

52. Verrengia M, Sachdeva P, Gaughan J, et al. Variation of symptoms during the menstrual cycle in female patients with gastroparesis. Neurogastroenterol Motil 2011;23:625–625.e254.
53. Hawthorne G. Maternal complications in diabetic pregnancy. Best Pract Res Clin Obstet Gynaecol 2011;25:77–90.
54. Singh A, Gull H, Singh RJ. Clinical significance of rapid (accelerated) gastric emptying. Clin Nucl Med 2003;28:658–62.
55. Balan K, Sonoda LI, Seshadri N, et al. Clinical significance of scintigraphic rapid gastric emptying. Nucl Med Commun 2011;32:1185–9.
56. Kaltenbach T, Crockett S, Gerson L. Are lifestyle measures effective in patients with gastroesophageal reflux disease? Arch Intern Med 2006;166:965–71.
57. DI B, Kaplan B, Spiegler J. Patient characteristics and lifestyle recommendations in the treatment of gastroesophageal reflux disease. J Fam Pract 1997;44: 266–72.
58. Heading RC, Monnikes H, Tholen A, et al. Prediction of response to PPI therapy and factors influencing treatment outcome in patients with GORD: a prospective pragmatic trial using pantoprazole. BMC Gastroenterol 2011;11:52.
59. Rossetti G, Limongelli P, Cimmino M, et al. Outcome of medical and surgical therapy of GERD: predictive role of quality of life scores and instrumental evaluation. Int J Surg 2014;12(Suppl 1):S112–6.
60. Yang Y, Lewis J, Epstein S, et al. Long-term proton pump inhibitor therapy and risk of hip fracture. JAMA 2006;296:2947–53.
61. Beck PE, Watson DI, Devitt PG, et al. Impact of gender and age on the long-term outcome of laparoscopic fundoplication. World J Surg 2009;33:2620–6.
62. Ip S, Tatsioni A, Conant A, et al. Predictors of clinical outcomes following fundoplication for gastroesophageal reflux disease remain insufficiently defined: a systematic review. Am J Gastroenterol 2009;104:752–8 [quiz: 759].
63. Nusrat S, Nusrat S, Bielefeldt K. Reflux and sex: what drives testing, what drives treatment? Eur J Gastroenterol Hepatol 2012;24:233–47.
64. Parkman HP, Carlson MR, Gonyer D. Metoclopramide nasal spray reduces symptoms of gastroparesis in women, but not men, with diabetes: results of a phase 2b randomized study. Clin Gastroenterol Hepatol 2015;13:1256–63.e1.
65. Anaparthy R, Pehlivanov N, Grady J, et al. Gastroparesis and gastroparesis-like syndrome: response to therapy and its predictors. Dig Dis Sci 2009;54:1003–10.
66. Parkman HP, Jacobs MR, Mishra A, et al. Domperidone treatment for gastroparesis: demographic and pharmacogenetic characterization of clinical efficacy and side-effects. Dig Dis Sci 2011;56:115–24.
67. Drici M, Knollmann B, Wang M, et al. Cardiac actions of erythromycin: influence of female sex. JAMA 1998;280:1774–6.
68. Parkman H, Mishra A, Jacobs M, et al. Clinical response and side effects of metoclopramide: associations with clinical, demographic, and pharmacogenetic parameters. J Clin Gastroenterol 2012;46:494–503.
69. Coleski R, Anderson MA, Hasler WL. Factors associated with symptom response to pyloric injection of botulinum toxin in a large series of gastroparesis patients. Dig Dis Sci 2009;54:2634–42.
70. Bromer M, Friedenberg FK, Miller L, et al. Endoscopic pyloric injection of botulinum toxin A for the treatment of refractory gastroparesis. Gastrointest Endosc 2005;61:833–9.
71. Heckert J, Sankineni A, Hughes WB, et al. Gastric electric stimulation for refractory gastroparesis: a prospective analysis of 151 patients at a single center. Dig Dis Sci 2016;61(1):168–75.

Complex Relationships Between Food, Diet, and the Microbiome

Laura A. Pace, MD, PhD, Sheila E. Crowe, MD, FRCPC*

KEYWORDS

- Celiac disease • Diet • Food • Functional GI disorders • Microbiome • Nutrition
- Obesity • Women's health

KEY POINTS

- Diet is a risk factor in several medically important disease states: obesity, cardiovascular disease, diabetes, celiac disease, and functional gastrointestinal disorders.
- Modification of diet can prevent, treat, or alleviate some of the symptoms associated with these diseases and improve general health.
- It is important to provide patients with simple dietary recommendations in order to increase the probability of successful implementation.
- Women can play an important role in maintaining family health by making informed dietary decisions.
- The gut microbiome may play a role in some gastrointestinal disorders. However, better designed studies are required to differentiate correlation from causation in this emerging area.

INTRODUCTION

For the vast majority of human evolution, our ancestors had been hunter-gatherers, migrating to take advantage of seasonal food availability from wild plants and animals. With the advent of agriculture approximately 10,000 to 12,000 years ago, humans began to take active roles in food production, which paved the way for major societal changes, such as the establishment of complex social organizations and the development of science, technology, and medicine. Since the dawn of agriculture, humans have been breeding plants and animals, actively selecting for particular, desirable traits of their food. However, recent major technological advances in food production—from agricultural practices, food harvesting, processing, preservation, and

The authors do not have any conflicts to disclose in relation to this article.
Division of Gastroenterology, Department of Medicine, University of California San Diego, 9500 Gilman Drive, La Jolla, CA 92093-0063, USA
* Corresponding author.
E-mail address: secrowe@ucsd.edu

distribution—have inadvertently led to the modern world's greatest threat to human health: obesity.

In the United States, greater than two-thirds of adults are classified as overweight (body mass index [BMI] of 25.0–29.9 kg/m^2), and more than one-third are classified as obese (BMI of 30 kg/m^2 and greater).[1] In 2010, the annual medical costs associated with obesity in the United States were estimated at 160 billion dollars, with indirect costs associated with obesity estimated at another 450 billion dollars. The obesity epidemic correlates closely with major changes in food production practices and consumption patterns. Currently, less than 20% of Americans consume what would be considered a healthful diet, which should include multiple daily servings of vegetables and fruits along with lean protein sources. Most Americans now consume most of their daily calories from processed foods, which includes the preponderance of prepared foods purchased from restaurants or grocery stores.[2]

Physicians are witnessing a significant change in another chronic disease that may also be related to alterations in dietary habits. Celiac disease is an immune-mediated enteropathy that manifests in some genetically susceptible individuals (HLA-DQ2 and/or HLA-DQ8) on exposure to dietary gluten: protein complexes found in wheat, rye, and barley. The prevalence rate of celiac disease in the 1950s was approximately 0.02%, and today is closer to 1% or greater.[3] Historically, celiac disease was diagnosed in childhood; however, now diagnosis is becoming more common at nearly any age. The explanation for this dramatic increase in prevalence remains unclear. There does not appear to have been an increase in overall wheat consumption during this period of time; however, major changes to the way in which cereal grains are processed for modern foods have led some to speculate that modifications associated with processing may be responsible for the increased prevalence of celiac disease. It is certain that changes in human population genetics cannot account for the increased prevalence, because celiac disease susceptibility genes remain at stable frequencies ($\sim$30%) within the US population.

Functional gastrointestinal disorders (FGIDs), which are defined as symptoms arising from the gastrointestinal tract without an identifiable structural or biochemical cause,[4] represent other processes that may also be related to diet. Irritable bowel syndrome (IBS) is the most common FGID, affecting an estimated 15% of the general population in Western countries and 11% worldwide.[5] The vast majority of afflicted individuals report at least one food trigger.[6,7] Women with IBS report more food items as potential triggers for their symptoms than men. Furthermore, individuals that report more food triggers have lower quality-of-life scores and more severe IBS symptoms.[6] An intriguing recent study by Fritscher-Ravens and colleagues[8] demonstrated real-time mucosal changes after exposure to certain food antigens using confocal laser endomicroscopy in IBS patients. In the group of individuals that experienced mucosal changes with food antigen application, dietary elimination of this specific food antigen led to dramatic improvement or complete resolution of their IBS symptoms that was durable at 1 year of follow-up. This work strongly suggests that food is playing a major role in the cause of IBS symptoms and provides a potential method to identify specific food triggers that could allow physicians to make better dietary recommendations for their patients.

Many patients seek guidance for dietary changes they can implement in an effort to alleviate their symptoms, but often lack the knowledge or motivation to implement these recommendations. Furthermore, because of the complexity of diet and food choices, getting people to embrace and adhere to major dietary changes is difficult. As a society, we seem to have lost sight of the fact that our diet is a major determinant of our health, health expectancy, life expectancy, and overall quality of life and can be a powerful tool in preventing disease and ameliorating symptoms of disease.

A review of the literature did not produce a consensus regarding the effects of gender on the response to specific dietary interventions or dietary adherence. However, for most households within the United States, food choices are primarily dictated by women, and women with greater food knowledge are better able to appropriately implement healthful dietary interventions.[9] Therefore, targeting women with dietary advice and nutrition-focused education has the potential to have far greater effects that could benefit the entire household.

In this article, the complex relationship of food and diet is discussed in the context of women's health. The authors encourage the reader to simplify the dietary recommendations suggested to patients in an effort to develop consistent messages about food and diet choices and increase compliance.

FOOD CONSUMPTION PATTERNS

Food consumption patterns in the United States have changed dramatically over the past few decades for multiple reasons. During this time period, there have been major advancements in food-processing and preservation technologies that have allowed for longer-term storage of prepared processed foods. This, combined with more women entering the out-of-home workforce, has created an environment in which food preparation within the home has significantly declined. Within most households, women traditionally have been responsible for food procurement and preparation, a pattern that has not changed significantly despite more women entering the out-of-home workforce.[2] As women entered the out-of-home workforce, this led to a decrease in time allotted for food preparation–related activities, and therefore, to greater demands for prepared or partially prepared processed foods that require less preparation time.[2] With these changes, there has also been a concomitant increase in consumption of higher calorie, lower nutrient-dense foods to the detriment of the consumption of fresh vegetables and fruits.

For many people, there is a lack of understanding of the important contribution food makes to overall health. Individuals no longer view food consumption as a necessary part of a healthy lifestyle and therefore are failing to see the direct consequences of poor food choices on their health and the development of disease.

CURRENT DIET TRENDS

The clinical definition of diet is simply the total food intake by an individual over a given time period. However, for many people, diet is defined as a short-term intervention to accomplish an objective such as weight loss. These types of diets are often associated with unsustainable or unhealthy food restrictions, which can reduce the long-term effectiveness of these interventions. For others, diet is a necessary medical therapy, such as those with celiac disease, who must commit to life-long avoidance of foods containing gluten in order to maintain health and minimize adverse outcomes from untreated disease. Some individuals consume certain diets because of a belief they represent a "healthier" way of eating, while other individuals avoid certain foods, such as meat, dairy, or eggs, due to religious restrictions or concerns for animal welfare and the environment.

Physicians encounter individuals that are interested in treating their ailments or preventing the development of disease with diet modification, yet most people in the United States do not consume a healthy diet. The reason for this contradiction is complicated. Physicians often fail to provide consistent messages about what constitutes a healthful diet, especially given the seemingly contradictory recommendations for patients with certain medical conditions. This problem is also confounded by the fact that an individual's motivation, level of knowledge, time, and finances all vary, as do their baseline nutritional state and medical comorbidities. Here, some of the more common dietary trends are reviewed, and it is argued that for most people simplified dietary recommendations can be made both to achieve overall better health and to treat a wide range of underlying medical conditions (**Table 1**).

Over the past few years, physicians have been recommending diets for several different conditions, such as weight loss, diabetes, cardiovascular disease, hypertension, or symptoms related to IBS. Examples include the low-carbohydrate diet for management of weight loss or diabetes, the low-fat diet for management of cardiovascular disease, the low-salt diet for management of hypertension, and the low-Fermentable Oligo-, Di-, Mono-Saccharides and Polyols (FODMAP) diet or the Mediterranean diet for management of IBS. Many physicians recommend these dietary interventions with little knowledge of what these diets entail or what burden this type of diet may place on their patients. Furthermore, when individuals are left to decipher the nuances of these particular diets themselves, they often become confused and frustrated with the conflicting information available to them.

For many physicians, time is also a factor in counseling patients regarding healthful food choices. The physician often refers the patient to nutritionists or dieticians and has little knowledge of the quality or validity of their recommendations or follow-up care. In this article, it is argued that simplification of nutritional recommendations will make physician counseling easier, less time-consuming, and less cumbersome for patients to implement.

In the following paragraphs, some of the more common diets that are encountered in clinical practice are reviewed. The basic nutritional principles that form the foundation of these diets are discussed, and some common pitfalls associated with them are described, providing the reader with the information required to educate their patients, empowering them to make healthful food choices.

LOW-CARBOHYDRATE DIET

The basic principle of the low-carbohydrate diet is to restrict the total daily calories from carbohydrate intake. The Institute of Medicine, Dietary Reference Index defines the consumption of between 45% and 65% of total daily calories from carbohydrates as normal.[10] Therefore, less than 45% of daily calories from carbohydrates can be considered a low-carbohydrate diet. When coupled with overall calorie restriction, these diets typically result in weight loss and beneficial metabolic changes.[11] However, some often interpret the focus of this diet solely on the carbohydrate restriction, without calorie restriction, and end up replacing the calorie reduction achieved from carbohydrate restriction with those from fat or protein consumption, which in turn can reduce or negate the positive health effects of this dietary intervention. The major pitfall of this diet is that, without concomitant calorie restriction, the health benefits of carbohydrate restriction are lost. Another pitfall of this diet is that it does not differentiate between carbohydrates from vegetables, fruits, and whole grains with those from processed foods, which have been shown to have differing effects on cardiometabolic parameters.[12]

LOW-FAT DIET

The basic principle of the low-fat diet is the restriction of total daily calories from fat intake. The Daily Reference Intakes from the Institutes of Medicine recommends that 20% to 35% of total daily calories should be from fat.[10] Therefore, a low-fat diet would constitute a diet of less than 20% of total calories. Fats from the diet are

Table 1
Comparison of current dietary trends

Diet	Major Principles	Major Pitfalls
Low-carbohydrate	Adherence to a diet low in total daily calories from carbohydrates, typically <45%. With concomitant total calorie reduction. Limitation of carbohydrates from processed foods.	Excess consumption of calories from fat. Failure to reduce overall calorie consumption. Failure to reduce carbohydrate consumption from processed foods.
Low-fat	Adherence to a diet low in total daily calories from fat, typically <20%. With concomitant total calorie restriction.	Excess consumption of calories from processed foods. Failure to reduce overall calorie consumption.
Low-FODMAP	Attempt to identify food triggers for IBS patients. Short-term avoidance of foods high in FODMAPS, followed by stepwise reintroduction of certain food groups. Long-term avoidance of identified food triggers.	Difficulty with implementation. Difficulty with food reintroduction. Requires assistance from a nutritionist. FODMAPS may not be source of symptoms. Reduction in FODMAPS may not improve metabolic parameters.
Mediterranean	Consumption of vegetables, fruits, legumes, nuts, and olive oil. Limitation of processed foods, meats, dairy.	At times complicated to follow because available information varies on what foods are part of this diet.
Paleolithic	Avoidance of processed foods. Consumption of vegetables, fruits, nuts, seeds, eggs, lean meats.	Requires knowledge of food preparation.
Gluten-free	Appropriate for treatment of celiac disease, dermatitis herpetiformis, and gluten ataxia. Avoidance of gluten-containing foods.	Excess consumption of calories from gluten-free alternative processed foods. No specific recommendations to limit consumption of processed foods. No specific recommendations about limiting fat consumption or dairy consumption. No specific recommendations advocating consumption of vegetables fruits, or lean meats.
Universal dietary recommendations	Prioritize the consumption of vegetables, fruits, lean proteins. Limit consumption of processed foods and dairy products. Intrinsic fiber content in foods leads to improved metabolic parameters and satiety. Consumption of lean protein sources aid in satiety.	—

a necessary energy source and aid in the absorption of fat-soluble food components, such as vitamins, A, D, E, and K. A diet too low in fat can lead to fat-soluble vitamin and other micronutrient deficiencies. The intention of this diet is to reduce total daily calorie consumption from fat and replace those calories with the consumption of vegetables, fruits, and lean protein sources, while also implementing overall daily calorie restriction. However, the major pitfall of this diet is that the calories avoided by fat consumption are often replaced by consumption of refined sugars and processed foods.[13]

LOW-FERMENTABLE OLIGO-, DI-, MONO-SACCHARIDES AND POLYOLS DIET

The low-FODMAP diet aims to limit foods containing Fermentable Oligo-, Di-, and Mono-saccharides And Polyols in an effort to treat IBS. Saccharides are simply sugars and can be either naturally occurring in food (intrinsic) or added during food processing or preparation (extrinsic). Glucose and fructose are examples of monosaccharides. Sucrose and lactose are examples of disaccharides. Sucrose comprises the monosaccharides, glucose and fructose, and when extracted and refined from cane, becomes common table sugar. Lactose comprises the monosaccharides, galactose and glucose, and is found primarily in mammalian milk sources. Lactose is broken down to its constituent monosaccharides by intestinal lactase. The persistence of intestinal lactase production into adulthood dates back approximately 4000 years to our European ancestors and correlates with increased consumption of dairy products into adulthood.[14] The terms, fructans, galactans, and inulins, refer to differing length oligosaccharides. Polyols are sugar alcohols, such as sorbitol and mannitol, intrinsic to fruits, such as apples, pears, and nectarines, and vegetables, such as cauliflower and mushrooms. Polyols can also be extrinsically added to processed foods as low-calorie sweeteners.

In several studies, the low-FODMAP diet has demonstrated significant improvement in the symptomatic treatment of IBS patients.[15–17] However, long-term adherence to a strict low-FODMAP diet is not recommended. The diet is complicated and can severely restrict food choices, especially when combined with other restrictive diets, such as a gluten-free diet. The goal of the low-FODMAP diet is to adhere to the diet in an effort to reduce symptoms. In individuals that respond to the strict low-FODMAP diet, a stepwise reintroduction of certain foods is undertaken, in an effort to identify their particular food triggers. Only the foods associated with trigger symptoms will need to be avoided long term. This diet typically requires the oversight from a nutritionist familiar with the diet and its nuances.[18] In addition, a recent small study evaluating the efficacy of dietary FODMAP restriction against standard dietary advice demonstrated similar rates of symptom reduction[19] without the complexities of the low-FODMAP diet.

MEDITERRANEAN DIET

The Mediterranean diet is primarily a plant-based diet. The Mediterranean diet emphasizes the consumption of vegetables, fruits, legumes, nuts, and "healthy" fats such as olive oil. There is also a focus on using spices and other seasonings to replace the use of salt. Another important component of the diet is the restriction of carbohydrates from processed foods. In a small study, women reported greater reductions in the desire to eat and sensation of hunger when following the Mediterranean diet compared with men following the same diet,[20] and this may be due to the increased fiber content of this diet. When properly followed, this diet is high in intrinsic fiber, low in fat from animal sources, low in carbohydrates from processed foods, and low in salt.

PALEOLITHIC DIET

The Paleolithic diet is based on the principle that humans should consume a diet close to that of their Stone Age hunter-gatherer ancestors. This diet emphasizes the avoidance of all processed foods, the consumption of vegetables, fruits, nuts, seeds, eggs, and lean meats. When properly followed, this diet is high in intrinsic fiber, low in fat (typically <25% of total daily calories), very low in carbohydrates from processed foods, and low in salt.

GLUTEN-FREE DIET

For people with celiac disease, gluten ataxia, and dermatitis herpetiformis, the avoidance of dietary gluten is essential for treatment of disease and maintenance of health. Gluten is a soluble complex of proteins found in wheat, barley, and rye. Gluten can also be added to medications as disintegrants, binders, or diluents. In processed foods such as breads, pastas, and pastries, gluten provides structure. There are now gluten-free alternatives to use in food production, such as flour from rice or corn, which has led to a cornucopia of gluten-free processed foods. A common pitfall of this diet is the consumption of large amounts of gluten-free processed food sources rather than consumption of fresh vegetables and fruits. In fact, many celiac disease patients are gaining weight while adhering to a gluten-free diet, which is a strong indication of the high rates of consumption of these gluten-free processed foods.

ORGANIC FOODS AND GENETICALLY MODIFIED FOODS

There are currently few known health benefits to eating organic versus conventionally grown vegetables and fruits.[21] Given the added expense of organic produce and the budgetary limitations of many patients, it is much more important that they are encouraged to consume more vegetables and fruits rather than subjecting them to the added expense of consuming organically produced foods. At this time, little is known about the health benefits of avoiding genetically modified foods, and therefore, the authors defer making recommendations on these foods.

DIETARY SUPPLEMENTS

Since the 1994 passage of the Dietary Supplement Health and Education Act, dietary supplements can be marketed with very little governmental oversight of manufacturing, contents, proof of safety, or proof of efficacy. Each year some dietary supplements are found to contain undeclared active pharmaceuticals, such as amphetamines, anabolic steroids, and toxins, such as heavy metals and bacteria.[22] The safety for many of these dietary supplements is presumed rather than proven, and therefore, it is only when these supplements reach the general market that their true dangers are revealed. Recently, the weight loss supplement, OxyElite Pro, was connected to nearly 100 cases of acute liver injury, 3 requiring liver transplantation and one resulting in death.[23] Dietary supplement contamination with gluten also remains a real hazard for individuals with true celiac disease, gluten ataxia, or dermatitis herpetiformis.

The National Institutes of Health, Office of Dietary Supplements, reports that Americans are spending more than 25 billion dollars annually on dietary supplements, including vitamins, minerals, probiotics, fish oils, and botanicals. For the vast majority of individuals without malabsorptive disorders, all nutrients required for optimal health can be easily obtained from a balanced diet. Nevertheless, most of the US population is underconsuming key nutrients, such as vitamin D, calcium, potassium, and fiber, from their diet, despite overconsumption of daily calories. Even higher rates of vitamin and micronutrient deficiencies are reported in obese individuals compared with normal weight individuals,[24–26] further supporting the fact that these individuals are consuming excess quantities of calorie-dense, nutrient-poor foods.

Therefore only individuals with documented nutritional deficiencies should be consuming dietary supplements, and when possible, these deficiencies should be supplemented through dietary interventions.

PROBIOTICS

There is a lot of excitement surrounding the recent advances in the understanding of the human gastrointestinal microbiome. A brief review of this data is discussed later in the article. However, despite these advances, this field of study remains in its infancy, and there are a few cautions that should be addressed here in regards to the use of dietary probiotics: (1) The strains typically selected for use in probiotics have not been reliably demonstrated to be key members of the healthy gastrointestinal microbiota. (2) There are real safety concerns, with several documented cases of bacteremia resulting from probiotic strains.[27] (3) There is a lack of understanding in how these supplemented microbes will affect the intact microbiota.[28] (4) There are issues pertaining to the quality and viability of the microbes within probiotics. (5) There are concerns with contamination from other pathogenic or antibiotic-resistant microbes along with other contaminants, such as gluten, despite gluten-free labeling.

At this time, no specific recommendations can be made as to the optimal composition of the human gastrointestinal microbiome. Therefore, in the absence of this crucial information and the safety concerns associated with probiotics, the authors do not broadly advocate for their use.

CANCER RISK

The working group from the International Agency for Research on Cancer released a statement in October of 2015, based on a review of 800 epidemiologic studies, stating there was an association between the consumption of red and processed meats and the development of cancer.[29] Although the exact mechanism for this association with the development of cancer is currently unknown, this supports the hypothesis that lifestyle choices directly contribute to cancer risk. Obesity has been attributed to approximately 6% of annual incident cancers in the United States,[30] with higher overall incidence rates reported in obese European women.[31] Obesity remains an important modifiable risk factor for the development of many diseases, including certain cancers, diabetes, and cardiovascular disease. Therefore, maintenance of optimal body weight must be emphasized as an important component of overall health and disease prevention. Proper food selection and consumption must be highlighted as the foundation for achievement of this goal.

UNIVERSAL DIET RECOMMENDATIONS

- Consume a diet primarily comprising fresh vegetables, fruits, and lean protein sources.
  - Increased fiber contributes to greater satiety and improved blood glucose parameters.
  - Lean protein sources also increase satiety.
- Limit intake of processed foods and extrinsic dietary sugars.
- Limit portion sizes.
- Avoid caloric intake from beverages.

A comparison of all the diets reviewed above reveals a central theme: increased consumption of vegetables, fruits, lean proteins, and a severely reduced consumption of processed foods leads to positive health benefits, which can be applied to a wide range of medical conditions. When implemented properly, any one of the reviewed diets will lead to improved health, along with improved cardiometabolic parameters.[32] The factors driving food choices by most people living in the United States tend to focus on quantity of food and ease of acquisition and preparation, over the content and quality of food. By prioritizing these factors, the idea that food is the energy source for our body, and therefore, an essential component of health, has been sadly lost. In turn, this has led to the mass consumption of high-calorie, low-nutrient-quality foods, which are directly contributing to the obesity epidemic.

Studies show that nearly 70% of processed foods contain extrinsic sugars, a trend that has increased over the past few decades.[33] During this same time period, portion size has increased as has the frequency of snacking, consumption of calories from beverages, and the caloric density of food.[34] Studies have shown that the calories consumed in sweetened beverages do not lead to a concomitant reduction in calorie consumption from food. Therefore, all of these factors have contributed to an increase in total daily caloric intake and concurrent weight gain.

A recent study in children demonstrated that isocaloric fructose restriction leads to improved cardiometabolic parameters in as little as 9 days of dietary intervention.[12] In this short-term intervention, dietary sugar was reduced from 28% to 10% of total daily calories and substituted with starch to maintain an isocaloric diet. The children in the study experienced improvements in diastolic blood pressure, low-density lipoprotein cholesterol, glucose tolerance, and hyperinsulinemia along with weight loss. Most of the children could not even consume all the food provided by the study because they reported higher rates of satiety.[12]

There has also been another unforeseen consequence of the prioritization of prepared foods in the diet that has resulted in the generational loss of food preparation knowledge. Typically, food preparation knowledge and skills have been passed between generations, with children growing up with the skills to prepare food as their parents and grandparents had. However, now there are adults with limited food preparation knowledge, and a lack of emphasis on food preparation as a necessary life skill. For the first time, there is a generation that does not understand the important link between food consumption choices and health or the skills necessary to implement this knowledge.

Because lack of time is cited as the greatest barrier to healthful food preparation,[2] we must strive to emphasize the importance of proper nutrition for health and must provide our patients with simple guidelines on proper nutrition, rather than focusing on specific diet recommendations unless medically indicated.

It would be interesting to evaluate if larger-scale interventions such as online classes focusing on simple, healthful food preparation combined with an emphasis on the health benefits of proper nutrition could help affect changes in food consumption patterns. Furthermore, a major limitation of food and nutrition–related studies is that they are often sponsored by the major producers of processed food products, the exact products we need to encourage less consumption of.

THE ROLE OF THE MICROBIOME IN HEALTH AND DISEASE

The human body is colonized by microbes on most surfaces that are topologically connected to the outside environment, including the skin, respiratory tract, gastrointestinal tract, and the vagina. Over the past decade, there has been an explosion of interest in understanding the structure, function, and ecology of the human microbiome. The aspirations of this research are to use this information to clinically diagnose disease states and eventually intelligently modify microbial communities to improve human health. Although progress has been made in certain areas, we are a long way from achieving these goals.

Microbial community structure is determined by the physical environment (such as the availability of nutrient sources, temperature, or presence of O_2) and interactions between community members (such as antibiotics and intercellular communication). Therefore, it is not surprising that microbial communities vary drastically along the length of the gastrointestinal tract and that mucosally adherent microbial communities differ significantly from the luminal bulk and stool communities.[35,36]

Physicians recognize that most nutrient processing and absorption occur within the small intestine and that many disease states, such as celiac disease, IBS symptoms triggered by food consumption, and inflammatory bowel disease, affect different areas along the length of the gastrointestinal tract. Therefore, it becomes necessary to directly interrogate the gastrointestinal microbiota from these specific regions. Unfortunately, the vast majority of work investigating the human gastrointestinal microbiome has been performed using stool samples. Several studies have shown that stool is an inadequate proxy for the entire gastrointestinal tract[35,36] and clearly not sufficient to understand the system as a whole.

A small prospective, crossover study evaluated the effects of diet on the stool microbiome and demonstrated that switching between a vegetarian diet and animal-based diet rapidly changes the composition of the stool microbiome.[37] Unfortunately, this study did not adequately control for the dramatic changes in fiber content that occurred with the particular dietary interventions. The fiber content of the vegetarian diet was 25.6 g fiber per 1000 kcal compared with 9.3 g fiber per 1000 kcal in the baseline diet and nearly 0 g of fiber with the animal-based diet. The observed changes in microbial community structure could be explained by the simple modification of dietary fiber content, as it is known that different micro-organisms ferment different nutrient sources. Furthermore, this study was limited in that it only evaluated the stool microbiome and did not investigate the microbiome of the mucosally adherent or luminal microbial communities along the length of the gastrointestinal tract.

Currently, the vast majority of gastrointestinal microbiome studies suffer from similar limitations that make it very difficult to distinguish between correlation and causation. Carefully controlled studies coupled with proper sampling are needed to address the complex interactions between the microbiome and human health and disease.

An excellent example of effective therapeutic microbial community modulation is that of fecal microbiota transplant for the treatment of *Clostridium difficile* colitis. Studies have shown that fecal microbiota transplant is an effective and safe treatment for recurrent and refractory *C. difficile* colitis,[38] and emerging data suggest it may also be effective in select patients for the treatment of toxic megacolon.[39] To date, fecal microbiota transplant has not demonstrated efficacy for the treatment of other disease states, such as inflammatory bowel disease or IBS. However, these treatment failures may be reflective of the source of the microbial communities being transplanted rather than the true efficacy of the treatment in these particular disease states.

SUMMARY

Food is literally the fuel for our bodies, and it is important that we recognize the effects that food choices have on overall health expectancy and life expectancy. Currently, two-thirds of the adult population within the United States is classified as overweight or obese, and this is a direct consequence of changing food consumption patterns. With the overconsumption of calorie-dense, nutrient-poor foods, there has been a paradoxic development of nutritional deficiencies in the face of calorie excess, a phenomenon that has never been witnessed before. Historically, nutritional deficiencies were only observed in cases of food instability that included calorie and protein malnutrition or diseases of malabsorption. However, now with less than 20% of individuals consuming a healthful diet, an emerging epidemic of vitamin and micronutrient deficiencies is again arising in the United States.

Furthermore, there are increasing rates of diseases, including metabolic disorders, cardiovascular disease, and certain cancers, that are directly attributable to obesity. Epidemiologic data report higher rates of cancer for obese women compared with normal body weight women. A recent large-scale cohort study that followed 1.3 million individuals for 30 years demonstrated that even aerobic fitness cannot completely mitigate the risk of early death due to obesity.[40]

Physicians are obligated to provide patients with consistent, easy-to-understand dietary recommendations to promote health. Therefore, we are advocating for a simplification of dietary recommendations that include the following components: (1) focus on consumption of primarily fresh vegetables and fruits; (2) consume reasonable amounts of lean proteins; (3) minimize consumption of processed foods; (4) avoid consuming calories from beverages; and (5) limit portion size.

REFERENCES

1. Ogden CL, Carroll MD, Kit BK, et al. Prevalence of childhood and adult obesity in the United States, 2011-2012. JAMA 2014;311(8):806–14.
2. Smith LP, Ng SW, Popkin BM. Trends in US home food preparation and consumption: analysis of national nutrition surveys and time use studies from 1965-1966 to 2007-2008. Nutr J 2013;12(1):45.
3. Rubio-Tapia A, Kyle RA, Kaplan EL, et al. Increased prevalence and mortality in undiagnosed celiac disease. Gastroenterology 2009;137(1):88–93.
4. Chey WD. The role of food in the functional gastrointestinal disorders: introduction to a manuscript series. Am J Gastroenterol 2013;108(5):694–7.
5. Ford AC, Moayyedi P, Lacy BE, et al. American College of Gastroenterology monograph on the management of irritable bowel syndrome and chronic idiopathic constipation. Am J Gastroenterol 2014;109(Suppl 1):S2–26 [quiz: S27].
6. Böhn L, Störsrud S, Törnblom H, et al. Self-reported food-related gastrointestinal symptoms in IBS are common and associated with more severe symptoms and reduced quality of life. Am J Gastroenterol 2013;108(5):634–41.
7. Hayes P, Corish C, O'Mahony E, et al. A dietary survey of patients with irritable bowel syndrome. J Hum Nutr Diet 2014;27(Suppl 2):36–47.
8. Fritscher-Ravens A, Schuppan D, Ellrichmann M, et al. Confocal endomicroscopy shows food-associated changes in the intestinal mucosa of patients with irritable bowel syndrome. Gastroenterology 2014;147(5):1012–20.e4.
9. Laz TH, Rahman M, Pohlmeier AM, et al. Level of nutrition knowledge and its association with weight loss behaviors among low-income reproductive-age women. J Community Health 2015;40(3):542–8.
10. Hellwig JP, Otten JJ, Meyers LD. Dietary reference intakes: the essential guide to nutrient requirements. Washington, DC: The National Academies Press; 2006.
11. Katz DL, Meller S. Can we say what diet is best for health? Annu Rev Public Health 2014;35:83–103.

12. Lustig RH, Mulligan K, Noworolski SM, et al. Isocaloric fructose restriction and metabolic improvement in children with obesity and metabolic syndrome. Obesity 2016;24(2):453–60.

13. Tobias DK, Chen M, Manson JE, et al. Effect of low-fat diet interventions versus other diet interventions on long-term weight change in adults: a systematic review and meta-analysis. Lancet Diabetes Endocrinol 2015;3(12):968–79.

14. Mathieson I, Lazaridis I, Rohland N, et al. Genome-wide patterns of selection in 230 ancient Eurasians. Nature 2015;528(7583):499–503.

15. Shepherd SJ, Parker FC, Muir JG, et al. Dietary triggers of abdominal symptoms in patients with irritable bowel syndrome: randomized placebo-controlled evidence. Clin Gastroenterol Hepatol 2008;6(7):765–71.

16. Halmos EP, Power VA, Shepherd SJ, et al. A diet low in FODMAPs reduces symptoms of irritable bowel syndrome. Gastroenterology 2014;146(1):67–75.e5.

17. Roest RH, Dobbs BR, Chapman BA, et al. The low FODMAP diet improves gastrointestinal symptoms in patients with irritable bowel syndrome: a prospective study. Int J Clin Pract 2013;67(9):895–903.

18. Gibson PR, Shepherd SJ. Evidence-based dietary management of functional gastrointestinal symptoms: the FODMAP approach. J Gastroenterol Hepatol 2010;25(2):252–8.

19. Böhn L, Störsrud S, Liljebo T, et al. Diet low in FODMAPs reduces symptoms of irritable bowel syndrome as well as traditional dietary advice: a randomized controlled trial. Gastroenterology 2015;149(6):1399–407.e2.

20. Bédard A, Hudon A-M, Drapeau V, et al. Gender differences in the appetite response to a satiating diet. J Obes 2015;2015:140139.

21. Bourn D, Prescott J. A comparison of the nutritional value, sensory qualities, and food safety of organically and conventionally produced foods. Crit Rev Food Sci Nutr 2002;42(1):1–34.

22. Cohen PA. American roulette–contaminated dietary supplements. N Engl J Med 2009;361(16):1523–5.

23. Cohen PA. Hazards of hindsight–monitoring the safety of nutritional supplements. N Engl J Med 2014;370(14):1277–80.

24. Kaidar-Person O, Person B, Szomstein S, et al. Nutritional deficiencies in morbidly obese patients: a new form of malnutrition? Part A: vitamins. Obes Surg 2008; 18(7):870–6.

25. Kaidar-Person O, Person B, Szomstein S, et al. Nutritional deficiencies in morbidly obese patients: a new form of malnutrition? Part B: minerals. Obes Surg 2008; 18(8):1028–34.

26. Via M. The malnutrition of obesity: micronutrient deficiencies that promote diabetes. ISRN Endocrinol 2012;2012:103472.

27. Bertelli C, Pillonel T, Torregrossa A, et al. Bifidobacterium longum bacteremia in preterm infants receiving probiotics. Clin Infect Dis 2015;60(6):924–7.

28. Michail S, Kenche H. Gut microbiota is not modified by randomized, double-blind, placebo-controlled trial of VSL#3 in diarrhea-predominant irritable bowel syndrome. Probiotics Antimicrob Proteins 2011;3(1):1–7.

29. Bouvard V, Loomis D, Guyton KZ, et al. Carcinogenicity of consumption of red and processed meat. Lancet Oncol 2015;16(16):1599–600.

30. Polednak AP. Estimating the number of U.S. incident cancers attributable to obesity and the impact on temporal trends in incidence rates for obesity-related cancers. Cancer Detect Prev 2008;32(3):190–9.

31. Renehan AG, Soerjomataram I, Tyson M. Incident cancer burden attributable to excess body mass index in 30 European countries. Int J Cancer 2010. http://dx.doi.org/10.1002/ijc.24803/pdf.
32. Sacks FM, Bray GA, Carey VJ, et al. Comparison of weight-loss diets with different compositions of fat, protein, and carbohydrates. N Engl J Med 2009; 360(9):859–73.
33. Popkin BM, Hawkes C. Sweetening of the global diet, particularly beverages: patterns, trends, and policy responses. Lancet Diabetes Endocrinol 2015;4(2): 174–86.
34. Piernas C, Popkin BM. Food portion patterns and trends among U.S. children and the relationship to total eating occasion size, 1977–2006. J Nutr 2011;141(6): 1159–64.
35. Stearns JC, Lynch MDJ, Senadheera DB, et al. Bacterial biogeography of the human digestive tract. Sci Rep 2011;1:170.
36. Yasuda K, Oh K, Ren B, et al. Biogeography of the intestinal mucosal and lumenal microbiome in the rhesus macaque. Cell Host Microbe 2015;17(3):385–91.
37. David LA, Maurice CF, Carmody RN, et al. Diet rapidly and reproducibly alters the human gut microbiome. Nature 2014;505(7484):559–63.
38. Kassam Z, Lee CH, Yuan Y, et al. Fecal microbiota transplantation for clostridium difficile infection: systematic review and meta-analysis. Am J Gastroenterol 2013; 108(4):500–8.
39. Costello SP, Chung A, Andrews JM, et al. Fecal microbiota transplant for Clostridium difficile colitis-induced toxic megacolon. Am J Gastroenterol 2015; 110(5):775–7.
40. Högström G, Nordström A, Nordström P. Aerobic fitness in late adolescence and the risk of early death: a prospective cohort study of 1.3 million Swedish men. Int J Epidemiol 2015. http://dx.doi.org/10.1093/ije/dyv321.

Gastrointestinal Diseases in Pregnancy

Nausea, Vomiting, Hyperemesis Gravidarum, Gastroesophageal Reflux Disease, Constipation, and Diarrhea

Cameron Body, MD, Jennifer A. Christie, MD*

KEYWORDS

- Pregnancy • Review • Vomiting • Hyperemesis gravidarum
- Gastroesophageal reflux disease (GERD) • Constipation • Diarrhea • Treatment

KEY POINTS

- Pregnant women are susceptible to nausea, vomiting, gastroesophageal reflux, constipation, and diarrhea at rates similar to or higher than the general population.
- Many of the pregnancy-induced gastrointestinal (GI) disorders result from the normal hormonal and structural changes associated with pregnancy.
- Although a vast majority of GI complaints are caused by normal pregnancy-related changes, other pathologic conditions and causes should be considered.
- When symptomatic remission cannot be achieved with nonpharmacologic therapy, pharmacologic treatment may be instituted, but the potential teratogenic side effects must be considered.
- Starting June 2015, the Food and Drug Administration (FDA) began replacing pregnancy categories A, B, C, D, and X with narrative statements regarding safety studies for all biological products and prescription drugs, which may result in improved understanding of fetal and maternal risk.

NAUSEA, VOMITING, AND HYPEREMESIS GRAVIDARUM

A majority of pregnant women experience nausea and vomiting during pregnancy.[1] The prevalence of nausea in this group is between 50% and 80% and for vomiting 50%.[2] These are the most common medical conditions during gestation, usually

Disclosure: Research support, Takeda Pharmaceuticals; Advisory Board, Synergy Pharmaceuticals.
Department of Internal Medicine, Division of Digestive Diseases, Emory University School of Medicine, 1365 Clifton Road, Suite 1264, Atlanta, GA 30322, USA
* Corresponding author. 1365 Clifton Road, Suite 1200, Atlanta, GA 30322.
E-mail address: Jennifer.Christie@emory.edu

beginning between weeks 4 and 6, peaking at approximately weeks 8 to 12, and often ceasing by week 20.[3]

Hyperemesis gravidarum (HG) is a severe and persistent form of nausea and vomiting.[2] Fortunately, it only affects approximately 1.2% of pregnant women.[3] Currently, there is no standard definition or diagnostic criteria for HG. Accepted definitions, however, combine the symptoms of protracted vomiting and nausea with the following findings: weight loss, ketonuria, electrolyte disturbances, dehydration, and/or hospitalization.[4]

Evaluation

In the setting of significant nausea and vomiting, other pathologic causes should be excluded. **Box 1** outlines other causes that may be considered.[2,5] If the work-up for

---

Box 1
Causes of nausea and vomiting in pregnancy

Gastrointestinal

Gastroenteritis
Biliary disease
Gastroparesis
Peptic ulcers
Pancreatitis
Hepatitis
Appendicitis
IBS

Genitourinary

Pyelonephritis
Uremia
Kidney stones

Miscellaneous

Drugs
Psychological

Metabolic

Diabetic ketoacidosis
Addison disease
Hyperthyroidism

Neurologic

Pseudotumor cerebri
Vestibular
Central nervous system tumors

Pregnancy Associated

Multifetal gestation
Gestational trophoblastic disease
Preeclampsia/HELLP
Acute fatty liver of pregnancy

Abbreviation: HELLP, Hemolysis, Elevated Liver Enzymes, and Low Platelets.
    Data from Refs.[2,5,6]

other causes is negative, a diagnosis of nausea and vomiting associated with pregnancy may be assigned.[2]

Pathophysiology

The exact cause of nausea and vomiting during pregnancy is not fully understood. Permeations in gastric tone and gastric motility due to elevations in progesterone are, however, thought to be involved.[7] Studies have shown that progesterone has an inhibitory effect on the smooth muscle of both the pylorus and the small bowel, which results in decreased GI contractility.[8] Other studies comparing the gastric emptying rates of premenopausal women to men and postmenopausal women have detected slower gastric emptying rates in the former, which further suggest a hormone-induced delayed gastric emptying.[7]

There are a few studies evaluating gastric function during pregnancy. However, studies have documented the presence of both tachygastria and bradygastria in pregnant women. Both of these gastric dysrhythmias have been associated with reports of nausea.[5]

Delayed small bowel transit may also contribute to nausea and vomiting. In humans, lactulose breath testing has confirmed delayed small bowel transit in the third trimester, which returns to normal after delivery. Similarly, animals studied have shown delayed gastric emptying in the third trimester that persists until postpartum day 4. Gastric emptying then returns to normal, suggesting that the motor dysfunction associated with pregnancy is not solely due to the presence of an enlarged uterus.[7]

Psychological factors may also have a role. Multiple studies report that nausea and vomiting can be worse in women who experience negative relationships with their mothers and in undesired pregnancies.[7] Other studies suggest a link between somatization and/or conversion disorders with nausea and vomiting. Also, anxiety and depression, which complicate up to one-third of pregnancies, are more common in patients with HG.[9]

Hyperemesis Gravidarum

As discussed previously, HG is a more severe form of nausea and vomiting. It is associated with a higher risk of negative pregnancy outcomes: preterm birth, low birth weight, and small-for-gestational-age infants. Risk factors for HG include female gender infant, young maternal age, previous pregnancy, and non-European heritage. Body mass index, smoking, and socioeconomic status are not risk factors for HG.[1]

Pathophysiology

The current body of literature suggests 3 pathoetiologies for HG: placental growth and function as reflected by free human chorionic gonadotropin (hCG), maternal endocrine function, and preexisting GI disease.[4] An observational study showed higher levels of free hCG in women with HG compared with controls. Higher maternal serum concentrations of hCG are seen in the first trimester when HG symptoms are often at their worse. Additionally, HG symptoms are more severe in molar pregnancies and multigestational pregnancy, conditions known to be associated with higher than normal hCG levels.[1] The exact mechanism, however, for how elevated levels of hCG leads to HG is unclear. One proposed mechanism involves the stimulatory effect of hCG on the secretory pathways in the upper GI tract.[10]

Other sex hormones and endocrine factors have been implicated in HG. A list of these hormones and their associated alterations is shown in **Table 1**. Theories on how these alterations lead to HG include higher levels of these hormones during early

Table 1	
Sex hormone and endocrine factors associated with hyperemesis gravidarum	
Factor	**Alteration**
Sex hormones	
Estrogens	Increased
Progesterone	Increased
Endocrine hormones	
Thyroid-stimulating hormone and thyroxine	Increased
Hypothalamic-pituitary-adrenal axis	Overactivity
Human growth hormone	Abnormal levels
Prolactin	Abnormal levels

Data from Verberg MF, Gillott DJ, Al-Fardan N, et al. Hyperemesis gravidarum, a literature review. Hum Reprod Update 2005;11(5):527–39.

pregnancy, an increased sensitivity to these hormones in patients with HG, and/or a different subtype or isoform of these hormones in women with HG.[10]

Multiple studies have also noted an association between *Helicobacter pylori* infection and HG. One study found that 95% of HG patients tested positive for *H pylori*, whereas only 50% of controls were positive. Additionally, the density of infection was higher in women with HG and correlated with the severity of symptoms. The cause for the increased incidence of *H pylori* in patients with HG is unclear and no causal relationship between HG and *H pylori* has been established.[1,10]

Management

After other physiologic causes for nausea and vomiting have been eliminated, nonpharmacologic treatment options should be instituted. These includes reassurance, dietary changes, and lifestyle modifications. Additionally, patients should be counseled to reduce stress and get adequate rest.[11] To prevent dehydration, daily consumption of 1 L to 1.5 L of either sports drinks or broth containing salt, glucose, and potassium is advised. Diet recommendations include small, frequent meals and the avoidance of fatty foods and fresh vegetables that may delay gastric emptying or have difficulty emptying from the stomach. High-protein liquid beverages have been shown to reduce gastric dysrhythmias and nausea in the first trimester.[5]

Given the concern for teratogenic effects of pharmacologic therapy, alternative therapies have been explored. Studies have shown that both thiamine (vitamin B_1) and pyridoxine (vitamin B_6) are efficacious in reducing nausea and vomiting. Therefore, both are indicated as routine supplements in patients with protracted vomiting.[11,12]

Zingiber officinale, the root of ginger, has also been studied in the treatment of nausea and vomiting. The antiemetic properties of ginger are due to the presence of gingerols and shogaols, which increase gastric motility, stimulate gastric antral contractions, and block the cholinergic M receptors as well as the serotonin receptor.[13,14] Multiple studies have reported a subjective decrease in nausea and an objective decrease in vomiting after daily consumption of 1 g of ginger.[11]

Due to the concern for teratogenic effects, judicious use of all pharmacologic therapy in pregnant women is indicated. Health care professionals should have thorough conversations with their patients regarding the potential risk and possible outcomes prior to starting medical therapy. To aid in this discussion, the Food and Drug

Administration (FDA) has classified many supplements as well as over-the-counter and prescription medications in 1 of 5 pregnancy categories (A, B, C, D, or X) based on the risk of developmental and reproductive adverse effects compared with the potential benefit (**Table 2**).[15]

This system has been in place since 1979, but both patients and heath care professionals found the pregnancy categories confusing and ineffective at communicating varying degrees of fetal risk. Therefore, the FDA issued a final rule in December 2014 to replace the pregnancy categories with a narrative structure to better convey potential teratogenic and reproductive risk based on human and/or animal safety data. Biological products and prescription drugs submitted after June 30, 2015, will immediately use the new format, whereas prescription drug labeling approved after or on June 30, 2001 will be gradually introduced. Labeling for over-the-counter medications will not change.[15] For historical purposes, subsequent tables regarding pharmacologic management of GI disease in pregnancy will contain the FDA pregnancy classification.

Regarding the pharmacologic treatment of nausea and vomiting, antiemetics should be used cautiously in pregnancy and should not be used before 12 to 14 weeks of gestation. The most commonly used agents include phenothiazines, histamine receptor blockers, and dopamine antagonists.[11] Of these, phenothiazines are considered the least safe in pregnancy due to their known ability to cross the placenta and their comparatively slower excretion from neonatal and fetal tissue.[7] Ondansetron, a 5-HT$_3$ antagonist, is particularly useful in the treatment of chemotherapy-induced nausea and vomiting.[11] Studies have shown, however, an increased risk of congenital heart defects when used in the first trimester.[6] Steroids, which are thought to relieve nausea via a central mechanism, are not routinely recommended in pregnancy due to concern for fetal growth impairment and increased risk of cleft palate.[11]

Metoclopramide, a dopamine antagonist, may be used in the treatment of nausea and vomiting during pregnancy. Although it crosses the placenta, there are no

Table 2	
Definition of Food and Drug Agency pregnancy classifications	
Class	**Definition**
A	Appropriately designed studies in pregnant women have not demonstrated fetal risk.
B	No fetal risk in animal reproduction studies; no well-controlled studies in pregnant women *OR* Adverse effect in animal studies, but studies in pregnant women failed to demonstrate fetal risk
C	Animal reproduction studies show adverse fetal effect but no well-controlled studies in humans. *OR* No animal reproduction studies and well-controlled studies in humans
D	Evidence of human fetal risk in investigational or marketing experience or studies in humans
X	Animals or humans studies have demonstrated fetal abnormalities. *OR* Evidence of fetal risk based on investigational and/or marketing experience

Data from Administration FaD. Content and format of labeling for human prescription drug and biological products; requirements for pregnancy and lactation labeling. Fed Regist vol. 2008:30831–68. Codified at 30821 CFR 30201.

reported teratogenetic effects in animals or humans.[7] Studies have shown that meto-clopramide and promethazine (a phenothiazine) have similar therapeutic effects, but metoclopramide has fewer side effects: less drowsiness, dizziness, and dystonia.[11]

Oral histamine receptor blockers, such as over-the-counter doxylamine, have proved efficacy and are considered first-line pharmacologic therapy in the treatment of pregnancy-associated nausea and vomiting.[6] There is no evidence of adverse fetal effects associated with the use of histamine antagonists.[7] A list of antiemetic medications, dosages, and their FDA classifications is in **Table 3**.

Management of HG may require intravenous fluids to correct or prevent dehydration and restore electrolyte balance. Additional nutritional support via nasogastric or enteral route may be considered for those with severe, intractable symptoms and/or weight loss in spite of appropriate therapy. These modalities, however, pose significant risk to both mother as well as fetus and should be reserved for the most severe cases.[11]

GASTROESOPHAGEAL REFLUX DISEASE

Gastroesophageal reflux disease (GERD) typically manifests as heartburn and is reported by 40% to 85% of pregnant women.[18] Pregnancy may be the first time a woman experiences GERD or it may exacerbate preexisting reflux disease.[19] **Box 2** lists the common symptoms of GERD, which typically begin in the later portion of the first trimester or early portion of the second trimester. When present, GERD usually lasts throughout gestation and may get progressively worse in the later months but typically resolves after delivery.[19] Although symptoms may be severe, erosive esophagitis, strictures, and bleeding are rare complications.[7] Risk factors for heartburn in pregnancy include multiparty, preexisting heartburn, and gestational age. Studies

Table 3		
Medical therapy for the treatment of nausea and vomiting		
Medication	Dosage	Food and Drug Administration Classification[a]
Alternative therapy		
Pyridoxine	10–25 mg Q8H	A
Thiamine	100 mg QD	A
Ginger	1 g QD	Not assigned
Histamine receptor blocker		
Doxylamine	12.5–25 mg Q4–6H	B
Dopamine antagonist		
Metoclopramide	10 mg Q8H	B
Phenothiazines		
Promethazine	25 mg Q8H	C
5-HT$_3$ antagonist		
Ondansetron	4 mg Q8H	C
Steroids		
Prednisone	40 mg QD	C

[a] Discontinued June 30, 2015, for biological products and prescription drugs; to be replaced by risk narratives based on human or animal studies.
Data from Refs.[7,11,16,17]

Box 2
Symptoms of gastroesophageal reflux disease

Heartburn
Nausea
Vomiting
Regurgitation
Epigastric pain
Anorexia
Dysphagia
Water brash
Cough
Hoarseness
Sore throat

Data from Ali RA, Egan LJ. Gastroesophageal reflux disease in pregnancy. Best Pract Res Clin Gastroenterol 2007;21(5):793–806.

---

have not shown an association between race, prepregnancy body mass index, or weight gain during pregnancy and the development of GERD.[19]

Evaluation

The clinical presentation for GERD is similar for both pregnant and nonpregnant patients, and the diagnosis can be made based on symptoms alone.[19] Barium radiography is unnecessary and should be avoided due to concern for fetal radiation exposure. Esophageal manometry and pH monitoring may be safely performed but rarely are necessary. For intractable reflux symptoms and/or complications, upper GI endoscopy is the procedure of choice and it may be safely performed with fetal monitoring, judicious use of sedation, and close monitoring of blood pressure and oxygenation.[19]

Pathophysiology

Both mechanical and hormonal factors are thought to play a role in the etiology and pathophysiology of GERD in pregnancy.[7,18] In the presence of estrogen, progesterone leads to lower esophageal sphincter (LES) relaxation.[18] Numerous studies have demonstrated progressively decreasing LES pressure throughout pregnancy, and this reduction has been associated with heartburn.[18] In the first trimester, however, basal LES pressure has not changed but is less responsive to normal physiologic and hormonal stimuli that increase LES tone (a protein meal, methacholine, and edrophonium).[18,19]

Hormonally induced alterations in gastric motility have also been implicated. Pregnancy hormones are thought to effect the function of the enteric nervous system and musculature that leads to a decrease in GI motility, which may promote GERD.[18] Researchers have hypothesized that increasing abdominal pressure due to the enlarging gravid uterus contribute to the symptoms of GERD. However, subsequent studies did not find evidence to support this notion. Additionally, because heartburn is typically reported early in pregnancy, it is less likely that increased intra-abdominal pressure plays primary role.[18]

Management

Because heartburn and dyspepsia are so common during pregnancy, many patients and obstetricians view it as a normal occurrence during pregnancy. Initial management tends to focus on lifestyle modification, dietary changes, and potential medication adjustment (**Box 3**, **Fig. 1**).[19]

When symptoms persist despite conservative therapy, pharmacologic therapy may be considered. Unfortunately, many of the medications used to treat GERD in pregnancy have not been tested in randomized clinical trials in this patient population. Therefore, recommendations for medical therapy are derived from expert opinion, retrospective cohort studies, and case reports (**Table 4**). In general, pharmacologic agents that are not absolutely required should be avoided 31 to 71 days from the last menstrual period as this is the most critical time of organogenesis.[18,19] Also, because gastric acidity facilitates iron absorption, all agents that decrease gastric acidity should be used with caution in those with iron deficiency.[18]

Because they are considered nonsystemic drug therapy, antacids are a logical first-line medical therapy.[7] Additionally, because they are fast acting and effective at providing quick symptomatic relief, antacids are often preferred by patients. Those containing calcium, aluminum, and magnesium are considered safe in pregnancy at the usual doses.[18,19] Antacids containing magnesium trisilicate, however, have been associated with cardiovascular impairment, respiratory distress, hypotonia, and neph-rolithiasis when used at high doses for extended periods of time.[18] Additionally, compounds containing sodium bicarbonate should be avoided because they may precipitate fluid overload and metabolic alkalosis in both the mother and fetus.[7]

Sucralfate, another nonabsorbable agent, has been studied in a randomized controlled trial during pregnancy. Sucralfate, one gram 3 times daily, has been shown more effective in inducing symptomatic remission than lifestyle management alone. No adverse maternal or fetal events were reported. In animal studies, sucralfate has no effect on fertility and is not teratogeneic with doses up to 50 times the recommended human dose.[7,18,19]

Histamine type 2 receptor antagonists (H_2RAs) are often next-line therapy. Both cimetidine and ranitidine have been used in pregnancy for more than 30 years and have excellent safety profiles. Ranitidine has been specifically studied in pregnancy and has proved efficacy over conservative management and antacids. Although cimetidine has weak antiandrogenic effect in animals and has been associated with gynecomastia in adult men, there are no reports of sexual abnormalities in infants after exposure to cimetidine or other H_2RAs.[18,19]

In general, proton pump inhibitors (PPIs) are the most effective medical therapy for symptom control and esophageal healing in GERD.[19] Similarly, in pregnancy, studies have shown that PPIs are more effective than other medical therapy.[18] They are not, however, extensively used. Omeprazole, the first PPI developed for clinical use, is classified as a category C drug due to dose-related fetal and embryonic mortality in

---

Box 3
Medications associated with decreased lower esophageal sphincter tone

Anticholinergics
Calcium channel antagonist
Theophylline
Antipsychotics
Antidepressants

Data from Ali RA, Egan LJ. Gastroesophageal reflux disease in pregnancy. Best Pract Res Clin Gastroenterol 2007;21(5):793–806.

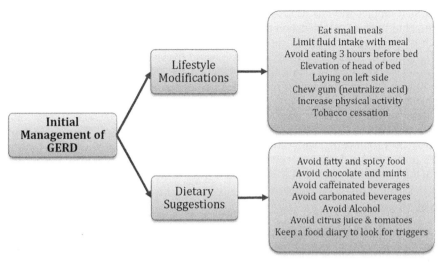

Fig. 1. Initial recommendations for the management of GERD. (*Data from* Refs.[16–18])

Table 4
Medical therapy for the treatment of gastroesophageal reflux disease

Medication	Food and Drug Administration Classification[a]	Comments
Antacids		
Calcium carbonate	C	Generally considered safe
Aluminum hydroxide	B	Generally considered safe
Magnesium hydroxide	B	Generally considered safe
Magnesium trisilicates	None	Should be avoided
Sodium bicarbonate	C	May cause metabolic alkalosis and fluid overload
Nonabsorbable drug		
Sucralfate	B	Good safety profile in humans and animals
H₂RAs		
Cimetidine	B	Antiandrogenic in adults; no fetal abnormalities
Famotidine	B	Considered safe
Ranitidine	B	Only H₂RA with proved efficacy in pregnancy
PPIs		
Lansoprazole	B	Considered safe
Omeprazole	C	Dose-related fetal toxicity in early animal studies
Pantoprazole	B	Limited human safety data; considered safe
Dopamine antagonist		
Metoclopramide	B	No reported teratogenic effects in humans or animals

[a] Discontinued June 30 2015, for biological products and prescription drugs; to be replaced by risk narratives based on human and/or animal studies.
Data from Refs.[17–20]

pregnant rabbits and rats. Subsequent human studies have not shown a teratogenic effect, but the FDA classification has not changed.[19] Other PPIs are FDA class B, but their use in pregnancy is reserved for those with known complications of GERD or symptoms not responding to other therapies. In these cases, lansoprazole is often the preferred agent because it has the most safety data.[7] Animal studies using up to 40 times the recommended human dose of lansoprazole have not demonstrated fetal toxicity.[18]

Metoclopramide, a promotility agent, is primarily used in the treatment of pregnancy associated nausea and vomiting. Nonetheless, it can also improve the symptoms of GERD by promoting gastric emptying, improving acid clearance, and increasing LES pressure. No congenital malformations or fetal toxicities have been associated with the use of metoclopramide in pregnancy.[18,19]

CONSTIPATION

Constipation is the second most common GI complaint in pregnancy.[21] After modifying the duration of symptoms (1 month instead of 3 months), Bradley and colleagues[22] used many elements of the Rome III Diagnositic Criteria for Functional Constipation to define constipation as the presence of at least 2 of the following 6 symptoms during at least 25% of defecations: having fewer than 3 bowel movements per week, straining, hard or lumpy stools, sensation of anorectal blockade/obstruction, sensation of incomplete emptying, or using manual maneuvers to assist with defecation. Using this definition, they found that up to 25% of pregnant women experience constipation at some point during their pregnancy.[22] Other studies, however, report constipation in up to 40% of pregnancies.[23]

Typically, the symptoms of constipation are most prevalent in the first and second trimesters and decrease in the third. For unknown reasons, subsequent pregnancies have a higher risk for constipation. Risk factors for constipation include a sedentary lifestyle, bed rest, low fiber intake, and inadequate fluid intake. Medications, such as iron, may also contribute to constipation.[21]

Evaluation

A vast majority of pregnant women who present with constipation are found to have functional constipation. Nonetheless, an evaluation to rule out other mechanical or systemic etiologies is indicated. When obtaining the history, practitioners should inquire about the frequency and consistency of stool, the presence of blood in the stool, abdominal pain, and bloating. The latter 2 symptoms may suggest irritable bowel syndrome (IBS). On the other hand, straining and the use of digital manipulation and/or perineal pressure to facilitate defecation may suggest pelvic floor dysfunction. Information regarding use of laxatives, enemas, and over-the-counter and prescription medications should also be obtained.[23]

The physical examination should focus on clinical signs of hypothyroidism and diabetes, which may contribute to constipation. Additionally, evaluation of the perineum and anal canal is particularly important. The perineum should be observed during retention maneuvers and simulation of defecation to evaluate for prolapse of the anorectal mucosa. Assessment of sphincter tone and anal canal can be accomplished via digital rectal examination. Upon completion of digital rectal examination, the patient should be asked to expel the examiner's finger as the inability to do so may suggest dyssynergic defecation.[23]

Laboratory investigation is focused on excluding endocrine and electrolyte abnormalities as the cause for constipation.[23] When associated with bleeding or anorectal lesions are suspected, flexible sigmoidoscopy or anoscopy may be indicated.[24] In patients with a history of gastric bypass or bowel surgery, small bowel obstruction may be considered. Other rare causes of constipation include neurologic disorders, polyps, and neoplasms.[21]

Pathophysiology

The cause of constipation in pregnancy is often multifactorial. Because constipation is more prevalent in early pregnancy, sex hormones are thought to be involved.[23] During normal pregnancy, serum concentrations of progesterone are elevated and progressively rise. Numerous animal studies have shown that progesterone inhibits gastric, small bowel, and colonic contractility via its dose-dependent regulation of intracellular calcium.[24] Pregnancy-induced permeations in serum levels of motilin and relaxin, hormones known to affect GI motility, may also contribute.[23,24]

Additionally, the formation of hard, scybalous stool may be caused by aldosterone-mediated increased colonic water absorption. Elevated levels of progesterone cause increased concentrations of aldosterone.[23] Additionally, decreased colonic smooth muscle contractility prolongs colonic transit time, which could also contribute to stool dehydration. **Fig. 2** summarizes these and other etiologies that may contribute to constipation in pregnancy.[23,24]

Management

The initial treatment of constipation in pregnancy is similar to that of the general population: dietary and lifestyle modifications.[25] Strenuous exercise may worsen constipation, but light physical activity can promote normal bowel function. Dietary adjustments include increasing fluid intake (>8 glasses per day) and fiber consumption (>20–35 g per day).[25] Intermittent iron supplementation can be as effective as daily dosing in the treatment of anemia but may reduce constipation.[21]

When lifestyle and diet modifications do not provide adequate symptomatic relief, bulk-forming agents are usually considered.[21] Because they are not systemically absorbed, these medications are thought to be safe in pregnancy and may be used for long durations. Because the therapeutic effect of these agents may not be seen for several days, they are not helpful for acute symptom relief.[23]

Lactulose and polyethylene glycol (PEG) are osmotic laxatives that stimulate the accumulation of fluid in the GI lumen.[21,25] Studies have shown that PEG can accelerate colorectal transit, increase the frequency of bowel movements, and improve defecation in patients with constipation refractory to dietary fiber.[25] Although this class of medication has poor systemic absorption and no known fetal risk, some medications in this class are FDA class C.[21]

Stimulant laxatives, such as sennosides and bisacodyl, are also minimally systemically absorbed but FDA class C.[16,21] These agents are associated with an increased risk of side effects, including diarrhea and abdominal pain. Both stimulating and osmotic laxatives should be used with caution and only for a short duration due to concern for electrolyte abnormalities. Additionally, for improved efficacy, fluid intake should be maximized when taking these agents.[21]

Medications not recommended in pregnancy include mineral oil, castor oil, and saline hyperosmotic agents. Mineral oil is associated with reduced maternal absorption of fat-soluble vitamins, which could lead to hemorrhage and neonatal hypoprothrombinemia.[23,25] Due to concern for premature uterine contractions induced by castor oil and fluid retention from hyperosmotic saline products, these agents are not recommended.[25]

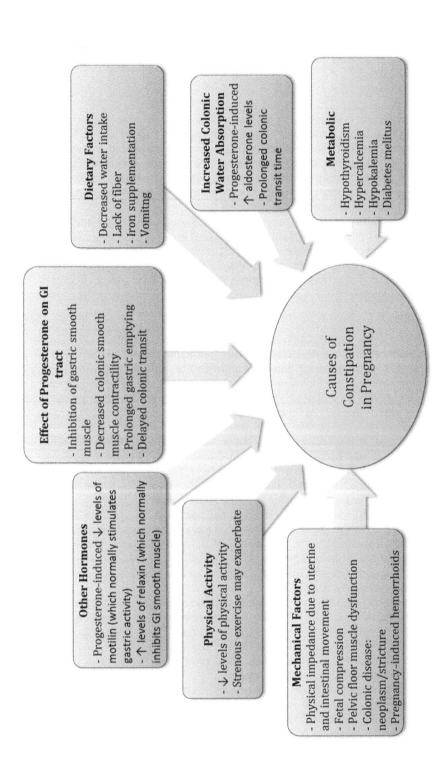

Fig. 2. Etiology of constipation in pregnancy. (*Data from* Zielinski R, Searing K, Deibel M. Gastrointestinal distress in pregnancy: prevalence, assessment, and treatment of 5 common minor discomforts. J Perinat Neonatal Nurs 2015;29(1):23–31; and Bradley CS, Kennedy CM, Turcea AM, et al. Constipation in pregnancy: prevalence, symptoms, and risk factors. Obstet Gynecol 2007;110(6):1351–57.)

Lubiprostone, a fatty acid derivative prostaglandin E_1, causes increased ion and fluid secretion inside the GI lumen.[26] Safety in human pregnancies has not been evaluated, but animal studies show that it may cause harm.[17] Therefore, it should be used with caution in pregnancy. **Table 5** lists some of the common medications used in the treatment of constipation and contains information regarding their safety in pregnancy.

DIARRHEA

Compared with other GI disorders in pregnancy, there is significantly less literature on diarrhea in pregnancy. There are no recent studies documenting the prevalence of diarrhea in pregnancy, and GI motility has not been evaluated in pregnant women who report diarrhea.[24,25] Previous studies from the 1970s reported an increased frequency of bowel movements in 34% of pregnant women.[27] Diarrhea that develops at or near term may be a precursor to labor.[21]

Etiology of Acute Diarrhea

In an otherwise healthy pregnant individual, the etiology of an abrupt onset of diarrhea is likely infectious. In developed countries, viruses are the most common cause of

Table 5
Medical therapy for the treatment constipation

Medication	Food and Drug Administration Classification[a]	Comments
Bulk-forming agent		
Methylcellulose	B	Generally considered safe; may cause bloating and cramping
Psyllium	C	Generally considered safe; may cause bloating and cramping
Osmotic agents		
Lactulose	B	No adverse events in animal studies
PEG	C	Limited data; good option for constipation in pregnancy
Saline hyperosmotic	X	May cause fluid retention
Stimulating agents		
Sennosides	C	Not associated with increased risk of abnormalities
Bisacodyl	C	Safe, but use limited by cramping
Emolients/lubricants		
Mineral oil	X	Reduced maternal absorption of fat soluble vitamins
Castor oil	X	Premature uterine contractions
Prokinetic agents		
Lubiprostone	C	No human studies; increased fetal risk in animal studies
Linaclotide	C	Adverse events in animal reproduction studies

[a] Discontinued June 30, 2015, for biological products and prescription drugs, to be replaced by risk narratives based on human and/or animal studies.
Data from Refs.[16,17,21,23,25]

acute diarrhea. The second most common cause is bacteria: *Escherichia coli, Salmonella, Shigella,* and *Campylobacter*. If there is a history of recent antibiotic usage, there should be an increased suspicion for *Clostridium difficile*. In developing countries, *Entamoeba histolytica, Cryptosporidium,* and *Giardia* are common causes. Lastly, diarrhea along with flulike symptoms with or without a recent outbreak of foodborne illness, should raise suspicion for *Listeria*.[21,25]

Evaluation

Further evaluation of acute diarrhea is warranted if any of the following symptoms are present: persistent diarrhea, weight loss, malnutrition, fever, or signs of volume depletion.[21,25] Stool should be assessed for an infectious cause and additional work-up to rule out noninfectious causes may also be indicated.[25] A list of the common causes for diarrhea in pregnancy is shown in **Box 4**. If necessary, a flexible sigmoidoscopy may be performed to evaluate the colonic mucosa.[24] Flexible sigmoidoscopy has demonstrated safety in pregnancy and is not associated with the induction of labor or congenital malformations.[28]

Pathophysiology

Based on current medical knowledge, the only known physiologic alteration that could induce diarrhea in pregnancy is through the effect of prostaglandins on smooth muscle. Prostaglandins cause smooth muscle contractions, which can increase GI expulsion forces.[25] In menstruating women, elevated levels of prostaglandins have been associated with abdominal discomfort, diarrhea, nausea, and vomiting, which improve after administration of prostaglandin synthesis inhibitors.[24]

Management

When antidiarrheal agents are needed to decrease the frequency of stool, loperamide is often considered. Once an FDA class B medication, loperamide was reclassified as

---

Box 4
Common causes of diarrhea in pregnancy

Infectious
  Viral
  Bacterial
  Protozoal

Food intolerance
  Fructose
  Lactose
  Mannitol
  Sorbitol

Accelerated GI transit
  Medications
  Increased prostaglandins

Irritable Bowel Syndrome

Inflammatory bowel disease

Malabsorption

Data from Christie J, Rose S. Constipation, diarrhea, hemorrhoids, and fecal incontinence. Pregnancy in gastrointestinal disorders. Bethesda (MD): ACG Monograph American College of Physicians; 2007. p. 4–9. Available at: https://www.acg.gi.org.

category C due to follow-up studies that showed an increased risk of hypospadias, caesarean section, placenta previa, and large-for-gestational-age infants in women who reported using loperamide in early pregnancy.[29]

Other common antidiarrheal agents, including diphenoxylate with atropine and bismuth subsalicylate, are contraindicated in pregnancy. Bismuth subsalicylate is contraindicated due to the potential for salicylate absorption.[24] Subsalicylates are known teratogens and have been associated with prolonged labor and gestation, increased perinatal mortality, decreased birth weight, and neonatal hemorrhage.[24,25] Diphenoxylate with atropine is teratogenic in both animals and humans after the first trimester of pregnancy.[24]

Many of the antibiotics used to treat infectious diarrhea are contraindicated throughout or during specific periods of gestation; these include the quinolones, tetracyclines, sulfa preparations, and metronidazole. In severe cases of infectious diarrhea, however, antibiotic therapy may be necessary. In these cases, antibiotics with a safer pregnancy profile, such as erythromycin and ampicillin, should be considered.[24]

Although IBS is common in women of childbearing age, there are no large studies following women with IBS throughout pregnancy. Similar to nonpregnant patients, medical therapy focuses on the treatment of diarrhea along with the abdominal pain and bloating commonly associated with IBS. In addition to the antidiarrheal agents discussed previously, cholestyramine, a bile-acid sequestrant, is sometimes used as an antidiarrheal agent in IBS. Due to the potential to cause malabsorption of fat-soluble vitamins, however, it is not recommended in pregnancy. Additionally, the

Table 6
Medical therapy for the treatment of diarrhea and irritable bowel syndrome

Medication	Food and Drug Administration Classification[a]	Comments
Antidiarrheal agents		
Loperamide	C	Contraindicated in blood diarrhea
Diphenoxylate with atropine	C	Should be avoided in pregnancy
Bismuth subsalicylate	C	Salicylates are contraindicated in pregnancy
Cholestyramine	C	May interfere with vitamin absorption
IBS medications		
Antispasmodics		
Dicyclomine	B	No adverse events in animal studies
Hyoscyamine	C	Only use during pregnancy if clearly needed
Tricyclic antidepressants		
Amitriptyline	C	Limb deformities and developmental delay
Nortriptyline	D	Inconclusive animal reproduction studies
Desipramine	C	Generally not recommended
Selective serotonin reuptake inhibitors		
Fluoxetine	C	Adverse events in animal studies
Paroxetine	D	Known fetal teratogenic effects

[a] Discontinued June 30, 2015, for biological products and prescription drugs, to be replaced by risk narratives based on human and/or animal studies.
   Data from Refs.[16,17,21,25,30]

use of antispasmodics, tricyclic antidepressants, and selective serotonin reuptake inhibitors should only be used in pregnant women who are severely symptomatic.[30] **Table 6** lists medications commonly used to treat diarrhea and IBS and contains information regarding their safety in pregnancy.

In summary, pregnancy-induced hormonal and/or anatomic changes may induce or exacerbate many of the common GI complaints of the general population: nausea and vomiting, GERD, constipation, and diarrhea. Fortunately, many of these bowel disturbances respond to lifestyle modifications and conservative medical management. When more aggressive medical therapy is needed, understanding the underlying pathophysiology is necessary so that appropriate therapy can be initiated. The FDA pregnancy categories are being replaced by narrative safety statements based on animal and human safety studies. These narratives should more accurately and effectively convey the teratogenic and reproductive risks associated with drug exposure and facilitate both clinician and patient understanding of the varying degrees of fetal risk. Although it is difficult to acquire prospective risk data in pregnant women, the search must be continued for the most effective and safe therapies to maximize maternal as well as fetal health and well-being.

REFERENCES

1. McCarthy FP, Lutomski JE, Greene RA. Hyperemesis gravidarum: current perspectives. Int J Womens Health 2014;6:719–25.
2. Matthews A, Haas DM, O'Mathuna DP, et al. Interventions for nausea and vomiting in early pregnancy. Cochrane Database Syst Rev 2014;(3):CD007575.
3. Einarson TR, Piwko C, Koren G. Prevalence of nausea and vomiting of pregnancy in the USA: a meta analysis. J Popul Ther Clin Pharmacol 2013;20(2):e163–70.
4. Niemeijer MN, Grooten IJ, Vos N, et al. Diagnostic markers for hyperemesis gravidarum: a systematic review and metaanalysis. Am J Obstet Gynecol 2014; 211(2):150.e1–15.
5. Koch KL. Gastrointestinal factors in nausea and vomiting of pregnancy. Am J Obstet Gynecol 2002;186(5 Suppl Understanding):S198–203.
6. Castillo MJ, Phillippi JC. Hyperemesis gravidarum: a holistic overview and approach to clinical assessment and management. J Perinat Neonatal Nurs 2015;29(1):12–22 [quiz: E11].
7. Richter JE. Heartburn, nausea, and vomiting during pregnancy. In: Pregnancy in gastrointestinal disorders. Bethesda (MD): ACG Monograph American College of Physicians; 2007. p. 18–25. Available at: https://www.acg.gi.org.
8. Verrengia M, Sachdeva P, Gaughan J, et al. Variation of symptoms during the menstrual cycle in female patients with gastroparesis. Neurogastroenterol Motil 2011;23(7):625–625.e254.
9. Jahangiri F, Hirshfeld-Cytron J, Goldman K, et al. Correlation between depression, anxiety, and nausea and vomiting during pregnancy in an in vitro fertilization population: a pilot study. J Psychosom Obstet Gynaecol 2011;32(3):113–8.
10. Verberg MF, Gillott DJ, Al-Fardan N, et al. Hyperemesis gravidarum, a literature review. Hum Reprod Update 2005;11(5):527–39.
11. Wegrzyniak LJ, Repke JT, Ural SH. Treatment of hyperemesis gravidarum. Rev Obstet Gynecol 2012;5(2):78–84.
12. Pope E, Maltepe C, Koren G. Comparing pyridoxine and doxylamine succinate-pyridoxine HCl for nausea and vomiting of pregnancy: a matched, controlled cohort study. J Clin Pharmacol 2015;55(7):809–14.

13. Hosseini FS, Adib-Hajbaghery M. Ginger essence effect on nausea and vomiting after open and laparoscopic nephrectomies. Nurs Midwifery Stud 2015;4(2): e28625.
14. Giacosa A, Morazzoni P, Bombardelli E, et al. Can nausea and vomiting be treated with ginger extract? Eur Rev Med Pharmacol Sci 2015;19(7):1291–6.
15. Food and Drug Administration, HHS. Content and format of labeling for human prescription drug and biological products; requirements for pregnancy and lactation labeling. Final rule. Fed Regist 2014;79(233):72063–103.
16. Epocrates [online]. San Francisco (CA): Epocrates Inc; 2015. Available at: http://www.epocrates.com. Accessed October 21, 2015.
17. Post T, editor. UpToDate. Waltham (MA): UpToDate; 2015. Available at: www.uptodate.com. Accessed October 7, 2015.
18. Ali RA, Egan LJ. Gastroesophageal reflux disease in pregnancy. Best Pract Res Clin Gastroenterol 2007;21(5):793–806.
19. Richter JE. Review article: the management of heartburn in pregnancy. Aliment Pharmacol Ther 2005;22(9):749–57.
20. Black RA, Hill DA. Over-the-counter medications in pregnancy. Am Fam Physician 2003;67(12):2517–24.
21. Zielinski R, Searing K, Deibel M. Gastrointestinal distress in pregnancy: prevalence, assessment, and treatment of 5 common minor discomforts. J Perinat Neonatal Nurs 2015;29(1):23–31.
22. Bradley CS, Kennedy CM, Turcea AM, et al. Constipation in pregnancy: prevalence, symptoms, and risk factors. Obstet Gynecol 2007;110(6):1351–7.
23. Cullen G, O'Donoghue D. Constipation and pregnancy. Best Pract Res Clin Gastroenterol 2007;21(5):807–18.
24. Bonapace ES Jr, Fisher RS. Constipation and diarrhea in pregnancy. Gastroenterol Clin North Am 1998;27(1):197–211.
25. Christie J, Rose S. Constipation, diarrhea, hemorrhoids, and fecal incontinence. In: Pregnancy in gastrointestinal disorders. Bethesda (MD): ACG Monograph American College of Physicians; 2007. p. 4–9. Available at: https://www.acg.gi.org.
26. Wilson N, Schey R. Lubiprostone in constipation: clinical evidence and place in therapy. Ther Adv Chronic Dis 2015;6(2):40–50.
27. Levy N, Lemberg E, Sharf M. Bowel habit in pregnancy. Digestion 1971;4(4): 216–22.
28. Cappell MS, Colon VJ, Sidhom OA. A study at 10 medical centers of the safety and efficacy of 48 flexible sigmoidoscopies and 8 colonoscopies during pregnancy with follow-up of fetal outcome and with comparison to control groups. Dig Dis Sci 1996;41(12):2353–61.
29. Kallen B, Nilsson E, Otterblad Olausson P. Maternal use of loperamide in early pregnancy and delivery outcome. Acta Paediatr 2008;97(5):541–5.
30. Thukral C, Wolf JL. Therapy insight: drugs for gastrointestinal disorders in pregnant women. Nat Clin Pract Gastroenterol Hepatol 2006;3(5):256–66.

Pregnancy and the Patient with Inflammatory Bowel Disease

Fertility, Treatment, Delivery, and Complications

 CrossMark

Ryan A. McConnell, MD[a], Uma Mahadevan, MD[b],*

KEYWORDS

- Inflammatory bowel disease • Crohn disease • Ulcerative colitis • Fertility
- Pregnancy • Obstetric delivery • Breast feeding
- Drug-related side effects and adverse reactions

KEY POINTS

- Inflammatory bowel disease increases the risk of pregnancy complications and adverse pregnancy outcomes. Active disease exacerbates these risks. Universal high-risk obstetric monitoring is recommended.
- Active disease and pelvic surgery reduce female fertility. Fertility is preserved with quiescent disease. Patient misperceptions about fertility, disease risks, and medication safety contribute to voluntary childlessness.
- Most medications have a favorable safety profile for use during pregnancy and breastfeeding to induce and maintain remission. This includes the aminosalicylates, thiopurines, and biologics.
- There are potential fetal risks with intrauterine exposure to corticosteroids, certain antibiotics, methotrexate, and thiopurine-biologic combination therapy. Risk/benefit assessments should be individualized.
- Patients should be counseled about the importance of medication adherence to optimize preconception disease control and maintain remission throughout pregnancy.

Conflicts of Interest: Dr U. Mahadevan has served as a consultant for or received research support from Abbvie, Janssen, UCB, Takeda, and Prometheus Labs. Dr R.A. McConnell has no conflicts of interest or funding sources.
Source of Funding: None.
[a] Division of Gastroenterology, University of California, San Francisco, 1701 Divisadero Street, #120, San Francisco, CA 94115, USA; [b] Division of Gastroenterology, UCSF Center for Colitis and Crohn's Disease, 1701 Divisadero Street, #120, San Francisco, CA 94115, USA
* Corresponding author.
E-mail address: uma.mahadevan@ucsf.edu

INTRODUCTION

Inflammatory bowel disease (IBD) incidence peaks during the years of childbearing potential, with half of patients diagnosed before age 32.[1] By nature of this age distribution at IBD onset, the complexities of family planning and IBD management often coincide. Although most IBD patients have successful pregnancies, women with IBD have fewer children than the general population because of voluntary childlessness.[2] Apprehension and misperceptions about fertility, medication safety, and the potential for adverse pregnancy outcomes may explain this phenomenon.[3,4] There is ample opportunity for knowledgeable providers to positively impact IBD pregnancy outcomes by optimizing disease control, mitigating medication-related risks, and enhancing patient education.

FERTILITY
Women

Fear of infertility is common among patients with IBD and may adversely impact family planning decisions.[5] In reality, women with quiescent IBD and no prior pelvic surgery have similar infertility rates (5%–14%) as the general population.[3,6] Active disease does impair fertility,[7,8] likely via multifactorial mechanisms, such as pelvic inflammation, poor nutrition, decreased libido, dyspareunia, and depression.[9] A small study demonstrated decreased ovarian reserve in women with Crohn disease, especially those with active disease.[10] Pelvic surgery significantly increases female infertility due to scarring and adhesions. A meta-analysis of ileal pouch anal anastomosis (IPAA) surgery in ulcerative colitis found a 48% postoperative infertility rate, threefold higher than the 15% rate in medically treated patients.[11] Laparoscopic total proctocolectomy with IPAA may preserve fertility compared with open surgery.[12] Abdominal surgeries that spare the pelvis, such as colectomy with ileorectal anastomosis, may also preserve female fertility.[13] Women of childbearing potential should be counseled before surgery about the infertility risk of IPAA, and less invasive procedures may be considered. However, given the retrospective nature of the studies and older techniques, true rates of infertility following IPAA are not known. IPAA does not appear to impact success rates of in vitro fertilization.[14]

Women who experience difficulty conceiving or spontaneous abortion should be assessed for occult disease activity, hypovitaminosis D, and celiac disease, all of which are associated with infertility.[15,16] If women remain unable to conceive after 6 months of calculated attempts, reproductive endocrinology referral is warranted.

Men

Less is known about male fertility in IBD. Zinc deficiency in Crohn disease may impair sperm function.[17] Certain medications have been shown to affect sperm quantity and quality. Sulfasalazine causes reversible infertility due to dose-dependent oligospermia, reduced sperm motility, and altered sperm morphology.[18] Methotrexate may reduce sperm quality, although any such effects are reversible when the drug is discontinued.[19] Some experts recommend that men stop methotrexate at least 3 months before attempting conception. Antitumor necrosis factor α (anti-TNF) medications may accelerate germ cell apoptosis in the seminiferous tubules,[20] which might theoretically decrease sperm count. However, a small study of 10 men did not find a decrement in sperm concentration following infliximab infusion.[21] It remains unknown whether medication-induced changes in sperm quality have any effect on fertility, and additional research is needed.

COMPLICATIONS

The interaction between IBD and pregnancy is bidirectional: IBD impacts pregnancy, and pregnancy may impact IBD. A robust comprehension of this interplay provides the framework for patient education and development of an individualized treatment strategy to mitigate risks.

Inflammatory Bowel Disease Detrimentally Impacts Pregnancy

Women with IBD, including those in remission, experience a higher rate of adverse pregnancy outcomes than the general population. A recent meta-analysis including 15,007 women with IBD found increased odds of preterm birth (odds ratio [OR] 1.85, 95% confidence interval [CI] 1.67–2.05), small for gestational age infants (OR 1.36, 95% CI 1.16–1.60), and still birth (OR 1.57, 95% CI 1.03–2.38).[22] The risk of congenital anomalies was also increased (OR 1.29, 95% CI 1.05–1.58), although there was evidence of publication bias. Multiple recent population-based studies failed to detect an increased risk of congenital anomalies in IBD pregnancies.[23,24] IBD is associated with higher rates of pregnancy complications, such as preeclampsia, preterm premature rupture of membranes, and venous thromboembolism.[25–27] Inadequate maternal weight gain has been identified as a predictor of adverse outcomes.[28,29] Additional hypothesized mediators of increased risk include inflammation, anemia, hypoalbuminemia, poor nutrition, and medication exposures. Based on these findings, all IBD pregnancies should be monitored by a maternal-fetal medicine specialist. Serial ultrasonography should be considered in the third trimester to assess fetal growth.

Active disease further compounds risk

Disease activity is the strongest predictor of adverse pregnancy outcomes. Active disease at conception increases the risk of spontaneous abortion and preterm birth,[7,30] whereas disease exacerbation during pregnancy increases the risk of preterm birth,[23,31–33] still birth,[34] and low birth weight.[33,35] The risk of low birth weight doubles with an ulcerative colitis flare and triples with a Crohn flare.[34] These observations emphasize the critical importance of maintaining remission throughout pregnancy, beginning in the preconception period.

Quiescent disease reduces risk

When patients conceive during IBD remission and maintain quiescent disease throughout pregnancy, the risks of preterm birth and low birth weight are similar to matched non-IBD controls.[25,36] We recommend that women achieve and sustain remission for at least 3 to 6 months before conception to maximize the chances of a successful and healthy pregnancy.

Pregnancy May Impact Inflammatory Bowel Disease

It remains uncertain whether pregnancy itself adversely affects the course of IBD. Among women in remission at conception, the risk of subsequent disease exacerbation during pregnancy is 20% in Crohn disease and 33% in ulcerative colitis.[37] The ongoing prospective, multicenter Pregnancy in Inflammatory Bowel Disease and Neonatal Outcomes (PIANO) registry of more than 1475 pregnant women with IBD also found a higher rate of ulcerative colitis activity relative to Crohn activity.[38] Overlapping immune pathways, such as placental production of proinflammatory cytokines, have been hypothesized as a potential explanation for this finding.[39] Alternatively, this may reflect less aggressive ulcerative colitis treatment, as most of these patients were on mesalamine monotherapy. A meta-analysis of 1720 patients with IBD found that disease activity during pregnancy strongly correlates with disease activity at the time of conception.[40] Active disease affected 46% to 55% of pregnancies commenced during active disease, compared with 23% to 29% of pregnancies conceived during remission. Overall, IBD relapse rates during pregnancy are similar to rates for nonpregnant women.[7,25,30]

Disease behavior during pregnancy and the postpartum period is likely confounded by the frequent and inappropriate discontinuation of maintenance medications, which increases the risk of flare.[41,42] Providers must educate patients about the risk of disease to the pregnancy and the importance of medication adherence to optimize preconception disease control and maintain remission throughout pregnancy.

Mode of delivery
The mode of delivery in IBD pregnancies is largely determined by obstetric indications and patient preference. Cesarean delivery is more common among women with IBD compared with the general population.[43] For example, 44% of women in the PIANO registry delivered via cesarean, often for elective reasons.[44] Theoretic concerns that vaginal delivery might trigger perianal disease are not supported by a recent cohort study, which found no association between mode of delivery and IBD natural history.[45] Cesarean delivery is typically recommended for women with active perianal disease, though evidence conflicts regarding the trajectory of active perianal disease following vaginal delivery.[46] Some colorectal surgeons also recommend cesarean delivery following IPAA to protect the pouch and preserve anal sphincter integrity. However, a systemic review found no increased risk of pouch dysfunction with vaginal delivery.[47] Finally, the mode of delivery does not appear to be a factor in the risk of childhood IBD.[48] Rather, heritability studies estimate that a child has a 2% to 5% chance of developing IBD if a single parent has the disease[49] and a 36% chance when both parents have IBD.[50]

TREATMENT

Before initiating IBD therapy in a woman of childbearing age, the patient's desire and timeline for pregnancy should be discussed. Preconception counseling about the low risk of most medications may improve medication adherence during pregnancy.[51] As a general rule, active disease poses a greater risk to the fetus than IBD therapies. This principle forms the basis for IBD treatment decisions in pregnancy.

Medications

With the exception of methotrexate and thalidomide, most medications used to treat IBD are considered low risk and may be continued during pregnancy and breastfeeding (**Table 1**). Of note, the US Food and Drug Administration recently implemented a revised medication labeling rule that removes the previously used pregnancy categories (A, B, C, D, X).[52] We will not reference the pregnancy categories in the following discussion.

Corticosteroids
Corticosteroid safety is discussed later in this article in the context of IBD exacerbations.

Aminosalicylates
The 5-aminosalicylates (balsalazide, mesalamine, olsalazine, and sulfasalazine) are considered safe in pregnancy.[53] The coating of delayed release mesalamine in Asacol HD (Actavis) contains dibutyl phthalate (DBP), which has been associated with

Table 1
Medication safety for use during pregnancy and lactation

Medication	Pregnancy Safety	Breastfeeding Safety
Aminosalicylates		
Balsalazide	Low risk	Compatible; enters breast milk Potential risk of infantile diarrhea
Mesalamine	Low risk Dibutyl phthalate coating in Asacol HD may be teratogenic in animals	Compatible; enters breast milk Potential risk of infantile diarrhea
Olsalazine	Low risk	Compatible; enters breast milk Potential risk of infantile diarrhea
Sulfasalazine	Low risk; give with folic acid 2 mg daily Reversible oligospermia in men	Compatible; enters breast milk Potential risk of infantile diarrhea
Immunomodulators		
Cyclosporine	Limited data; possible risk of pregnancy complications, preterm birth, low birthweight	Contraindicated; enters breast milk
Methotrexate	Contraindicated: teratogenic, abortifacient Supplement with folic acid Discontinue 3–6 mo before conception	Contraindicated; enters breast milk
Thiopurines (azathioprine, 6-mercaptopurine)	Low risk in monotherapy Delayed infant infections in combination therapy	Compatible; clinically insignificant concentration enters breast milk Wait 4 h after ingestion if able
Tofacitinib	Limited human data	Unknown; no human data
Biologics		
Adalimumab	Low risk in monotherapy	Compatible; clinically insignificant concentration enters breast milk
Certolizumab pegol	Low risk Does not actively cross placenta	Compatible; clinically insignificant concentration enters breast milk
Golimumab	Low risk in monotherapy	Compatible; undetectable
Infliximab	Low risk in monotherapy	Compatible; clinically insignificant concentration enters breast milk
Natalizumab	Low risk in monotherapy	Compatible; undetectable
Ustekinumab	Limited human data	Likely compatible; limited human data
Vedolizumab	Low risk in monotherapy; limited data	Likely compatible; no human data

(continued on next page)

Table 1 (continued)		
Medication	**Pregnancy Safety**	**Breastfeeding Safety**
Corticosteroids		
Budesonide	Low risk	Compatible; clinically insignificant concentration enters breast milk
Prednisone	Moderate risk; possible orofacial cleft (first trimester exposure), adrenal insufficiency, gestational diabetes, premature rupture of membranes, preterm birth, infant infections	Compatible; clinically insignificant concentration enters breast milk
Antibiotics		
Amoxicillin with clavulanic acid	Low risk; preferred antibiotic during pregnancy	Compatible; enters breast milk
Ciprofloxacin	Low risk; affinity for cartilage	Compatible; enters breast milk
Metronidazole	Low risk; avoid in first trimester due to possible risk of orofacial clefts	Contraindicated; enters breast milk

congenital anomalies in animals at doses more than 190 times the therapeutic human dose.[54] All agents aside from Asacol HD do not have DBP in their coating, and multiple human studies have failed to identify mesalamine teratogenicity. Women taking sulfasalazine should receive supplemental folic acid 2 mg daily to prevent folate deficiency. Aminosalicylates enter breast milk but are considered compatible with use during breastfeeding. There is a rare association with diarrhea in the infant, which resolves on breastfeeding cessation.[55] Mesalamine enemas and suppositories may be continued without any known pregnancy risk.

Immunomodulators
Methotrexate Methotrexate is an abortifacient, teratogenic inhibitor of DNA synthesis and is contraindicated during conception and pregnancy. Women should not attempt conception within 3 to 6 months of methotrexate use due to the drug's long half-life. Although there are limited data pertaining to the lower doses commonly used to modulate the immunogenicity of biologic medications,[56] it is recommended that methotrexate be given only to those women of childbearing potential who practice 1 to 2 methods of contraception and take supplemental folic acid. Methotrexate is also contraindicated in breastfeeding. Although it is excreted in breast milk at levels below 10% of maternal plasma concentration,[57] the long half-life allows accumulation in neonatal tissue.

Thiopurines Like methotrexate, the thiopurines (azathioprine and 6-mercaptopurine) inhibit DNA synthesis. High doses are teratogenic in animals.[58] The metabolite 6-thioguanine crosses the human placenta and has been associated with newborn anemia.[59] However, most studies of thiopurine safety during pregnancy are confounded by unmeasured disease activity. Nearly 25% of women in a recent study discontinued thiopurines early in pregnancy, highlighting the uncertainty surrounding thiopurine management during pregnancy.[24]

Recent large studies of thiopurine-exposed pregnancies failed to detect an elevated risk of congenital anomalies.[24,60] A population-based study that attempted to account for disease activity found that thiopurine exposure increased the risk of preterm delivery irrespective of disease activity.[34] Conversely, a multicenter study comparing the disease activity and outcomes of pregnant women treated with thiopurines, anti–tumor necrosis factor (TNF) drugs, or neither medication class found no difference in pregnancy complications among the groups.[61] In multivariate analysis, thiopurine treatment was actually associated with favorable global pregnancy outcome. Two meta-analyses found that thiopurine use was associated with preterm delivery (relative risk [RR] 1.67; 95% CI 1.2–2.4), but disease activity was not directly assessed in any of the included studies.[62,63] The risk of congenital anomalies was increased compared with healthy women (RR 1.45; 95% CI 1.07–1.96), but there was no difference compared with unexposed IBD controls.[63]

Among more than 335 thiopurine-exposed pregnancies in the PIANO registry, there is no heightened risk of congenital anomalies or pregnancy complications.[38] After adjusting for disease activity, thiopurine-exposed infants have equivalent or better achievement of developmental milestones compared with unexposed infants.[64] However, infections at 9 to 12 months of age were more common among the 107 infants exposed to thiopurine plus anti-TNF combination therapy (RR 1.50; 95% CI 1.08–2.09).[38]

It is reasonable to continue thiopurine monotherapy during pregnancy to maintain remission, as the risks of active disease likely outweigh the risks associated with thiopurine use. Due to the potential for delayed infant infections, a woman in durable remission using a thiopurine in combination with a biologic may consider stopping the thiopurine before conception. Thiopurines generally should not be initiated during pregnancy due to their slow onset of action and the risks of bone marrow suppression and pancreatitis.

Clinically insignificant thiopurine concentrations in breast milk peak within 4 hours of maternal ingestion.[65] Lactating mothers might consider breastfeeding avoidance during this interval.

Biologics
Anti–tumor necrosis factor agents Of the 4 anti-TNF medications approved for IBD, infliximab and adalimumab provide most pregnancy safety information. Although mainly limited to case series, available data on the anti-TNF class suggest low risk for use during pregnancy.[66] However, the long-term implications of intrauterine exposure remain unknown, especially with respect to immune system development and function.

Series with more than 100 IBD pregnancies each exposed to infliximab,[67] adalimumab,[68] and certolizumab pegol[69] found no adverse effect on pregnancy outcomes. Golimumab is predicted to have a similar safety profile. More than 500 women in the PIANO registry have been exposed to anti-TNF medications during pregnancy: more than 260 infliximab, more than 150 adalimumab, more than 65 certolizumab pegol, and 29 multiple agents.[38] There is no increased risk of congenital anomalies compared with the unexposed IBD cohort. A systematic review including more than 1500 anti-TNF exposed pregnancies found no pattern of adverse pregnancy outcomes or congenital anomalies.[70] A recent meta-analysis showed a similar rate of unfavorable pregnancy outcomes between women taking anti-TNF therapy and unexposed controls (OR 1.00; 95% CI 0.72–1.41), including preterm delivery (OR 1.00; 95% CI 0.62–1.62), low birth weight (OR 1.05; 95% CI 0.62–1.78), and congenital anomalies (OR 1.10; 95% CI 0.58–2.09).[71]

Combination therapy with an anti-TNF and thiopurine may be associated with a higher risk of preterm birth (OR 2.4; 95% CI 1.3–4.3) and any pregnancy complication (OR 1.7; 95% CI 1.0–2.2), in addition to the risk of delayed infant infections described previously.[38]

There is clinically insignificant anti-TNF excretion into breast milk, with milk concentrations less than 1% of maternal plasma concentrations. Furthermore, antibodies ingested orally are unlikely to be bioavailable. In the PIANO registry, breastfed infants exposed to anti-TNF monoclonal antibodies have similar rates of growth and milestone achievement compared with unexposed breastfed infants, with no increased risk of infection.[72]

Transplacental drug transfer Monoclonal immunoglobulin G1 (IgG1) medications (infliximab, adalimumab, golimumab) are actively transported across the placenta along with other maternal antibodies, beginning in the second trimester.[73] Fetal IgG1 concentrations increase logarithmically, with 80% of transfer occurring in the third trimester.[74] Cord blood infliximab and adalimumab concentrations at birth exceed maternal levels by up to fourfold,[73] and these agents remain detectable in infants for up to 12 months.[75] This raises concern about potential adverse effects on neonatal immune system development.[76] In the PIANO registry, third trimester anti-TNF exposure did not detrimentally affect infant growth rate, immune development, number of infections, or achievement of developmental milestones.[44,64] A small study of 25 anti-TNF exposed children reported appropriate serologic response to vaccination and normal cellular immunity.[77]

Until the implications of intrauterine anti-TNF exposure are better understood, it is reasonable for women in sustained remission to consider third trimester dosing adjustments to reduce neonatal exposure (**Table 2**).[78,79] Therapeutic drug monitoring with trough serum concentrations in the late second or early third trimester may also help guide dosing before delivery.[66] However, any decision to alter medication dosing schedule should be individualized and balanced against the risks, which include triggering active disease or maternal immunization with diminished future drug effectiveness.

Infants exposed to anti-TNF agents should not receive live vaccines for at least the first 6 months of life or until drug levels are undetectable. All other childhood vaccinations may be given on schedule. This recommendation does not apply to certolizumab pegol, which as a Fab' fragment is not actively transported across the placenta and does not reach significant levels in the infant.[73] Pediatricians should be notified of intrauterine anti-TNF exposure so that vaccinations and any potential infections can be appropriately managed.

Anti-integrin agents Natalizumab (IgG4) and vedolizumab (IgG1) are both monoclonal antibodies that would be expected to actively cross the placenta. Among several hundred natalizumab-exposed pregnancies, largely in patients with multiple sclerosis, there is no observed increased risk of preterm birth, low birth weight, or congenital anomalies.[80] The half-life of vedolizumab is more than 3 times longer than that of infliximab, which may have implications for infant drug exposure and dosing adjustment considerations during pregnancy. Available vedolizumab pregnancy safety data are extremely limited.[81] The PIANO registry contains data from 6 natalizumab-exposed pregnancies, with no observed increased rates of congenital anomalies, growth impairment, or developmental delay.[38]

Emerging therapies
Anti-interleukin 12 to 23 Ustekinumab is an IgG1 monoclonal antibody approved for psoriasis and psoriatic arthritis that showed benefit in a phase III Crohn disease

Table 2
Checklist for managing the patient with inflammatory bowel disease before, during, and after pregnancy

Time Period	Task
Preconception	Establish care with multidisciplinary team: primary care physician, gastroenterologist, obstetrician, maternal-fetal medicine specialist Update health care maintenance, vaccinations, and surveillance colonoscopy as appropriate Check baseline laboratories (complete blood count, iron studies, B12, folate, vitamin D) and correct any nutrient deficiencies Assess disease activity • Consider baseline fecal calprotectin or colonoscopy if appropriate Optimize disease control • Adjust medications to achieve steroid-free remission • Discontinue methotrexate and switch to an alternate agent Develop medication plan for pregnancy and postpartum period • Communicate plan to all providers • Ensure patient understands and is in agreement
First trimester	Continue maintenance medications
Second trimester	Continue maintenance medications Consider therapeutic drug monitoring of biologics and dosing adjustments
Third trimester	Continue maintenance medications Consider adjusting biologic medication dosing schedule to reduce placental transfer Last dose: • Infliximab: week 30–32 • Adalimumab: week 36–38 • Certolizumab pegol: no adjustment • Golimumab: week 34–36 • Natalizumab: week 36 • Vedolizumab: week 30–32 Consider serial ultrasonographic assessment of fetal growth beginning at week 26–28, especially with active disease or inadequate maternal weight gain
Delivery	Mode of delivery determined by obstetric considerations • Active perianal disease is an indication for cesarean delivery
Postpartum	Resume biologic therapy if interval appropriate and no infection • 24 h after vaginal delivery • 48 h after cesarean delivery Review safety of continuing most medications during lactation Inform pediatrician of in utero biologic medication exposures Avoid live vaccines for at least 6 mo or until infant drug level becomes undetectable (applies to all biologic agents except certolizumab pegol)

trial. A series of 26 exposed pregnancies reported a spontaneous abortion rate similar to the general population rate.[82] Clinically insignificant breast milk concentrations were detected in 1 of 3 women.[72]

Oral janus kinase inhibitors Tofacitinib is approved for rheumatoid arthritis and phase II trial data support efficacy in ulcerative colitis. Animal studies demonstrate teratogenicity at doses more than 10 times higher than the maximum recommended human dose. Human pregnancy outcome data are sparse and confounded by frequent concomitant methotrexate use.[83]

Managing Inflammatory Bowel Disease Exacerbations in Pregnancy

Managing disease flares during pregnancy follows similar evaluation and treatment algorithms as for the nonpregnant patient, with response rates to standard medical therapy exceeding 80%.[33] Several considerations are unique to pregnancy (**Box 1**).

Corticosteroids

Corticosteroids may be used to treat disease flares, although their use is associated with an increased risk of pregnancy complications. A meta-analysis of older literature reported a 3.4-fold increased risk of orofacial clefts with first trimester corticosteroid exposure.[84] A more recent nationwide cohort study of 51,973 pregnancies with first-trimester exposure showed no such risk (OR 1.05, 95% CI 0.80–1.38).[85] In the PIANO registry, corticosteroid use was associated with gestational diabetes (OR 2.8, 95% CI 1.3–6.0), preterm birth (OR 1.8, 95% CI 1.0–3.1), and low birth weight (OR 2.8, 95% CI 1.3–6.1). There was a nonsignificant increase in infant infections in the first 4 months of life (OR 1.5, 95% CI 0.9–2.7).[86] In a separate retrospective study, these risks were not seen with budesonide.[87] Although the risks are likely outweighed by the benefits of controlling active disease, corticosteroid use during pregnancy should be limited to the lowest effective dose and shortest duration. Both prednisone and budesonide are compatible with breastfeeding, with one study reporting breast milk drug levels less than 0.05% of the maternal dose.[88]

Cyclosporine

A systematic review comprising mainly transplant patients found increased rates of pregnancy complications, preterm birth, and low birthweight in cyclosporine-exposed pregnancies.[89] Whether these findings reflect maternal illness, cyclosporine toxicity, or both is unknown. A small case-control study reported successful cyclosporine treatment of severe, steroid-refractory colitis in 5 pregnant patients with IBD.[33] Cyclosporine use for fulminant colitis during pregnancy should be limited to specialized centers. Cyclosporine is incompatible with breastfeeding, as therapeutic cyclosporine levels have been observed in breastfeeding infants.

Box 1
Managing inflammatory bowel disease exacerbations during pregnancy

Evaluation
  Rule out *Clostridium difficile* infection, which is more prevalent in the peripartum period.
  Interpret laboratory tests with caution: low albumin, low hemoglobin, and elevated erythrocyte sedimentation rate are common in pregnancy and may not reflect inflammation.
  Unsedated flexible sigmoidoscopy to assess disease severity can be performed safely in any trimester.
  Full colonoscopy is rarely necessary and requires anesthesia with fetal monitoring.
  MRI is preferred over computed tomography to avoid fetal radiation exposure. Gadolinium is a potential teratogen and should be avoided in the first trimester.

Treatment
  Use corticosteroids at the lowest effective dose and for the shortest necessary duration. Consider budesonide when clinically appropriate.
  Stress dosing may be necessary during labor and delivery to avoid adrenal insufficiency.
  Aminosalicylates, corticosteroids, and biologics may be used for induction therapy in pregnancy.
  If an antibiotic is needed, amoxicillin-clavulanic acid has a favorable safety profile.
  Nonemergent surgery should be performed in the second trimester.

Antibiotics

Ciprofloxacin and metronidazole are perhaps the most commonly used antibiotics in IBD management. A meta-analysis of first trimester quinolone exposure did not detect any increased risk of adverse pregnancy outcomes.[90] Although ciprofloxacin is excreted in breast milk, the American Academy of Pediatrics considers it compatible with breastfeeding. Metronidazole should be avoided in the first trimester due to a possible increased risk of orofacial clefts,[91] and is incompatible with breastfeeding due to potential toxicities. Amoxicillin-clavulanic acid is our preferred antibiotic during pregnancy, with a favorable safety profile and breastfeeding compatibility.[92]

Surgery

Indications for surgery do not differ in the pregnant patient and include bowel obstruction, perforation, and medically refractory disease. Nonemergent surgery should preferentially be performed during the second trimester.[93] Maternal and fetal outcomes after colectomy for fulminant disease may be improving, in contrast to historic data showing high maternal and fetal morbidity and mortality.[94]

BREASTFEEDING

The benefits of breastfeeding are substantial and may include protection against pediatric IBD.[95] Most IBD medications are compatible with breastfeeding (see **Table 1**). The PIANO registry found no increased risk of infection or developmental delay among nursing infants whose mothers took thiopurines or anti-TNF agents.[72] Even so, women taking these medications are less likely to breastfeed compared with women not on these medications, citing concern for drug transfer to the infant. Targeted patient education is needed, along with additional research to confirm long-term breastfeeding safety.

SUMMARY

- Women with IBD are at risk for pregnancy complications and adverse outcomes, and should be managed as high-risk obstetric patients.
- Active disease is the greatest threat to fertility and maternal and fetal health. Sustained remission maximizes the chance of a successful and healthy pregnancy.
- With the exception of methotrexate, most medications are compatible with continued use during pregnancy and lactation.
- Medication adjustments to reduce fetal exposure, such as thiopurine withdrawal from combination therapy and third trimester biologic dosing manipulation, may be considered on an individualized basis in quiescent disease.
- Patients require counseling about the importance of medication adherence to optimize and maintain disease control, beginning in the preconception period.
- Close monitoring by a multidisciplinary team is essential, with attention to specific tasks during each pregnancy stage (see **Table 2**).

REFERENCES

1. Kappelman MD, Rifas-Shiman SL, Kleinman K, et al. The prevalence and geographic distribution of Crohn's disease and ulcerative colitis in the United States. Clin Gastroenterol Hepatol 2007;5:1424–9.

2. Marri SR, Ahn C, Buchman AL. Voluntary childlessness is increased in women with inflammatory bowel disease. Inflamm Bowel Dis 2007;13:591–9.

3. Tavernier N, Fumery M, Peyrin-Biroulet L, et al. Systematic review: fertility in non-surgically treated inflammatory bowel disease. Aliment Pharmacol Ther 2013;38: 847–53.

4. Selinger CP, Eaden J, Selby W, et al. Inflammatory bowel disease and pregnancy: lack of knowledge is associated with negative views. J Crohns Colitis 2013;7: e206–13.

5. Mountifield R, Bampton P, Prosser R, et al. Fear and fertility in inflammatory bowel disease: a mismatch of perception and reality affects family planning decisions. Inflamm Bowel Dis 2009;15:720–5.

6. Ording Olsen K, Juul S, Berndtsson I, et al. Ulcerative colitis: female fecundity before diagnosis, during disease, and after surgery compared with a population sample. Gastroenterology 2002;122:15–9.

7. Nielsen OH, Andreasson B, Bondesen S, et al. Pregnancy in ulcerative colitis. Scand J Gastroenterol 1983;18:735–42.

8. Ban L, Tata LJ, Humes DJ, et al. Decreased fertility rates in 9639 women diagnosed with inflammatory bowel disease: a United Kingdom population-based cohort study. Aliment Pharmacol Ther 2015;42:855–66.

9. Timmer A, Bauer A, Dignass A, et al. Sexual function in persons with inflammatory bowel disease: a survey with matched controls. Clin Gastroenterol Hepatol 2007; 5:87–94.

10. Senates E, Colak Y, Erdem ED, et al. Serum anti-Mullerian hormone levels are lower in reproductive-age women with Crohn's disease compared to healthy control women. J Crohns Colitis 2013;7:e29–34.

11. Waljee A, Waljee J, Morris AM, et al. Threefold increased risk of infertility: a meta-analysis of infertility after ileal pouch anal anastomosis in ulcerative colitis. Gut 2006;55:1575–80.

12. Beyer-Berjot L, Maggiori L, Birnbaum D, et al. A total laparoscopic approach reduces the infertility rate after ileal pouch-anal anastomosis: a 2-center study. Ann Surg 2013;258:275–82.

13. Mortier PE, Gambiez L, Karoui M, et al. Colectomy with ileorectal anastomosis preserves female fertility in ulcerative colitis. Gastroenterol Clin Biol 2006;30: 594–7.

14. Pabby V, Oza SS, Dodge LE, et al. In vitro fertilization is successful in women with ulcerative colitis and ileal pouch anal anastomosis. Am J Gastroenterol 2015;110: 792–7.

15. Paffoni A, Ferrari S, Vigano P, et al. Vitamin D deficiency and infertility: insights from in vitro fertilization cycles. J Clin Endocrinol Metab 2014;99:E2372–6.

16. Choi JM, Lebwohl B, Wang J, et al. Increased prevalence of celiac disease in patients with unexplained infertility in the United States. J Reprod Med 2011;56: 199–203.

17. El-Tawil AM. Zinc deficiency in men with Crohn's disease may contribute to poor sperm function and male infertility. Andrologia 2003;35:337–41.

18. Toovey S, Hudson E, Hendry WF, et al. Sulphasalazine and male infertility: reversibility and possible mechanism. Gut 1981;22:445–51.

19. French AE, Koren G. Effect of methotrexate on male fertility. Can Fam Physician 2003;49:577–8.

20. Suominen JS, Wang Y, Kaipia A, et al. Tumor necrosis factor-alpha (TNF-alpha) promotes cell survival during spermatogenesis, and this effect can be blocked by infliximab, a TNF-alpha antagonist. Eur J Endocrinol 2004;151:629–40.

21. Mahadevan U, Terdiman JP, Aron J, et al. Infliximab and semen quality in men with inflammatory bowel disease. Inflamm Bowel Dis 2005;11:395–9.

22. O'Toole A, Nwanne O, Tomlinson T. Inflammatory bowel disease increases risk of adverse pregnancy outcomes: a meta-analysis. Dig Dis Sci 2015;60:2750–61.

23. Stephansson O, Larsson H, Pedersen L, et al. Congenital abnormalities and other birth outcomes in children born to women with ulcerative colitis in Denmark and Sweden. Inflamm Bowel Dis 2011;17:795–801.

24. Ban L, Tata LJ, Fiaschi L, et al. Limited risks of major congenital anomalies in children of mothers with IBD and effects of medications. Gastroenterology 2014;146: 76–84.

25. Mahadevan U, Sandborn WJ, Li DK, et al. Pregnancy outcomes in women with inflammatory bowel disease: a large community-based study from Northern California. Gastroenterology 2007;133:1106–12.

26. Boyd HA, Basit S, Harpsoe MC, et al. Inflammatory bowel disease and risk of adverse pregnancy outcomes. PLoS One 2015;10:e0129567.

27. Broms G, Granath F, Linder M, et al. Complications from inflammatory bowel disease during pregnancy and delivery. Clin Gastroenterol Hepatol 2012;10: 1246–52.

28. Oron G, Yogev Y, Shcolnick S, et al. Inflammatory bowel disease: risk factors for adverse pregnancy outcome and the impact of maternal weight gain. J Matern Fetal Neonatal Med 2012;25:2256–60.

29. Bengtson M, Martin CF, Aamodt G, et al. Insufficient weight gain during pregnancy in maternal IBD predicts adverse pregnancy outcomes: results from the PIANO and Norwegian registry [abstract]. Gastroenterology 2015;148:S-238.

30. Nielsen OH, Andreasson B, Bondesen S, et al. Pregnancy in Crohn's disease. Scand J Gastroenterol 1984;19:724–32.

31. Norgard B, Fonager K, Sorensen HT, et al. Birth outcomes of women with ulcerative colitis: a nationwide Danish cohort study. Am J Gastroenterol 2000;95: 3165–70.

32. Norgard B, Hundborg HH, Jacobsen BA, et al. Disease activity in pregnant women with Crohn's disease and birth outcomes: a regional Danish cohort study. Am J Gastroenterol 2007;102:1947–54.

33. Reddy D, Murphy SJ, Kane SV, et al. Relapses of inflammatory bowel disease during pregnancy: in-hospital management and birth outcomes. Am J Gastroenterol 2008;103:1203–9.

34. Broms G, Granath F, Linder M, et al. Birth outcomes in women with inflammatory bowel disease: effects of disease activity and drug exposure. Inflamm Bowel Dis 2014;20:1091–8.

35. Bush MC, Patel S, Lapinski RH, et al. Perinatal outcomes in inflammatory bowel disease. J Matern Fetal Neonatal Med 2004;15:237–41.

36. Bortoli A, Pedersen N, Duricova D, et al. Pregnancy outcome in inflammatory bowel disease: prospective European case-control ECCO-EpiCom study, 2003-2006. Aliment Pharmacol Ther 2011;34:724–34.

37. Pedersen N, Bortoli A, Duricova D, et al. The course of inflammatory bowel disease during pregnancy and postpartum: a prospective European ECCO-EpiCom Study of 209 pregnant women. Aliment Pharmacol Ther 2013;38:501–12.

38. Mahadevan U, Martin CF, Sandler RS, et al. PIANO: a 1000 patient prospective registry of pregnancy outcomes in women with IBD exposed to immunomodulators and biologic therapy [abstract]. Gastroenterology 2012;142:S-149.

39. Nasef NA, Ferguson LR. Inflammatory bowel disease and pregnancy: overlapping pathways. Transl Res 2012;160:65–83.

40. Abhyankar A, Ham M, Moss AC. Meta-analysis: the impact of disease activity at conception on disease activity during pregnancy in patients with inflammatory bowel disease. Aliment Pharmacol Ther 2013;38:460–6.
41. Julsgaard M, Norgaard M, Hvas CL, et al. Self-reported adherence to medical treatment, breastfeeding behaviour, and disease activity during the postpartum period in women with Crohn's disease. Scand J Gastroenterol 2014;49:958–66.
42. Ujihara M, Ando T, Ishiguro K, et al. Importance of appropriate pharmaceutical management in pregnant women with ulcerative colitis. BMC Res Notes 2013; 6:210.
43. Nguyen GC, Boudreau H, Harris ML, et al. Outcomes of obstetric hospitalizations among women with inflammatory bowel disease in the United States. Clin Gastroenterol Hepatol 2009;7:329–34.
44. Mahadevan U, Martin CF, Dubinsky M, et al. Exposure to anti-TNFα therapy in the third trimester of pregnancy is not associated with increased adverse outcomes: results from the PIANO registry [abstract]. Gastroenterology 2014;146:S-170.
45. Ananthakrishnan AN, Cheng A, Cagan A, et al. Mode of childbirth and long-term outcomes in women with inflammatory bowel diseases. Dig Dis Sci 2015;60: 471–7.
46. Cheng AG, Oxford EC, Sauk J, et al. Impact of mode of delivery on outcomes in patients with perianal Crohn's disease. Inflamm Bowel Dis 2014;20:1391–8.
47. Cornish JA, Tan E, Teare J, et al. The effect of restorative proctocolectomy on sexual function, urinary function, fertility, pregnancy and delivery: a systematic review. Dis Colon Rectum 2007;50:1128–38.
48. Bruce A, Black M, Bhattacharya S. Mode of delivery and risk of inflammatory bowel disease in the offspring: systematic review and meta-analysis of observational studies. Inflamm Bowel Dis 2014;20:1217–26.
49. Yang H, McElree C, Roth MP, et al. Familial empirical risks for inflammatory bowel disease: differences between Jews and non-Jews. Gut 1993;34:517–24.
50. Bennett RA, Rubin PH, Present DH. Frequency of inflammatory bowel disease in offspring of couples both presenting with inflammatory bowel disease. Gastroenterology 1991;100:1638–43.
51. Mountifield R, Andrews JM, Bampton P. It IS worth the effort: patient knowledge of reproductive aspects of inflammatory bowel disease improves dramatically after a single group education session. J Crohns Colitis 2014;8:796–801.
52. Food and Drug Administration. Content and format of labeling for human prescription drug and biological products; requirements for pregnancy and lactation labeling [Federal Register Web site]. 2014. Available at: http://federalregister. gov/a/2014-28241. Accessed October 24, 2015.
53. Norgard B, Fonager K, Pedersen L, et al. Birth outcome in women exposed to 5-aminosalicylic acid during pregnancy: a Danish cohort study. Gut 2003;52:243–7.
54. Gallinger ZR, Nguyen GC. Presence of phthalates in gastrointestinal medications: is there a hidden danger? World J Gastroenterol 2013;19:7042–7.
55. Nelis GF. Diarrhoea due to 5-aminosalicylic acid in breast milk. Lancet 1989;1: 383.
56. Martinez Lopez JA, Loza E, Carmona L. Systematic review on the safety of methotrexate in rheumatoid arthritis regarding the reproductive system (fertility, pregnancy, and breastfeeding). Clin Exp Rheumatol 2009;27:678–84.
57. Johns DG, Rutherford LD, Leighton PC, et al. Secretion of methotrexate into human milk. Am J Obstet Gynecol 1972;112:978–80.
58. Polifka JE, Friedman JM. Teratogen update: azathioprine and 6-mercaptopurine. Teratology 2002;65:240–61.

59. Jharap B, de Boer NK, Stokkers P, et al. Intrauterine exposure and pharmacology of conventional thiopurine therapy in pregnant patients with inflammatory bowel disease. Gut 2014;63:451-7.
60. Coelho J, Beaugerie L, Colombel JF, et al. Pregnancy outcome in patients with inflammatory bowel disease treated with thiopurines: cohort from the CESAME Study. Gut 2011;60:198-203.
61. Casanova MJ, Chaparro M, Domenech E, et al. Safety of thiopurines and anti-TNF-alpha drugs during pregnancy in patients with inflammatory bowel disease. Am J Gastroenterol 2013;108:433-40.
62. Akbari M, Shah S, Velayos FS, et al. Systematic review and meta-analysis on the effects of thiopurines on birth outcomes from female and male patients with inflammatory bowel disease. Inflamm Bowel Dis 2013;19:15-22.
63. Hutson JR, Matlow JN, Moretti ME, et al. The fetal safety of thiopurines for the treatment of inflammatory bowel disease in pregnancy. J Obstet Gynaecol 2013;33:1-8.
64. Mahadevan U, Martin CF, Chambers C, et al. Achievement of developmental milestones among offspring of women with inflammatory bowel disease: the PIANO registry [abstract]. Gastroenterology 2014;146:S-1.
65. Christensen LA, Dahlerup JF, Nielsen MJ, et al. Azathioprine treatment during lactation. Aliment Pharmacol Ther 2008;28:1209-13.
66. McConnell RA, Mahadevan U. Use of immunomodulators and biologics before, during, and after pregnancy. Inflamm Bowel Dis 2016;22(1):213-23.
67. Lichtenstein GR, Feagan BG, Cohen RD, et al. Serious infection and mortality in patients with Crohn's disease: more than 5 years of follow-up in the TREAT registry. Am J Gastroenterol 2012;107:1409-22.
68. Jurgens M, Brand S, Filik L, et al. Safety of adalimumab in Crohn's disease during pregnancy: case report and review of the literature. Inflamm Bowel Dis 2010;16:1634-6.
69. Mahadevan U, Vermeire S, Wolf DC, et al. Pregnancy outcomes after exposure to certolizumab pegol: updated results from safety surveillance [abstract]. Gastroenterology 2015;148:S-858-9.
70. Nielsen OH, Loftus EV Jr, Jess T. Safety of TNF-alpha inhibitors during IBD pregnancy: a systematic review. BMC Med 2013;11:174.
71. Narula N, Al-Dabbagh R, Dhillon A, et al. Anti-TNFalpha therapies are safe during pregnancy in women with inflammatory bowel disease: a systematic review and meta-analysis. Inflamm Bowel Dis 2014;20:1862-9.
72. Matro R, Martin CF, Wolf DC, et al. Detection of biologic agents in breast milk and implication for infection, growth and development in infants born to women with inflammatory bowel disease: results from the PIANO registry [abstract]. Gastroenterology 2015;148:S-141.
73. Mahadevan U, Wolf DC, Dubinsky M, et al. Placental transfer of anti-tumor necrosis factor agents in pregnant patients with inflammatory bowel disease. Clin Gastroenterol Hepatol 2013;11:286-92.
74. Kane SV, Acquah LA. Placental transport of immunoglobulins: a clinical review for gastroenterologists who prescribe therapeutic monoclonal antibodies to women during conception and pregnancy. Am J Gastroenterol 2009;104:228-33.
75. Julsgaard M, Christensen LA, Gibson PR, et al. Adalimumab and infliximab levels in neonates (ERA Study) [abstract]. Gastroenterology 2015;148:S-108.
76. Arsenescu R, Arsenescu V, de Villiers WJ. TNF-alpha and the development of the neonatal immune system: implications for inhibitor use in pregnancy. Am J Gastroenterol 2011;106:559-62.

77. Bortlik M, Duricova D, Machkova N, et al. Impact of anti-tumor necrosis factor alpha antibodies administered to pregnant women with inflammatory bowel disease on long-term outcome of exposed children. Inflamm Bowel Dis 2014;20: 495–501.

78. Mahadevan U, Cucchiara S, Hyams JS, et al. The London Position Statement of the World Congress of Gastroenterology on Biological Therapy for IBD with the European Crohn's and Colitis Organisation: pregnancy and pediatrics. Am J Gastroenterol 2011;106:214–23 [quiz: 224].

79. Zelinkova Z, van der Ent C, Bruin KF, et al. Effects of discontinuing anti-tumor necrosis factor therapy during pregnancy on the course of inflammatory bowel disease and neonatal exposure. Clin Gastroenterol Hepatol 2013;11: 318–21.

80. Ebrahimi N, Herbstritt S, Gold R, et al. Pregnancy and fetal outcomes following natalizumab exposure in pregnancy. A prospective, controlled observational study. Mult Scler 2015;21:198–205.

81. Dubinsky M, Mahadevan U, Vermeire S, et al. Vedolizumab exposure in pregnancy: outcomes from clinical studies in inflammatory bowel disease [abstract]. J Crohns Colitis 2015;9:S361–2.

82. Schaufelberg BW, Horn E, Cather JC, et al. Pregnancy outcomes in women exposed to ustekinumab in the psoriasis clinical development program [abstract]. J Am Acad Dermatol 2014;70:AB178.

83. Marren A, Chen Y, Frazier D, et al. Pregnancy outcomes in the tofacitinib RA safety database through April 2014 [abstract]. Ann Rheum Dis 2015;74: 256–7.

84. Park-Wyllie L, Mazzotta P, Pastuszak A, et al. Birth defects after maternal exposure to corticosteroids: prospective cohort study and meta-analysis of epidemiological studies. Teratology 2000;62:385–92.

85. Hviid A, Molgaard-Nielsen D. Corticosteroid use during pregnancy and risk of orofacial clefts. CMAJ 2011;183:796–804.

86. Lin K, Martin CF, Dassopoulos T, et al. Pregnancy outcomes amongst mothers with inflammatory bowel disease exposed to systemic corticosteroids: results of the PIANO registry [abstract]. Gastroenterology 2014;146:S-1.

87. Truta B. Potential risks of immunosuppressant drugs to the pregnant patient [abstract]. Honolulu (HI): American College of Gastroenterology; 2015.

88. Greenberger PA, Odeh YK, Frederiksen MC, et al. Pharmacokinetics of prednisolone transfer to breast milk. Clin Pharmacol Ther 1993;53:324–8.

89. Paziana K, Del Monaco M, Cardonick E, et al. Ciclosporin use during pregnancy. Drug Saf 2013;36:279–94.

90. Bar-Oz B, Moretti ME, Boskovic R, et al. The safety of quinolones–a meta-analysis of pregnancy outcomes. Eur J Obstet Gynecol Reprod Biol 2009;143:75–8.

91. Czeizel AE, Rockenbauer M. A population based case-control teratologic study of oral metronidazole treatment during pregnancy. Br J Obstet Gynaecol 1998; 105:322–7.

92. Czeizel AE, Rockenbauer M, Sorensen HT, et al. Augmentin treatment during pregnancy and the prevalence of congenital abnormalities: a population-based case-control teratologic study. Eur J Obstet Gynecol Reprod Biol 2001;97: 188–92.

93. ACOG Committee on Obstetric Practice. ACOG committee opinion No. 474: nonobstetric surgery during pregnancy. Obstet Gynecol 2011;117:420–1.

94. Dozois EJ, Wolff BG, Tremaine WJ, et al. Maternal and fetal outcome after colectomy for fulminant ulcerative colitis during pregnancy: case series and literature review. Dis Colon Rectum 2006;49:64–73.
95. Barclay AR, Russell RK, Wilson ML, et al. Systematic review: the role of breastfeeding in the development of pediatric inflammatory bowel disease. J Pediatr 2009;155:421–6.

Caring for Women with Inflammatory Bowel Disease

Linda A. Feagins, MD[a], Sunanda V. Kane, MD, MSPH[b],*

KEYWORDS

- Inflammatory bowel disease • Gender • Women

KEY POINTS

- Women with inflammatory bowel disease (IBD) consistently report lower quality of life (QOL) and sexual function than men.
- Women with IBD on immunosuppressants have an increased risk of cervical cancer and should be encouraged to undergo regular screening.
- IBD can affect the regularity of a woman's menstrual cycle and IBD symptoms may worsen before and during menstruation.

INTRODUCTION

Ulcerative colitis (UC) and Crohn disease are chronic inflammatory diseases with typical onset in early adulthood. These diseases, therefore, can affect a woman throughout the many stages of her life, including menstruation, sexuality, pregnancy, and menopause. Unique health issues face women during these stages and can affect the course of IBD as well as treatment strategies and health maintenance. This article covers the non–pregnancy-related issues that are important in caring for women with IBD. The topics of pregnancy and fertility are covered in a separate review.

GENDER DIFFERENCES IN PRESENTATION OF INFLAMMATORY BOWEL DISEASE
Incidence

Older data had suggested that there was a slight female predominance in developing Crohn disease and a slight male predominance in developing UC.[1] A recent large

Conflicts of Interest: L.A. Feagins has no relevant conflicts of interest. S.V. Kane is a consultant to UCB Pharma.
[a] Division of Gastroenterology and Hepatology, VA North Texas Healthcare System, University of Texas Southwestern Medical Center, 4500 S. Lancaster Rd (111B1), Dallas, TX 75216, USA;
[b] Division of Gastroenterology and Hepatology, Mayo Clinic, 200 First Street Southwest, Rochester, MN 55905, USA
* Corresponding author.
E-mail address: kane.sunanda@mayo.edu

Gastroenterol Clin N Am 45 (2016) 303–315
http://dx.doi.org/10.1016/j.gtc.2016.02.007
0889-8553/16/$ – see front matter

systematic review, however, that included gender-specific incidence rates for Crohn disease (59 studies) and UC (50 studies) reported a female-to-male ratio varying from 0.51 to 1.58 for UC and 0.34 to 1.65 for Crohn disease, suggesting no true gender-specific difference in the incidence of UC or Crohn disease.[2] Few studies are available that differentiate between the disease distribution for Crohn disease and UC between men and women. One study in children, however, evaluated for gender differences regarding clinical phenotypes, disease behavior, and treatment and found no differences between girls and boys.[3]

Differential Diagnosis

When evaluating a patient with suspected IBD, there are several entities to consider in the differential for female patients. Endometriosis, similar to IBD, is a chronic inflammatory disorder with a typical onset in younger women and is common, affecting 5% to 10% of reproductive age women.[4] Less commonly, it can affect the bowel (75% affecting the rectosigmoid and 25% the ileocecal/appendix) and could be confused with Crohn disease. Histology is often helpful in differentiating these diseases but occasionally can show marked inflammatory and architectural mucosal changes, making the distinction more difficult.[5] Moreover, the diseases are not mutually exclusive and it has been reported that the risk of developing IBD is increased in patients with endometriosis (standardized incidence ratio = 1.5)[6] and for those with both endometriosis and Crohn disease, a stricturing phenotype of Crohn disease is more common (odds ratio [OR] = 11.8).[7]

Behçet disease is a rare chronic inflammatory disease that can be confused with IBD because they share many common features, including affecting patients in young adulthood, intestinal inflammation with diarrhea and bleeding, inflammatory arthritis, and skin manifestations like erythema nodosum.[8] Additional features that may help set Behçet apart from IBD include genital ulcers and central nervous system and large vessel vasculidities. Although Behçet is rare in the United States, it is somewhat more common in Japanese and Korean women and Middle Eastern men.

Lastly, irritable bowel syndrome (IBS) is commonly confused with IBD and, moreover, can occur in combination with IBD. IBS is common in population-based studies, with an 11% prevalence in 1 study[9] and more common in women than men, with a 2:1 female-to-male ratio.[10] IBS is commonly diagnosed in patients with IBD and studies have revealed that IBS is even more common in patients with IBD than non-IBD controls, with a prevalence of 39% and an OR of close to 5 (4.89).[11] This is an important overlap to recognize to avoid escalating immunosuppression for symptoms that are gastrointestinal (GI) but not truly from active inflammation.

Extraintestinal Manifestations of Inflammatory Bowel Disease

IBD can affect many systems outside the GI tract, including the eyes, skin, joints, and bile ducts. These manifestations, overall, are more commonly seen in women than in men.[12] A study of approximately 400 patients with IBD found that cutaneous manifestations (namely, erythema nodosum and pyoderma gangrenosum) were more common in women than men (15% vs 4%).[13] Moreover, in women, skin manifestations of Crohn disease rarely may present as vulvar lesions. Although perianal disease with fistulas are common in Crohn disease, it is important to remember metastatic Crohn disease of the skin in the differential for vulvar lesions because perianal disease rarely extends to the genital area.[14] A biopsy revealing noncaseating epithelioid cell granuloma establishes the diagnosis; however, it is not always seen on all biopsies of metastatic Crohn disease and clinical suspicion must remain high.

Moreover, some women may present with vulvar involvement with Crohn disease as their initial presentation before having bowel symptoms. Two features that should raise concern for metastatic Crohn disease of the vulva include painless vulvar swelling and concomitant perianal lesions (like skin tags, anorectal strictures, and fissures).[14]

TREATMENT DIFFERENCES BETWEEN MEN AND WOMEN

Several reasons exist why men and women may respond to medical therapies differently. From a pharmacokinetic standpoint, drug distribution is different simply based on differences in weight (men are generally heavier), body composition (women have a higher percentage of body fat), glomerular filtration rate (women have lower glomerular filtration rate than men even after adjusting for weight), and differences in metabolism of various drugs.[15] The data assessing these differences between men and women, specifically for the drugs used to treat IBD, are sparse. A pharmacokinetic analysis was done for the UC patients treated with infliximab who participated in the large Active Ulcerative Colitis Trials 1 and 2 trials.[16] Drug clearance was found 33% lower in women than men and the central volume of drug distribution was 16% lower for men. Because men have both higher weight and increased drug clearance, however, it is difficult to completely separate these changes from differences in weight. Another study that specifically looked at inflammatory patients (IBD, rheumatoid arthritis, and psoriasis) started on biologics conversely suggested that at the same extent of disease, women had more subjective complaints regarding disease activity, possibly indicating undertreatment or simply greater disease effect.[17] Another study evaluated adverse events in patients with Crohn disease who used thiopurines and found that women over age 40 had a higher risk of adverse event, leading to discontinuation of their thiopurine.[18] Lastly, a recent meta-analysis reported that the most reliable predictor for nonadherence to anti–tumor necrosis factor use was female gender but without convincing rationale.[19]

When planning surgery for women with UC, consideration must be given to their plans for future childbearing. It has been clearly shown that fertility is reduced after ileoanal pouch anastomosis (IPAA). A meta-analysis revealed that infertility was increased 3-fold after IPAA, from baseline 15% to 48%.[20] This reduction in fertility seems related, however, to the dissection into the pelvis that accompanies proctectomy, because fertility is preserved in patients who undergo other surgeries without removal of the rectum.[21] Physicians need to discuss the options of a conventional IPAA, performing only the first stage of the IPAA with completion after childbearing and ileorectal anastomosis in context of disease control and fertility. Moreover, when counseling women prior to surgery, it is important to relay that there have been differences observed between men and women after surgery. A large study of more than 3400 patients from the Cleveland Clinic showed higher rates of long-term complications after IPAA for women.[22] They reported female patients were significantly more likely to experience bowel obstruction (21% vs 17%) and pouch-related fistulas (11% vs 8%); had more daily bowel movements, urgency, and seepage after surgery; and reported more dietary and work restrictions after surgery compared with men. Although the reasons for these differences remain incompletely understood, some experts hypothesize that estrogens may affect the formation of abdominal adhesions and potentially explain the increased risk for bowel obstruction. Moreover, in the Cleveland Clinic study, baseline anal manometry prior to surgery revealed lower resting and squeeze pressures for women and it was postulated this may be representative of physiologic differences between men and women and may account for the difference in bowel movements, urgency, and seepage after surgery. Lastly, for women with Crohn disease, several older studies have shown that the risk of disease recurrence after intestinal resection is higher for women than men (OR = 1.2) and occurs earlier (4.8 years vs 6.5 years).[23,24] Possible explanations for this finding may be the effect of tobacco smoke or hormones on bowel, because surgical technique was not different and these studies were done in the era of laparoscopic procedures.

QUALITY OF LIFE

QOL is important for all people, but even more so for patients who are diagnosed with a chronic disease, often at a young age, that will affect them for their entire lives. Multiple studies have shown that women with IBD have overall lower health-related QOL (HRQL) compared with men with IBD.[25–28] A study from Croatia found that women have a lower HRQL and more emotional disturbances related to their disease compared with men, and this was especially true in women with higher levels of depression and anxiety.[27] Moreover, in a Swedish population-based cohort, Crohn disease had a greater negative impact on HRQL than did UC, and this was more pronounced for women.[29] It is unclear if these differences between men and women are due to perceived differences in disease symptoms or if this is a gender-related difference caused by the disease itself. The good news however, is that a large European cohort of patients reported that a majority of patients had improvements in QOL with specific treatment of their disease.[30]

Comorbid depression and anxiety are diseases that can greatly affect QOL for patients with IBD, similar to patients with other chronic diseases. Multiple studies have evaluated the presence of anxiety and depression in patients with IBD and have found that the rate of depression is at least 2-fold higher than in the general population.[31] Therefore, gastroenterologists should be aware of this and include screening for depression and anxiety in clinics and, when identified, refer for or begin appropriate treatment.

SEXUAL HEALTH

Sexual health is defined by the World Health Organization as a state of physical, emotional, mental, and social well-being in relation to sexuality, not merely the absence of disease, dysfunction, or infirmity.[32] Gastroenterologists, when addressing sexual health (if they even do), focus more on sexual dysfunction, which encompasses predominantly the physical aspects of sexuality, and often neglect to address the other areas of sexual health. The impact that IBD, however, can have on sexual health when caring for women with IBD, who are often young and in the midst of their reproductive years, is important.

Sexual Dysfunction

Sexual function can be influenced by several factors, including increasing age, psychological problems like depression or anxiety, relationship problems, body image, and chronic medical problems. Similar to HRQL, women report a greater negative impact of IBD on multiple aspects of sexuality than do men.[33] A German study reported strikingly low levels of sexual interest and activity in a cohort of 336 women with IBD. In this study, 80% of women reported no activity or only low activity during the 4 weeks preceding the survey.[34] In an Australian cohort with IBD, women reported a greater disease-related decrease in sexual activity and decrease in libido than men.[33] Another group found that women with Crohn disease had more concerns with sexual performance and intimacy than men with Crohn disease.[35] Moreover, several studies have shown that a poorer body image[33,35] and depression[36,37] both contribute greatly to reduced sexual function in women.

For chronic medical problems like IBD, medications, surgery, and, in particular, disease activity can all contribute to sexual dysfunction. There are few data regarding the impact of medical therapy for IBD on sexual function. In a questionnaire study, patients associated steroid use with low pleasure and orgasm scores[34]; however, it is difficult to separate the use of steroids from the impact from presumably active disease as the indication for steroids. Other studies have reported that although a majority of patients did not believe that their IBD medications affected their sexual function, a small portion (9.7%) did stop their medications for this reason.[33] The specific medications that patients attributed to negative effects on sexual function in this study, however, were not reported. Surgery can affect sexual function by disturbing the innervation to the genitalia or by distorting anatomy in the pelvis. Dyspareunia, a frequent complaint, can occur after surgery due to altered anatomy or sympathetic nerve injury, which may cause decreased lubrication or decreased vaginal proprioception. Fecal incontinence during intercourse has also been reported and is obviously distressing to patients.[38] On the other hand, a study of patients undergoing IPAA found that although male sexual function did not change after surgery, for women, sexual function improved within 12 months of surgery.[39] Disease activity is likely the most important component of IBD that affects sexual function with associated depression worsening symptoms. Active disease symptoms, whether diarrhea, pain, or even active perianal disease, affects feelings of sexual attractiveness and desire and can cause associated discomfort during intercourse.

Body Image

Body image is an important factor that plays into QOL and sexual function. Body image is a person's own sense of how he or she appears physically in addition to the impression of how other people see his or her body. A negative body image has been associated with low self-esteem and depression.[40] Moreover, chronic illness has been found a predictor of body image dissatisfaction.[41]

For women with IBD, studies report higher rates of body image dissatisfaction than men.[42,43] Furthermore, dissatisfaction with body image has been associated with active disease and with being treated with steroids (but not other immunosuppressives).[42,44] Moreover, body image dissatisfaction in patients with IBD was also linked to lower self-esteem, higher rates of anxiety and depression, and less sexual satisfaction.[44]

In addition to medication side effects and active disease, scars and ostomies left after surgery can affect body image and thus sexual function. An Australian study of approximately 350 IBD patients found that more patients who had undergone surgery reported an impaired body image compared with patients who had not undergone surgery (81% vs 51%).[33] Patients with Crohn disease who underwent laparoscopic surgery as opposed to open surgery reported a better body image after surgery as well as QOL.[45] On the other hand, in a group of men and women who underwent IPAA, there was no significant difference found in body image between those who underwent open versus laparoscopic IPAA, although there was a trend toward lower self-esteem postoperatively for women compared with men. Moreover, they also found a trend toward better body image in the women who underwent laparoscopic compared with open IPAA.[46]

Disease aspects in patients with IBD that may affect body image
Active disease
Weight loss
Hair loss
Cutaneous manifestations of IBD (pyoderma gangrenosum and erythema nodosum)
Fistulas to skin or perineum
Arthritis
Medication side effects
Weight gain, lipodystrophy, hair growth, acne, skin thinning (corticosteroids)
Hair loss, photosensitivity (6-mercaptopurine/azathioprine)
Hair loss (methotrexate)
Psoriasis (anti–tumor necrosis factor)
Surgery
Stomas
Surgical scars

CERVICAL CANCER RISK, SCREENING, AND PREVENTION

The most widely accepted risk factor for cervical cancer is chronic infection with high-risk oncogenic types of human papilloma virus (HPV).[47] Although many HPV infections are cleared spontaneously, others become chronic and may progress to cancer. It remains unclear, however, why some people spontaneously clear and others progress. In addition to HPV infections, other risk factors for the development of cervical cancer include early onset of sexual activity, multiple sexual partners, a history of sexually transmitted diseases (ie, early and/or higher probability for HPV exposure), and impaired ability to clear HPV infections (ie, immunosuppression).[48] For the authors' patients with IBD, the frequent use of immunosuppressants to treat their disease or even the immunologic changes that occur in the disease itself may be risk factors for an increased risk of cervical cancer in this population. Initial studies reported an increased risk of abnormal cytology (Papanicolaou smears) in women with IBD (42.5% in women with IBD vs 7% in controls) and this risk was increased more so in women with a history of immunosuppressant use.[49] Other studies did not find any increased risk for cervical dysplasia in women with IBD on immunosuppressants but did find that the risk was increased if they were current smokers, exposed to oral contraceptive use, or used combinations of corticosteroids and immunosuppressants.[50,51] Most recently, a meta-analysis of the available studies (5 cohort studies and 3 case-control studies) revealed that IBD patients on immunosuppressive medications did have an increased risk of cervical high-grade dysplasia and cancer compared with healthy controls (OR = 1.34; 95% CI, 1.23–1.46).[52]

Current guidelines for women in general recommend screening for cervical cancer with cytology every 3 years beginning at age 21.[53] For women aged 30 to 65, cotesting with cervical cytology and HPV testing every 5 years is preferred. Over age 65, provided women have been adequately screened previously, no further screening is recommended. Several studies have assessed rates of screening for cervical cancer specifically in women with IBD. One US study of a large insurance claims database found that 70% of women with IBD received cervical testing every 3 years whereas a large population-based study in Canada found that only 54% of their women with IBD had regular cervical cancer screening.[54,55] Predictors for lower utilization of cervical cancer screening included immunosuppressant use in both groups. Improved adherence to current guidelines for screening would improve prevention and early detection of cervical cancer for women with IBD and should be stressed as a part of routine IBD health maintenance. The American College of Obstetricians and Gynecologists recommends more frequent screening for patients with HIV and women who are immunocompromised (specifically solid organ transplant recipients) and, although there is no specific societal guidance for IBD, many experts advocate increased screening for women with IBD who are on immunosuppressants.[56,57]

Lastly, it is important for gastroenterologists to be aware of the recommendations for HPV vaccines, which have the potential to significantly reduce the burden of cervical dysplasia and cancer. Current vaccines for HPV include Gardasil (covers HPV types 6, 11, 16, and 18) and Cervarix (covers HPV 16 and 18) and the newly approved Gardasil 9 (covers HPV types 6, 11, 16, 18, 31, 33, 45, 52, and 58). Any of these is recommended as an option by the Advisory Committee on Immunization Practices for girls by age 11 or 12. They can be given, however, as early as 9 and the Gardasil and Gardasil 9 are also recommended for boys of the same age. For young women up to the age of 26 (or boys up to age 21) who were not previously vaccinated or did not receive the complete 3-shot series, a catch-up series of immunizations is recommended.

COLORECTAL CANCER RISK

Population-based studies of IBD-associated colorectal cancer (CRC) have been done in Ireland, France, Japan, and Denmark.[58–61] These studies report similar incidences of CRC in both men and women, with IBD-associated CRCs accounting for 0.2% to 0.7% of all of the CRC cases. A Swedish study, however, specifically evaluated gender differences in CRC development in patients with IBD and compared them with their general population. They found that women with IBD had a lower risk of developing CRC than men with IBD.[62] The reduced risk for women was almost completely attributed to women who were diagnosed with IBD before age 45 and found that men had a 60% greater chance of developing cancer then women. These results suggested that estrogen may have some protective effect in the carcinogenesis of CRC in IBD; however, it remains unclear how other factors, like degree of disease activity, medications, and adherence to surveillance programs, may have played in.

METABOLIC BONE DISEASE

Metabolic bone disease, specifically osteoporosis, increases the risk of fracture. Patients with IBD are at increased risk for metabolic bone disease due to glucocorticoid use, disease-related inflammation, malabsorption leading to poor absorption of calcium and vitamin D, avoidance of dairy products that may exacerbate IBD symptoms, and low body weight.[63] Moreover, other non-IBD specific risk factors for metabolic bone disease include advancing age, previous fracture, ongoing tobacco use, and excessive alcohol use. The prevalence of osteoporosis in patients with IBD has been reported in 1 study to be present in 2% to 15% of patients and of osteopenia in 37% to 39% of patients, with patients with Crohn disease at higher risk than UC patients (OR 2.9) and those who used steroids for multiple flares (OR 8.7) being higher risk.[64] Furthermore, although in the general population postmenopausal women are considered higher risk for metabolic bone disease, in patients with IBD, men and women have similar risk for osteoporosis.[65]

IBD patients at high risk for osteoporosis include those with at least 3 months of corticosteroid use, postmenopausal women and men greater than 50, those with hypogonadism, or those with history of prior fragility fracture, and they should be screened with bone mineral density testing.[65] Most important in preventing bone disease in the authors' patients with IBD is to minimize the use of glucocorticoids. Patients should be encouraged to avoid tobacco, limit alcohol intake, and incorporate regular weight-bearing exercise into their routines. Patients with osteopenia or osteoporosis should ensure adequate intake of calcium (1000–1500 mg/d) and vitamin D (400–800 U/d). Patients should be screened for hypogonadism and treated, if it is present, especially if they have had significant glucocorticoid exposure, because this increases the risk of hypogonadism. Lastly, in those with osteoporosis as well as men older than 50 years and postmenopausal women without osteoporosis but with high-risk World Health Organization Fracture Risk Assessment Tool scores, consideration should be given to the addition of specific therapy for the osteoporosis. The guidelines for treatment of osteoporosis in IBD patients, however, are not clearly delineated. Most experts use bisphosphonates first line and consider other options like parathyroid hormone, selective estrogen receptor modulators (postmenopausal women), and denosumab as second line, given there are few data for these agents in patient with IBD.

HORMONES AND INFLAMMATORY BOWEL DISEASE
Menstrual Cycle

It is important for gastroenterologists to be mindful that cyclic changes in GI symptoms (ie, diarrhea, abdominal pain, constipation, and nausea) have been associated with the menstrual cycle in patients with IBD, in particular Crohn disease. A retrospective study compared women with Crohn disease, UC, and IBS to healthy controls and found that women with IBD and IBS were more likely to report premenstrual and menstrual symptoms as well as changes in their bowel habits during these times.[66] Several studies have specifically found that women with Crohn disease have more diarrhea before and during menses.[66–68] Having patients track their symptoms in relation to their menstrual cycle can help shed light on a potential trigger for brief flare-ups. Patients can then be assured that these symptoms will remit once their cycle progresses and that alterations can be made to their drug regimens during this brief time (eg, increasing the dose of 5-aminosalicylic acid during that week); or, if symptoms are debilitating, even stopping their periods all together with hormone treatments can be considered. One study supports this later notion, reporting improvement in cyclic GI symptoms in IBD patients after treatment with estrogen-based contraceptives or levonorgestrel intrauterine devices (improved in 19% and 47% of patients queried, respectively), and only 5% of patients reporting worsening of their symptoms.[69]

Lastly, women with IBD more commonly experience abnormalities in their menstrual cycle (ie, oligomenorrhea, polymenorrhea, menorrhagia, metrorrhagia, irregular menses, and dysmenorrhea) than women without IBD.[70,71] Patients can be reassured, however, that these abnormalities often improve with longer duration of their IBD. A recent study evaluated menstrual cycle changes in women during the time just before they were diagnosed with IBD and thereafter. They reported that these women frequently experienced changes in their cycle (25% with changes in interval and 21% with changes in duration) the year preceding diagnosis, but that cycle regularity increased over time after diagnosis.[72]

Menopause and Hormone Replacement Therapy

Several factors can affect the timing of menopause, including genetics (family history), ethnicity, and smoking. Women with IBD, in particular Crohn disease, have been reported to have a slightly earlier onset of menopause. One study reported menopause in women with Crohn disease occurred at 47 years of age compared with 49 years in a similar control population.[73] Given that changes in hormones seem to affect GI symptoms, 1 study investigated disease activity in women premenopause and postmenopause. Although the investigators did not find any differences in rates of flare in patients premenopause or postmenopause, they did find that the use of hormone replacement therapy (in the postmenopausal state) afforded these women a protective effect regarding flare-ups (hazard ratio 0.18; 95% CI, 0.04–0.72) and the effect was dose dependent.[74] Conversely, a recent large study using data from the Nurses' Health Study found that the use of hormone replacement therapy was associated with an increased risk of incident UC but not Crohn disease.[75] Therefore, in the current era, where the use of hormone replacement therapy has become more controversial regarding cancer risk and cardiovascular benefit, the risks and benefits of these therapies must continue to be individualized.

SUMMARY

Numerous aspects of IBD can affect men and women differently (**Box 1**). Women not only may present differently with their disease but also may interpret their disease differently regarding symptom severity and it may have greater effects on their general QOL as well as their sexual health. Moreover, a woman's menstrual cycle may have an impact on her disease control, which is important to consider when making decisions regarding changes in treatment. Even subspecialists in gastroenterology often serve as primary care physicians for IBD patients and need to be aware of the effect of immunosuppression on cervical cancer risk and understand ways to help prevent this disease. Lastly, by being aware of these differences in the care of women, physicians will be able to make a more personalized plan of care and hopefully be able to have have a meaningful impact on patients' lives.

Box 1
Management considerations in female patients with inflammatory bowel disease

Extraintestinal manifestations
    More likely to have skin conditions
    More likely to have gallbladder issues
    Less likely to have primary sclerosing cholangitis

Sexual health
    Decreased libido
    Distorted body image

Altered fertility
    Secondary to chronic illness
    Secondary to surgery

Cancer screening
    Higher risk for cervical dysplasia
    Lower risk for colon cancer

Hormone use

REFERENCES

1. Loftus EV Jr, Schoenfeld P, Sandborn WJ. The epidemiology and natural history of Crohn's disease in population-based patient cohorts from North America: a systematic review. Aliment Pharmacol Ther 2002;16:51–60.
2. Molodecky NA, Soon IS, Rabi DM, et al. Increasing incidence and prevalence of the inflammatory bowel diseases with time, based on systematic review. Gastroenterology 2012;142:46–54.e42 [quiz: e30].
3. Herzog D, Buehr P, Koller R, et al. Gender differences in paediatric patients of the swiss inflammatory bowel disease cohort study. Pediatr Gastroenterol Hepatol Nutr 2014;17:147–54.
4. Bulun SE. Endometriosis. N Engl J Med 2009;360:268–79.
5. Guadagno A, Grillo F, Vellone VG, et al. Intestinal endometriosis: mimicker of inflammatory bowel disease? Digestion 2015;92:14–21.
6. Jess T, Frisch M, Jorgensen KT, et al. Increased risk of inflammatory bowel disease in women with endometriosis: a nationwide Danish cohort study. Gut 2012;61:1279–83.
7. Lee KK, Jharap B, Maser EA, et al. Impact of concomitant endometriosis on phenotype and natural history of inflammatory bowel disease. Inflamm Bowel Dis 2015;22(1):159–63.
8. Grigg EL, Kane S, Katz S. Mimicry and deception in inflammatory bowel disease and intestinal behcet disease. Gastroenterol Hepatol (N Y) 2012;8:103–12.
9. Hungin AP, Whorwell PJ, Tack J, et al. The prevalence, patterns and impact of irritable bowel syndrome: an international survey of 40,000 subjects. Aliment Pharmacol Ther 2003;17:643–50.
10. Mayer EA. Clinical practice. Irritable bowel syndrome. N Engl J Med 2008;358: 1692–9.
11. Halpin SJ, Ford AC. Prevalence of symptoms meeting criteria for irritable bowel syndrome in inflammatory bowel disease: systematic review and meta-analysis. Am J Gastroenterol 2012;107:1474–82.
12. Barreiro-de Acosta M, Dominguez-Munoz JE, Nunez-Pardo de Vera MC, et al. Relationship between clinical features of Crohn's disease and the risk of developing extraintestinal manifestations. Eur J Gastroenterol Hepatol 2007;19:73–8.
13. Ampuero J, Rojas-Feria M, Castro-Fernandez M, et al. Predictive factors for erythema nodosum and pyoderma gangrenosum in inflammatory bowel disease. J Gastroenterol Hepatol 2014;29:291–5.
14. Sides C, Trinidad MC, Heitlinger L, et al. Crohn disease and the gynecologic patient. Obstet Gynecol Surv 2013;68:51–61.
15. Whitley H, Lindsey W. Sex-based differences in drug activity. Am Fam Physician 2009;80:1254–8.
16. Fasanmade AA, Adedokun OJ, Ford J, et al. Population pharmacokinetic analysis of infliximab in patients with ulcerative colitis. Eur J Clin Pharmacol 2009;65: 1211–28.
17. Lesuis N, Befrits R, Nyberg F, et al. Gender and the treatment of immune-mediated chronic inflammatory diseases: rheumatoid arthritis, inflammatory bowel disease and psoriasis: an observational study. BMC Med 2012;10:82.
18. Moran GW, Dubeau MF, Kaplan GG, et al. Clinical predictors of thiopurine-related adverse events in Crohn's disease. World J Gastroenterol 2015;21:7795–804.
19. Lopez A, Billioud V, Peyrin-Biroulet C, et al. Adherence to anti-TNF therapy in inflammatory bowel diseases: a systematic review. Inflamm Bowel Dis 2013;19: 1528–33.

20. Waljee A, Waljee J, Morris AM, et al. Threefold increased risk of infertility: a meta-analysis of infertility after ileal pouch anal anastomosis in ulcerative colitis. Gut 2006;55:1575–80.
21. Mortier PE, Gambiez L, Karoui M, et al. Colectomy with ileorectal anastomosis preserves female fertility in ulcerative colitis. Gastroenterol Clin Biol 2006;30: 594–7.
22. Rottoli M, Remzi FH, Shen B, et al. Gender of the patient may influence perioperative and long-term complications after restorative proctocolectomy. Colorectal Dis 2012;14:336–41.
23. Bernell O, Lapidus A, Hellers G. Risk factors for surgery and postoperative recurrence in Crohn's disease. Ann Surg 2000;231:38–45.
24. Wagtmans MJ, Verspaget HW, Lamers CB, et al. Gender-related differences in the clinical course of Crohn's disease. Am J Gastroenterol 2001;96:1541–6.
25. Moradkhani A, Beckman LJ, Tabibian JH. Health-related quality of life in inflammatory bowel disease: psychosocial, clinical, socioeconomic, and demographic predictors. J Crohns Colitis 2013;7:467–73.
26. Tabibian A, Tabibian JH, Beckman LJ, et al. Predictors of health-related quality of life and adherence in Crohn's disease and ulcerative colitis: implications for clinical management. Dig Dis Sci 2015;60:1366–74.
27. Hauser G, Tkalcic M, Stimac D, et al. Gender related differences in quality of life and affective status in patients with inflammatory bowel disease. Coll Antropol 2011;35(Suppl 2):203–7.
28. Huppertz-Hauss G, Hoivik ML, Langholz E, et al. Health-related quality of life in inflammatory bowel disease in a European-wide population-based cohort 10 years after diagnosis. Inflamm Bowel Dis 2015;21:337–44.
29. Stjernman H, Tysk C, Almer S, et al. Unfavourable outcome for women in a study of health-related quality of life, social factors and work disability in Crohn's disease. Eur J Gastroenterol Hepatol 2011;23:671–9.
30. Ghosh S, Mitchell R. Impact of inflammatory bowel disease on quality of life: Results of the European Federation of Crohn's and Ulcerative Colitis Associations (EFCCA) patient survey. J Crohns Colitis 2007;1:10–20.
31. Graff LA, Walker JR, Bernstein CN. Depression and anxiety in inflammatory bowel disease: a review of comorbidity and management. Inflamm Bowel Dis 2009;15: 1105–18.
32. Satcher D, Hook EW 3rd, Coleman E. Sexual Health in America: improving patient care and public health. JAMA 2015;314:765–6.
33. Muller KR, Prosser R, Bampton P, et al. Female gender and surgery impair relationships, body image, and sexuality in inflammatory bowel disease: patient perceptions. Inflamm Bowel Dis 2010;16:657–63.
34. Timmer A, Kemptner D, Bauer A, et al. Determinants of female sexual function in inflammatory bowel disease: a survey based cross-sectional analysis. BMC Gastroenterol 2008;8:45.
35. Maunder R, Toner B, de Rooy E, et al. Influence of sex and disease on illness-related concerns in inflammatory bowel disease. Can J Gastroenterol 1999;13: 728–32.
36. Bel LG, Vollebregt AM, Van der Meulen-de Jong AE, et al. Sexual dysfunctions in men and women with inflammatory bowel disease: the influence of IBD-related clinical factors and depression on sexual function. J Sex Med 2015;12:1557–67.
37. Marin L, Manosa M, Garcia-Planella E, et al. Sexual function and patients' perceptions in inflammatory bowel disease: a case-control survey. J Gastroenterol 2013;48:713–20.

38. Ghazi LJ, Patil SA, Cross RK. Sexual dysfunction in inflammatory bowel disease. Inflamm Bowel Dis 2015;21:939–47.
39. Davies RJ, O'Connor BI, Victor C, et al. A prospective evaluation of sexual function and quality of life after ileal pouch-anal anastomosis. Dis Colon Rectum 2008; 51:1032–5.
40. Rosenstrom T, Jokela M, Hintsanen M, et al. Body-image dissatisfaction is strongly associated with chronic dysphoria. J Affect Disord 2013;150:253–60.
41. Rakhkovskaya LM, Holland JM. Body dissatisfaction in older adults with a disabling health condition. J Health Psychol 2015. [Epub ahead of print].
42. Saha S, Zhao YQ, Shah SA, et al. Body image dissatisfaction in patients with inflammatory bowel disease. Inflamm Bowel Dis 2015;21:345–52.
43. Jedel S, Hood MM, Keshavarzian A. Getting personal: a review of sexual functioning, body image, and their impact on quality of life in patients with inflammatory bowel disease. Inflamm Bowel Dis 2015;21:923–38.
44. McDermott E, Mullen G, Moloney J, et al. Body image dissatisfaction: clinical features, and psychosocial disability in inflammatory bowel disease. Inflamm Bowel Dis 2015;21:353–60.
45. Dunker MS, Stiggelbout AM, van Hogezand RA, et al. Cosmesis and body image after laparoscopic-assisted and open ileocolic resection for Crohn's disease. Surg Endosc 1998;12:1334–40.
46. Kjaer MD, Laursen SB, Qvist N, et al. Sexual function and body image are similar after laparoscopy-assisted and open ileal pouch-anal anastomosis. World J Surg 2014;38:2460–5.
47. Walboomers JM, Jacobs MV, Manos MM, et al. Human papillomavirus is a necessary cause of invasive cervical cancer worldwide. J Pathol 1999;189:12–9.
48. Vesco KK, Whitlock EP, Eder M, et al. Risk factors and other epidemiologic considerations for cervical cancer screening: a narrative review for the U.S. Preventive Services Task Force. Ann Intern Med 2011;155:698–705. W216.
49. Kane S, Khatibi B, Reddy D. Higher incidence of abnormal Pap smears in women with inflammatory bowel disease. Am J Gastroenterol 2008;103:631–6.
50. Lees CW, Critchley J, Chee N, et al. Lack of association between cervical dysplasia and IBD: a large case-control study. Inflamm Bowel Dis 2009;15: 1621–9.
51. Singh H, Demers AA, Nugent Z, et al. Risk of cervical abnormalities in women with inflammatory bowel disease: a population-based nested case-control study. Gastroenterology 2009;136:451–8.
52. Allegretti JR, Barnes EL, Cameron A. Are patients with inflammatory bowel disease on chronic immunosuppressive therapy at increased risk of cervical high-grade dysplasia/cancer? A meta-analysis. Inflamm Bowel Dis 2015;21:1089–97.
53. Wilt TJ, Harris RP, Qaseem A, et al. Screening for cancer: advice for high-value care from the American College of Physicians. Ann Intern Med 2015;162:718–25.
54. Long MD, Porter CQ, Sandler RS, et al. Suboptimal rates of cervical testing among women with inflammatory bowel disease. Clin Gastroenterol Hepatol 2009;7:549–53.
55. Singh H, Nugent Z, Demers AA, et al. Screening for cervical and breast cancer among women with inflammatory bowel disease: a population-based study. Inflamm Bowel Dis 2011;17:1741–50.
56. Nee J, Feuerstein JD. Optimizing the care and health of women with inflammatory bowel disease. Gastroenterol Res Pract 2015;2015:435820.
57. Committee on Practice B-G. ACOG Practice Bulletin Number 131: screening for cervical cancer. Obstet Gynecol 2012;120:1222–38.

58. Ali RA, Dooley C, Comber H, et al. Clinical features, treatment, and survival of patients with colorectal cancer with or without inflammatory bowel disease. Clin Gastroenterol Hepatol 2011;9:584–9.e1–e2.

59. Jensen AB, Larsen M, Gislum M, et al. Survival after colorectal cancer in patients with ulcerative colitis: a nationwide population-based Danish study. Am J Gastroenterol 2006;101:1283–7.

60. Peyrin-Biroulet L, Lepage C, Jooste V, et al. Colorectal cancer in inflammatory bowel diseases: a population-based study (1976-2008). Inflamm Bowel Dis 2012;18:2247–51.

61. Watanabe T, Konishi T, Kishimoto J, et al. Ulcerative colitis-associated colorectal cancer shows a poorer survival than sporadic colorectal cancer: a nationwide Japanese study. Inflamm Bowel Dis 2011;17:802–8.

62. Soderlund S, Granath F, Brostrom O, et al. Inflammatory bowel disease confers a lower risk of colorectal cancer to females than to males. Gastroenterology 2010; 138:1697–703.

63. Schulte CM. Review article: bone disease in inflammatory bowel disease. Aliment Pharmacol Ther 2004;20(Suppl 4):43–9.

64. Legido J, Gisbert JP, Mate J. Bone metabolism changes in 100 patients with inflammatory bowel disease. Gastroenterol Hepatol 2011;34:379–84 [in Spanish].

65. Bernstein CN, Leslie WD, Leboff MS. AGA technical review on osteoporosis in gastrointestinal diseases. Gastroenterology 2003;124:795–841.

66. Kane SV, Sable K, Hanauer SB. The menstrual cycle and its effect on inflammatory bowel disease and irritable bowel syndrome: a prevalence study. Am J Gastroenterol 1998;93:1867–72.

67. Bernstein MT, Graff LA, Targownik LE, et al. Gastrointestinal symptoms before and during menses in women with IBD. Aliment Pharmacol Ther 2012;36:135–44.

68. Parlak E, Dagli U, Alkim C, et al. Pattern of gastrointestinal and psychosomatic symptoms across the menstrual cycle in women with inflammatory bowel disease. Turk J Gastroenterol 2003;14:250–6.

69. Gawron LM, Goldberger A, Gawron AJ, et al. The impact of hormonal contraception on disease-related cyclical symptoms in women with inflammatory bowel diseases. Inflamm Bowel Dis 2014;20:1729–33.

70. Weber AM, Ziegler C, Belinson JL, et al. Gynecologic history of women with inflammatory bowel disease. Obstet Gynecol 1995;86:843–7.

71. Saha S, Midtling E, Roberson E, et al. Dysmenorrhea in women with Crohn's disease: a case-control study. Inflamm Bowel Dis 2013;19:1463–9.

72. Saha S, Zhao YQ, Shah SA, et al. Menstrual cycle changes in women with inflammatory bowel disease: a study from the ocean state Crohn's and colitis area registry. Inflamm Bowel Dis 2014;20:534–40.

73. Lichtarowicz A, Norman C, Calcraft B, et al. A study of the menopause, smoking, and contraception in women with Crohn's disease. Q J Med 1989;72:623–31.

74. Kane SV, Reddy D. Hormonal replacement therapy after menopause is protective of disease activity in women with inflammatory bowel disease. Am J Gastroenterol 2008;103:1193–6.

75. Khalili H, Higuchi LM, Ananthakrishnan AN, et al. Hormone therapy increases risk of ulcerative colitis but not Crohn's disease. Gastroenterology 2012;143: 1199–206.

Obesity in Women

The Clinical Impact on Gastrointestinal and Reproductive Health and Disease Management

Octavia Pickett-Blakely, MD, MHS[a],*, Laura Uwakwe, MD[b],
Farzana Rashid, MD[c]

KEYWORDS

• Overweight • Obesity • Women • Bariatric

KEY POINTS

• Obesity is a multifactorial disease process that affects women differently than men.
• Severe obesity is more common in women.
• Complicated gastroesophageal reflux disease (GERD) is less common in women.
• Obesity adversely affects fertility, conception, and maternal and fetal pregnancy outcomes.
• Obesity-related diet and exercise counseling should take into consideration gender differences in the epidemiology, pathophysiology, and clinical manifestations of obesity.

INTRODUCTION

Obesity is a well-known, chronic condition that affects individuals in all walks of life **(Table 1)**. Previously considered a disease of privilege, the worldwide obesity epidemic has had significant societal impact, ranging from the social stigma associated with obesity to costly, comorbid diseases. Research efforts have focused on all facets of obesity from the epidemiology to treatment strategies. Thus far, the work done in this area has revealed that, like other chronic diseases, intriguing gender differences exist between women and men. This article focuses on the epidemiologic and pathophysiologic features, clinical manifestations, and management of obesity-related disorders that are unique to women and pertinent to gastroenterologists.

Disclosures: All authors have nothing to disclose.
[a] Division of Gastroenterology and Hepatology, University of Pennsylvania, 3400 Civic Center Boulevard, 4 South, Philadelphia, PA 19104, USA; [b] Department of Medicine, Drexel University College of Medicine, 245 North 15th Street, New College Building, Suite 5104, Philadelphia, PA 19102, USA; [c] Division of Gastroenterology and Hepatology, University of Pennsylvania, 51 North, 39th Street, 218 Wright Building, Philadelphia, PA 19104, USA
* Corresponding author.
E-mail address: octavia.pickett-blakely@uphs.upenn.edu

Gastroenterol Clin N Am 45 (2016) 317–331
http://dx.doi.org/10.1016/j.gtc.2016.02.008
0889-8553/16/$ – see front matter © 2016 Elsevier Inc. All rights reserved.

Table 1
Gender-specific differences of obesity in women

	Obesity-Related Characteristics in Women
Epidemiology	• Prevalence similar to men • Higher prevalence of severe obesity
Sociology	• Greater dissatisfaction with weight and body • Positive correlation of body image and self-esteem
Pathophysiology	See **Fig. 1**
Comorbid GI illness	
GERD-related disease	GERD complications (erosive esophagitis, Barrett esophagus, and esophageal adenocarcinoma) less common
NAFLD	• Symptomatic improvement with lower degrees of weight loss • Lower prevalence in premenopausal women vs age-matched male controls
Gallstones	Higher prevalence common in women
Reproductive health	See **Table 2**
Treatment	
Behavioral modifications	• Greater likelihood of dieting • Effect of aerobic and aerobic-resistance exercise less pronounced
Bariatric surgery	• Greater proportion of bariatric surgery recipients • Lower bariatric surgery complication rates

EPIDEMIOLOGY

All demographic segments of society, including age, race/ethnicity, and gender, have been impacted by the obesity epidemic. Overall, the prevalence of obesity is similar in women and men, with approximately one-third of adults in the United States being obese.[1] Gender disparities in the prevalence of obesity have been described, however, in certain subpopulations. For example, when different racial groups are examined, obesity is more prevalent in non-Hispanic African American women than men (57% vs 37%, respectively).[1,2] This gender disparity is not observed, however, in non-Hispanic whites, Hispanics, or Asians. Obesity also seems more prevalent in older women (age >60) than men.[2] Furthermore, more severe forms of obesity affect women more commonly than men.[2] The reasons for the epidemiologic gender disparities in obesity are unclear but may result from the culmination of pathophysiologic and sociologic differences between genders.

PATHOPHYSIOLOGY

Obesity is thought to be the result of a multifactorial process driven primarily by excessive energy/caloric intake and inadequate physical activity. There are a minority of individuals affected by monogenetic disorders where a single gene mutation leads to obesity. Researchers have proposed gender-specific physiologic and biochemical differences, among other factors, to explain differences in excessive body weight in women and men.

Aspects of energy intake, utilization, and storage differ between women and men (**Fig. 1**).[3] Gender differences in energy metabolism have been reported, with studies showing a higher resting metabolic rate in men compared with women.[4] In terms of

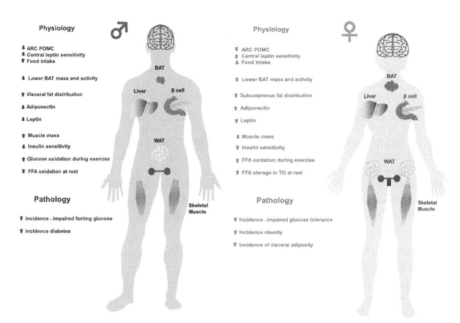

Fig. 1. Gender dimorphisms in metabolic homeostasis, diabetes, and obesity. Men are represented on the left and women represented on the right. ARC, arcuate nucleus; BAT, brown adipose tissue; FFA, free fatty acids; POMC, pro-opiomelanocortin; TG, triglycerides; WAT, white adipose tissue. (*From* Mauvais-Jarvis F. Sex differences in metabolic homeostasis, diabetes, and obesity. Biol Sex Differ 2015;6:14.)

fat storage, the less metabolically active form of fat, subcutaneous fat, is predominant in women. Meanwhile, visceral fat, which is more metabolically active, predominates in men.[3] These factors favor a propensity for fat storage in a distribution that favors obesity in women more so than men. Furthermore, biochemical differences, such as higher circulating levels of leptin and adiponectin, both of which are involved in the regulation of food intake and satiety, have been described in women.[3] Sex hormones may also play a role in the differential expression of obesity in women and men. Later in life, the proandrogen hormonal profile that is characterized by low levels of estrogen and increased levels of androgens has been observed in perimenopausal and post-menopausal women. This hormone shift favors body fat redistribution with increased visceral fat, a phenotype that is seen in men and correlates with the higher prevalence (although not statistically significant) of obesity in women over 60 years of age.[2,5]

Studies that examine eating behavior with respect to gender show that women exhibit significantly higher cognitive restraint, disinhibition scores, and hunger scores.[6,7] It has also been reported that a greater proportion of women tend to engage in dieting behavior than men.[7] Studies also show that in women, however, a history of dieting is positively associated with weight gain.[8,9] It is possible that certain eating behaviors, such as cognitive restraint, are difficult to maintain and may result in increased fat intake and bingeing.

SOCIOLOGY

Obesity is associated with a negative social stigma while societal standards of beauty have not evolved in parallel with the obesity epidemic.[10] In general, women tend to be held to a different beauty aesthetic than men, which may influence the aforementioned behaviors related to food intake. Although obesity is common, studies show that weight-related bias is pervasive in workplaces, health care systems, interpersonal relationships, and the media, although it is unclear if gender differences in weight-related bias exist.[10] The notion that weight is not modifiable contradicts the societal stigma of obesity. There are few data to confirm that society at large believes that weight is not modifiable, although a recent study showed that individuals who believed that weight is unchangeable had poor health practices.[11] Gender was not associated with belief in weight changeability or exercise/dietary behavior.[11] When compared with men, women are more likely to (1) be dissatisfied with their weight, (2) be dissatisfied with their body, and (3) associate body image with self-esteem.[12–14] Nonetheless, positive body image has been shown an indicator of positive mental and physical health indices in both women and men.[15] From a societal perspective, promoting the concept of self-acceptance and positive body image may ultimately translate into more widespread adoption of healthy lifestyle practices.

OBESITY-ASSOCIATED GASTROINTESTINAL DISEASE
Gastroesophageal Reflux Disease

Obesity is a known risk factor for GERD.[16] Given the established association between obesity and GERD, it is not surprising that the global obesity epidemic has been accompanied by an increased burden of symptomatic GERD and its complications.[17,18] Although the existing literature suggests a similar prevalence of symptomatic GERD in women and men, GERD complications, such as erosive esophagitis, Barrett esophagus, and esophageal adenocarcinoma, are less common in women.[19–21]

Of the factors that contribute to GERD, increased abdominal pressure is often present in obesity. Central or abdominal adiposity results in increased abdominal pressure and is a risk factor for GERD complications independent of body mass index (BMI). Central adiposity is less common in women than men and may explain the lower prevalence of such complications in women. The role of sex hormones has been implicated to explain the different manifestations of GERD in women and men. Menon and colleagues[19] showed, however, that increased estradiol levels were associated with physiologic GERD even when controlling for BMI.

Medical management, including behavioral modifications and acid suppressive therapy, is effective in ameliorating GERD symptoms. The association drawn between BMI and GERD has led to an emphasis on weight reduction as an important part of the behavioral modifications for GERD. One systematic review concluded that weight loss resulting from surgical or diet/lifestyle interventions can reduce or eliminate the symptoms of GERD while noting (1) a dose-response relationship between the degree of weight loss and resolution of GERD symptoms and (2) that women have a lower threshold for weight loss to achieve symptom improvement compared with men (5%–10% vs >10% weight reduction).[19]

Obesity is a risk factor for GERD, which is similar in prevalence in women and men. Women are less likely to develop complications of GERD, however, and more likely to derive benefit from smaller amounts of weight loss than men.

Nonalcoholic Fatty Liver Disease

Nonalcoholic fatty liver disease (NAFLD) is often described as the hepatic manifestation of the metabolic syndrome, which involves insulin resistance, lipid metabolism, and obesity. Studies show strong correlations between NAFLD and obesity in women.[22] In a large cohort study of more than 9300 women in China, 48% of obese women had NAFLD compared with 12.8% of the general population of women.[22] Although the prevalence of NAFLD is similar in women and men, NAFLD is less common in premenopausal women versus age-matched men, perhaps due to a pathologic process involving the hormonal effects on fat distribution.[23]

Although the pathogenesis of NAFLD remains an area of active research, it is known that the pattern of liver injury involves steatosis and cytotoxic liver injury.[24] In obese individuals, the biochemical effects of increased body weight depress certain molecular anti-inflammatory pathways in the liver, enabling NAFLD to progress.[25] Sex hormones are also linked to obesity and NAFLD. Perimenopausal and postmenopausal women have lower levels of estrogen and increased levels of androgens, a hormonal profile that favors the development of the metabolic syndrome and NAFLD via increased visceral fat deposition.[22] The suggested protective effect of female sex hormones is corroborated by the epidemiologic findings that (1) there is a lower prevalence of NAFLD in premenopausal women compared with men of the same age,[23] (2) women with NAFLD have significantly lower levels of serum estradiol compared with those without NAFLD,[26] and (3) women older than age 50 have a higher prevalence of NAFLD than those younger than 50.[22] It has been suggested that increased concentrations of estrogen inhibit the spontaneous secretion of proinflammatory cytokines, such as interleukin (IL)-1, IL-6, and tumor necrosis factor α,[26] and possibly exert an antifibrogenic effect on the liver.[27] Further studies of the pathophysiological link between obesity and gender may provide better insight into therapeutic targets for treating NAFLD.

Although studies suggest that hormone replacement therapy (HRT) may be beneficial in treating NAFLD, to date there have been no prospective studies investigating this therapy. Weight loss is typically recommended for obese patients with NAFLD; however, the impact on the natural history of the disease is unclear. Modest weight loss of 5% to 10% or more of body weight can correct abnormal liver chemistries and decrease liver size, fat content, and features of steatohepatitis.[28,29] Rapid weight loss after gastric bypass surgery, very-low-calorie diets, or prolonged fasting, however, lowers hepatic fat content but can induce hepatic inflammation, thereby worsening steatohepatitis.[30] Because women are more likely than men to diet and undergo bariatric surgery[31,32] gastroenterologists should be aware of their risk for this complication and emphasize the importance of slow, gradual as opposed to rapid, weight loss.

NAFLD in women is also linked to diabetes mellitus, the metabolic syndrome, low estrogen levels, and elevated androgen levels. Premenopausal women have a lower prevalence of NAFLD, likely due to the protective effect of estrogen. Effective treatment of NAFLD includes slow, gradual weight loss, which is favored over rapid weight loss that is seen with very-low-calorie diets.

Gallstone Disease

The link between gallstones and both women and obesity is well established.[33] Gallstone disease is approximately 2 to 3 times more common in women than in men.[33] The Nurses' Health Study showed that elevated BMI is strongly linked to gallstone disease in women.[34] Given the elevated risk for gallstone formation, particularly in obese women, researchers have worked to elucidate the pathways of gallstone formation in this high-risk group.

Cholesterol gallstones form with cholesterol saturation of bile and reduced gallbladder emptying.[35] In obesity, cholesterol saturation of bile may occur as a result of dietary intake. Low-calorie/low-fat diets are linked to an increased likelihood of gallstone formation compared with a low-calorie/high-fat diet with the same weight loss.[36] Although the weight loss process can increase the formation of gallstones, elevated

BMI is an independent risk factor for gallstone disease in women, and the successful reduction of BMI is associated with a lower the risk of future gallstone development.[36]

Similar to weight loss rates, hormonal influences have been linked to increased bile cholesterol saturation, which may result in gallstones. It is known that the gravidity of women is a predictor of gallstone formation. The high risk of gallstone formation in women is primarily observed in women of childbearing age.[33] Estrogen is known to increase biliary cholesterol secretion, causing cholesterol supersaturation of the bile. This hormonal link to gallstone formation has also been invoked to explain the increased incidence of gallstones in other states of high estrogen levels, such as in postmenopausal women on hormone replacement therapy as well as in women using oral contraceptives.[33] This relationship may be dose dependent, because women using low-estrogen oral contraceptives do not have an increased incidence of gallstones.[33]

In light of the risk of gallstone formation with obesity and rapid weight loss, women should be encouraged to strive for slow, gradual weight reduction (2.2 kg per week). Primary prevention of gallstones can be achieved with pharmacologic agents, such as ursodeoxycholic acid, and has been used by some during periods of rapid weight loss, like postbariatric surgery.[37,38] Because women are more likely than men to undergo postbariatric surgery,[32] some investigators advocate the use of ursodeoxycholic acid after bariatric surgery.[39]

Gallstone disease is significantly more prevalent in women than in men and is strongly linked to obesity. Both rapid weight loss and high estrogen levels are associated with the development of gallstones. Gradual weight loss and pharmacotherapy with ursodeoxycholic acid are both effective at preventing gallstone formation in obese women.

OBESITY IN REPRODUCTIVE HEALTH
Conception

Epidemiologic data suggest that obesity negatively affects reproductive health. One study showed that obesity was more prevalent in a cohort of women seeking medical attention to become pregnant.[40] In addition, the time required to achieve a spontaneous pregnancy is longer and pregnancy rates are lower in obese women, including obese women with regular ovulation.[41,42] The risk of infertility is 3-fold higher in obese women than in nonobese women in both natural and assisted conception cycles.[43,44] Although weight loss can improve fertility, the benefits of weight loss are best seen in women under 35 years old.[45–47]

The pathophysiologic impact of obesity on reproduction is a complex, multifactorial process and ranges from menstrual dysfunction to infertility. Specifically, obesity is associated with (1) oligo-ovulation/anovulation, (2) abnormal oocyte recruitment/ovulation and poor oocyte quality, (3) poor embryo quality and development, and (4) decreased uterine receptivity and embryo implantation.[45,48] Several biochemical alterations in obese women may explain the physical manifestations. First, white adipose tissue regulates energy homeostasis and metabolism by secreting adipokines, leading to insulin resistance.[49] The resulting hyperinsulinemia stimulates ovarian androgen production and increases peripheral aromatization of sex hormones. Conversion of excess androgens to estrogens in adipose tissue leads to increased free estrogen, which impairs the hypothalamic-pituitary-gonadal axis.[49] The hypothalamic-pituitary-gonadal axis is further impaired by decreased luteinizing hormone, androstenedione, estrone, insulin, triglycerides, and very low-density lipoprotein.[50] These factors may alter gonadotropin-releasing hormone secretion (via negative feedback), altering follicular development and leading to irregular or anovulatory cycles.[49,51]

Pregnancy

As seen in the general population, the prevalence of obesity in pregnant women has dramatically increased since the early 1990s,[52] and now 28% of pregnant women are obese.[53] Obesity affects both maternal and fetal pregnancy outcomes (**Table 2**).

Pregnancy outcome is influenced by obesity and is associated with an increased risk of first-trimester and recurrent miscarriage.[54] Specifically, a meta-analysis showed that a BMI over 25 kg/m^2 carries a higher risk of miscarriage independent of mode of conception.[55] The exact pathophysiology for the link between obesity and miscarriage is unclear but may involve poor oocyte quality, deranged ovarian function, and/or endometrial function. A strong link has also been seen between obesity and stillbirth. Late, unexplained stillbirth is associated with increasing BMI in obese women compared with normal weight women.[54,56] Although the data vary, a recent meta-analysis reported a 20% increased risk of stillbirth in obese women that increased with greater degree of obesity.[57] The risk of fetal and neonatal death is also increased in obese women.[57] Obesity is associated with prolonged and post-term pregnancy (beyond 41 weeks' gestation and at or beyond 42 weeks' gestation, respectively),[53,58] which may be explained by inaccurate estimation of gestational dating in obese women. Another possibility is that elevated estrogen levels in obese women compared with nonobese women may hinder the onset of spontaneous labor.

Hypertensive disorders of pregnancy are more common with increased maternal weight. Observational studies demonstrate a 2.5-fold to a 3.2-fold increased risk of hypertensive disorders in obese women.[53] In particular, obesity is linked to preeclampsia[53] with elevated prepregnancy BMI a dose-dependent, independent risk factor for preeclampsia.[53,54] Although unclear, the pathogenesis of preeclampsia

Table 2	
Maternal and fetal complications of pregnancy in overweight and obese women	
Preconceptual period	• Subfertility/infertility • Menstrual disorder
Antenatal period	• Miscarriage (including recurrent) • Stillbirth • Fetal anomalies • Difficulty with ultrasound assessment of fetus • GDM • Preeclampsia
Intrapartum	• Prolonged pregnancy • Need for induction of labor • Stillbirth (unexplained) • Caesarean section • Anesthesia difficulties • Postpartum hemorrhage • Difficulty with fetal monitoring • Fetal macrosomia • Shoulder dystocia • Fetal distress • Perinatal morbidity and mortality • Birth injury
Postpartum	• Thromboembolism • Wound infection • Difficulty with breastfeeding
Long term	Risk for long-term diabetes mellitus, hypertension, cardiovascular disease

may involve insulin resistance, endotheial cell activation, dyslipidemia, and elevated cytokines, such as tumor necrosis factor.

Likewise, gestational diabetes mellitus (GDM) is more common in obese women and the risk of GDM increases in a dose-dependent fashion as well.[53,54]

GDM and suboptimal glycemic control can lead to fetal macrosomia and an increased risk of caesarean delivery and birth trauma (eg, perineal tears, shoulder dystocia, and asphyxia).[59] Furthermore, GDM increases maternal risk for developing diabetes mellitus later in life and is a predictor of developing the metabolic syndrome by 10 years postpartum.[39] Lastly, obese women are at increased risk for venous thromboembolism during pregnancy. Obesity compounds the pregnancy-related hypercoagulable state through its effect on clotting factors, impeding venous return through adipose tissue deposition and immobility, and endothelial cell damage.[54]

The preconception, pregnancy, and postpartum periods can influence the mother and the infant. Gestational weight gain (GWG) usually persists postpartum in women and increases with increasing parity. Persistent GWG can result in central adiposity, dyslipidemia, and glucose intolerance, leading to obesity, type 2 diabetes mellitus, the metabolic syndrome, and potentially cardiovascular disease (**Fig. 2**).[39] In addition, excessive maternal gain between the first and second pregnancies is associated with increased risks of preeclampsia, large-for-gestational-age birth, caesarean delivery, and future GDM.[60]

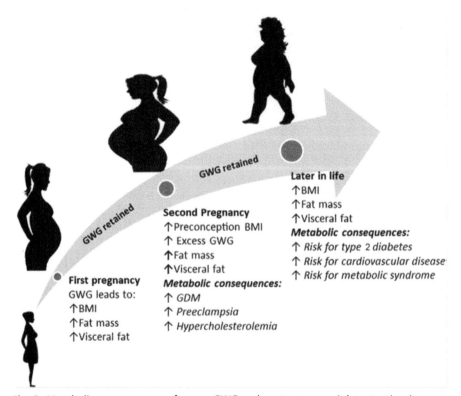

Fig. 2. Metabolic consequences of excess GWG and postpartum weight retention in reproductive age women. (*Adapted from* Gilmore LA. Pregnancy as a window to future health: excessive gestational weight gain and obesity. Semin Perinatol 2015;39:301; with permission.)

Maternal obesity is associated with an increased risk of fetal anomalies, including neural tube defects, spina bifida, congenital heart defects, orofacial clefts, anorectal atresia, hydrocephaly, limb reduction defects, diaphragmatic hernia, and omphalocele.[53,54] Congenital anomalies are perhaps more likely in gestational obesity due to undiagnosed diabetes mellitus, reduced dietary folate intake, and/or the technical limitations of visualizing defects by prenatal ultrasound.[61]

Obesity is also a risk factor for fetal macrosomia (even in the absence of diabetes mellitus) and intrauterine fetal growth restriction.[53,54] Furthermore, greater degrees of maternal weight gain during pregnancy are associated with increased infant birth weight.[62]

In the intrapartum period, monitoring contractions and assessing the progression of labor can be challenging in obese women. Manual palpation and/or external tocodynamometry are difficult, and fetal scalp electrode monitoring is frequently needed. To this end, maternal obesity is linked to longer labor inductions, longer or dysfunctional labor, failure of regional anesthesia, and increased risk of emergent and complicated cesarean delivery.[53]

In the postpartum period and beyond, initiation and duration of breastfeeding reduced gestational obesity.[63,64] Difficulty obtaining correct positioning and impaired prolactin response to suckling have been proposed mechanisms for this phenomenon.[65] Long term, there is a growing body of literature suggesting that the in utero environment can predict future neonatal, child, and adult health.[66] Infants born to obese mothers are at increased risk of developing childhood obesity and type 2 diabetes mellitus.[67] In a large cohort of more than 8400 children, Whitaker[68] showed that children of obese mothers were twice as likely to be obese by age 2.

Menopause

Menopause refers to the last physiologic menstrual period in a woman's life, during which time the loss of ovarian estrogen causes vasomotor symptoms of hot flushes, night sweats, insomnia, depression, vaginal dryness, and dyspareunia. The age at menopause and body mass are not clearly associated.[69] Some studies report later age of natural menopause with increased BMI and upper body fat distribution[70,71] whereas others refute this association.[72,73]

Women with more abdominal adiposity are more likely to report vasomotor symptoms during the transition to menopause.[74] One possible explanation is that adipose tissue functions as an insulator, thereby affecting normal thermoregulatory mechanisms of heat dissipation.[69] Another explanation is that adipose tissue may have an endocrine function that influences vasomotor symptoms.[75] Vulvovaginal atrophy is another common symptom of menopause that is related to estrogen deficiency that more commonly causes vaginal dryness, dyspareunia, itching, and irritation in obese women.[76]

Weight gain and changes in the distribution of adipose tissue after menopause may be, in part, due to the dramatic fall in serum estrogen levels and relative hyperandrogenism. Weight gain and obesity in midlife women, however, seem related more to age and a more sedentary lifestyle rather than to menopause.[51,69] Results from human studies show that postmenopausal women had significantly greater reductions in their physical activity compared with their premenopausal controls.

TREATMENT/MANAGEMENT OF OBESITY

Despite the widely recognized obesity epidemic and its societal impact, obesity tends to be underdiagnosed by health care providers, with only one-third of obese patients receiving a diagnosis.[77] Female gender, however, is a positive predictor of being diagnosed as obese.[77] Diet, behavioral modifications, and exercise are the mainstays of treatment of obesity, undoubtedly because of the known positive impact of modifiable health behaviors on overall morbidity and mortality.[78] Although an obesity diagnosis is a positive predictor of receipt of diet/nutrition, exercise, and weight reduction counseling from a health care provider, such counseling is provided to only a minority (20%–30%) of obesity individuals and there seems a difference between women in men in receipt of counseling.[77] One study did, however, show that diet/nutrition and exercise counseling is more likely to occur in male gender concordant patient provider pairs compared with female gender concordant pairs, a finding perhaps explained by the perception by health care providers that women are more sensitive about weight and less amenable to weight-related discussions.[79,80]

Diet/Exercise/Behavioral Modifications

Some literature suggests that women are more likely to engage in positive health behaviors, like eating a healthy diet.[81] Likewise, the concept of dieting is more common in women and is not surprising because women are more likely to be dissatisfied with their body and weight.[31] It is unclear from the existing literature that exercise practices are different between genders, but limited data suggest that the effect of exercise may differ with respect to gender and exercise type.[82] For example, aerobic exercise has been shown to lead to greater weight loss in men.[83] In a randomized control trial, Sanal and colleagues[83] recently showed that aerobic-resistance exercise was effective in reducing the fat free mass in the upper/whole body and trunk in men, whereas fat free mass was only reduced in the lower body of women. Such data can be used as a guide for prescribing gender-specific, tailored exercise regimens.

Bariatric Surgery

Bariatric surgery is a well-established means of weight loss that is both effective and durable.[84] Although obesity is equally prevalent in women and men, and men have greater obesity-related comorbidities, women comprise the majority of the bariatric surgery population.[32,85] One study noted that women who underwent bariatric surgery had a lower baseline BMI and mean age.[85] In terms of outcomes, there is no reported difference in weight loss between genders during the first 3-year after bariatric surgery. In 1 study, however, male patients who underwent laparoscopic adjustable gastric banding had greater BMI reduction than female patients (-8.2 ± 4.3 kg/m^2 vs -3.9 ± 1.9 kg/m^2; $P = .02$).[85–87] Furthermore, complications of bariatric surgery are also reportedly higher in men compared with women[86] but it is unclear that this finding influences the selection of bariatric surgery candidates.

SUMMARY

Although on the surface obesity affects women and men in similar proportions, there are stark differences in how obesity develops and manifests itself in the 2 genders. More severe forms of obesity affect women at a higher rate, which underscores the need for health care providers, and gastroenterologists in particular, to identify and recommend treatment of obese women.

Comorbid gastrointestinal diseases like GERD and NAFLD affect women differentially, whereas gallstone disease is highly prevalent in women. Obesity similarly has adverse effects on the reproductive health of women as well ranging from impaired fertility and conception to pregnancy complications, such as preeclampsia, GDM, fetal anomalies, and macrosomia.

Lastly, given the impact of obesity, efforts should focus not only on understanding the pathophysiologic mechanisms but also on effective, gender-specific treatment strategies that begin with accurate diagnosis of obesity and, thereafter, offering weight-related counseling and referrals for bariatric surgery when appropriate. Given the female predominance of the bariatric surgery population, gastroenterologists must be well versed in the care of patients after bariatric surgery. In light of the known gender-specific biochemical differences in dietary intake, metabolism, and storage of energy, gastroenterologists are uniquely positioned to influence the management of obese patients.

REFERENCES

1. Ogden CL, Carroll MD, Kit BK, et al. Prevalence of obesity among adults: United states, 2011-2012. NCHS Data Brief 2013;(131):1–8.
2. Ogden CL, Carroll MD, Flegal KM. Prevalence of obesity in the United States. JAMA 2014;312(2):189–90.
3. Mauvais-Jarvis F. Sex differences in metabolic homeostasis, diabetes, and obesity. Biol Sex Differ 2015;6:14.
4. McMurray RG, Soares J, Caspersen CJ, et al. Examining variations of resting metabolic rate of adults: a public health perspective. Med Sci Sports Exerc 2014;46(7):1352–8.
5. Crowell MD, Dubin NH, Robinson JC, et al. Functional bowel disorders in women with dysmenorrhea. Am J Gastroenterol 1994;89(11):1973–7.
6. Ernst B, Wilms B, Thurnheer M, et al. Eating behaviour in treatment-seeking obese subjects - influence of sex and BMI classes. Appetite 2015;95:96–100.
7. Provencher V, Drapeau V, Tremblay A, et al. Eating behaviors and indexes of body composition in men and women from the quebec family study. Obes Res 2003;11(6):783–92.
8. Korkeila M, Rissanen A, Kaprio J, et al. Weight-loss attempts and risk of major weight gain: a prospective study in finnish adults. Am J Clin Nutr 1999;70(6):965–75.
9. Doucet E, St-Pierre S, Almeras N, et al. Evidence for the existence of adaptive thermogenesis during weight loss. Br J Nutr 2001;85(6):715–23.
10. Sikorski C, Luppa M, Kaiser M, et al. The stigma of obesity in the general public and its implications for public health - a systematic review. BMC Public Health 2011;11:661.
11. Parent MC, Alquist JL. Born fat: the relations between weight changeability beliefs and health behaviors and physical health. Health Educ Behav 2015. [Epub ahead of print].
12. Green KL, Cameron R, Polivy J, et al. Weight dissatisfaction and weight loss attempts among canadian adults. canadian heart health surveys research group. CMAJ 1997;157(Suppl 1):S17–25.
13. Furnham A, Badmin N, Sneade I. Body image dissatisfaction: gender differences in eating attitudes, self-esteem, and reasons for exercise. J Psychol 2002;136(6):581–96.
14. Elgin J, Pritchard M. Gender differences in disordered eating and its correlates. Eat Weight Disord 2006;11(3):e96–101.
15. Gillen MM. Associations between positive body image and indicators of men's and women's mental and physical health. Body Image 2015;13:67–74.
16. Nadaleto BF, Herbella FA, Patti MG. Gastroesophageal reflux disease in the obese: pathophysiology and treatment. Surgery 2015;159(2):475–86.

17. Nilsson M, Lundegardh G, Carling L, et al. Body mass and reflux oesophagitis: an oestrogen-dependent association? Scand J Gastroenterol 2002;37(6):626–30.

18. Jacobson BC, Somers SC, Fuchs CS, et al. Body-mass index and symptoms of gastroesophageal reflux in women. N Engl J Med 2006;354(22):2340–8.

19. Menon S, Prew S, Parkes G, et al. Do differences in female sex hormone levels contribute to gastro-oesophageal reflux disease? Eur J Gastroenterol Hepatol 2013;25(7):772–7.

20. Locke GR 3rd, Talley NJ, Fett SL, et al. Prevalence and clinical spectrum of gastroesophageal reflux: a population-based study in olmsted county, minnesota. Gastroenterology 1997;112(5):1448–56.

21. Sandler RS, Everhart JE, Donowitz M, et al. The burden of selected digestive diseases in the united states. Gastroenterology 2002;122(5):1500–11.

22. Wang Z, Xu M, Hu Z, et al. Prevalence of nonalcoholic fatty liver disease and its metabolic risk factors in women of different ages and body mass index. Menopause 2015;22(6):667–73.

23. Arun J, Clements RH, Lazenby AJ, et al. The prevalence of nonalcoholic steatohepatitis is greater in morbidly obese men compared to women. Obes Surg 2006; 16(10):1351–8.

24. Schuppan D, Schattenberg JM. Non-alcoholic steatohepatitis: pathogenesis and novel therapeutic approaches. J Gastroenterol Hepatol 2013;28(Suppl 1):68–76.

25. Di Naso FC, Porto RR, Fillmann HS, et al. Obesity depresses the anti-inflammatory HSP70 pathway, contributing to NAFLD progression. Obesity (Silver Spring) 2015;23(1):120–9.

26. Gutierrez-Grobe Y, Ponciano-Rodriguez G, Ramos MH, et al. Prevalence of non alcoholic fatty liver disease in premenopausal, posmenopausal and polycystic ovary syndrome women. the role of estrogens. Ann Hepatol 2010;9(4):402–9.

27. Florentino GS, Cotrim HP, Vilar CP, et al. Nonalcoholic fatty liver disease in menopausal women. Arq Gastroenterol 2013;50(3):180–5.

28. Promrat K, Kleiner DE, Niemeier HM, et al. Randomized controlled trial testing the effects of weight loss on nonalcoholic steatohepatitis. Hepatology 2010;51(1): 121–9.

29. Zelber-Sagi S, Ratziu V, Oren R. Nutrition and physical activity in NAFLD: an overview of the epidemiological evidence. World J Gastroenterol 2011;17(29): 3377–89.

30. Papandreou D, Andreou E. Role of diet on non-alcoholic fatty liver disease: an updated narrative review. World J Hepatol 2015;7(3):575–82.

31. Pingitore R, Spring B, Garfield D. Gender differences in body satisfaction. Obes Res 1997;5(5):402–9.

32. Pickett-Blakely OE, Huizinga MM, Clark JM. Sociodemographic trends in bariatric surgery utilization in the USA. Obes Surg 2012;22(5):838–42.

33. Novacek G. Gender and gallstone disease. Wien Med Wochenschr 2006; 156(19–20):527–33.

34. Pi-Sunyer X. The medical risks of obesity. Postgrad Med 2009;121(6):21–33.

35. Gustafsson U, Benthin L, Granstrom L, et al. Changes in gallbladder bile composition and crystal detection time in morbidly obese subjects after bariatric surgery. Hepatology 2005;41(6):1322–8.

36. Stokes CS, Gluud LL, Casper M, et al. Ursodeoxycholic acid and diets higher in fat prevent gallbladder stones during weight loss: a meta-analysis of randomized controlled trials. Clin Gastroenterol Hepatol 2014;12(7):1090–100.e2 [quiz: e61].

37. Everhart JE. Contributions of obesity and weight loss to gallstone disease. Ann Intern Med 1993;119(10):1029–35.

38. Uy MC, Talingdan-Te MC, Espinosa WZ, et al. Ursodeoxycholic acid in the prevention of gallstone formation after bariatric surgery: a meta-analysis. Obes Surg 2008;18(12):1532–8.
39. Gilmore LA. Pregnancy as a window to future health: excessive gestational weight gain and obesity. Semin Perinatol 2015;3(9):296–303.
40. Vahratian A, Smith YR. Should access to fertility-related services be conditional on body mass index? Hum Reprod 2009;24:1532–7.
41. Gesink Law DC, Maclehose RF, Longnecker MP. Obesity and time to pregnancy. Hum Reprod 2007;22:414–20.
42. Wise LA, Rothman KJ, Mikkelsen EM, et al. An internet-based prospective study of body size and time-to-pregnancy. Hum Reprod 2010;25:253–64.
43. Zaadstra BM, Seidell JC, Van Noord PA, et al. Fat and female fecundity: prospective study of effect of body fat distribution on conception rates. BMJ 1993;306:484–7.
44. Crosignani PG, Ragni G, Parazzini F, et al. Anthropometric indicators and response to gonadotrophin for ovulation induction. Hum Reprod 1994;9:420–3.
45. Jungheim E, Travieso J, Hopeman M. Weighing the impact of obesity on female reproductive function and fertility. Nutr Rev 2013;71:3–8.
46. Luke B, Brown MB, Missmer SA, et al. The effect of increasing obesity on the response to and outcome of assisted reproductive technology: a national study. Fertil Steril 2011;96:820–5.
47. Sneed ML, Uhler ML, Grotjan HE, et al. Body mass index: impact on IVF success appears age-related. Hum Reprod 2008;23:1835–9.
48. Bellver J, Melo MA, Bosch E, et al. Obesity and poor reproductive outcome: the potential role of the endometrium. Fertil Steril 2007;88:446–51.
49. Dag ZO, Dilbaz B. Impact of obesity on infertility in women. J Turk Ger Gynecol Assoc 2015;16:111–7.
50. Parihar M. Obesity and infertility. Rev Gynecol Pract 2003;3:120–6.
51. Rachon D, Teede H. Ovarian function and obesity—Interrelationship, impact on women's reproductive lifespan and treatment option. Mol Cell Endocrinol 2010;316:172–9.
52. Heslehurst N, Ells LJ, Simpson H, et al. Trends in maternal obesity incidence rates, demographic predictors, and health inequalities in 36,821 women over a 15-year period. BJOG 2007;114(2):187–94.
53. Mission JF, Marshall NE, Caughey AB, et al. Pregnancy risks associated with obesity. Obstet Gynecol Clin North Am 2015;42:335–53.
54. Thannon O, Gharaibeh A, Mahmood T, et al. The implications of obesity on pregnancy outcome. Obstetrics Gynaecol Reprod Med 25(4):102–5.
55. Metwally M, Ong KJ, Ledger WL, et al. Does high body mass index increase the risk of miscarriage after spontaneous and assisted conception? A meta-analysis of the evidence. Fertil Steril 2008;90(3):714–26.
56. Flenady V, Koopmans L, Middleton P, et al. Major risk factors for still birth in high-income countries: a systematic review and meta-analysis. Lancet 2011;377(9774):1331–40.
57. Aune D, Saugstad OD, Henriksen T, et al. Maternal body mass index and the risk of fetal death, stillbirth, and infant death: a systematic review and metaanalysis. JAMA 2014;311(15):1536–46.
58. Denison FC, Price J, Graham C, et al. Maternal obesity, length of gestation, risk of postdates pregnancy and spontaneous onset of labour at term. BJOG 2008;115(6):720–5.

59. Marshall NE, Guild C, Cheng YW, et al. The effect of maternal body mass index on perinatal outcomes in women with diabetes. Am J Perinatol 2014;31(3): 249–56.

60. Villamor E, Cnattingius S. Interpregnancy weight change and risk of adverse pregnancy outcomes: a population-based study. Lancet 2006;368:1164–70.

61. Chung JH, Pelayo R, Hatfield TJ, et al. Limitations of the fetal anatomic survey via ultrasound in the obese obstetrical population. J Matern Fetal Neonatal Med 2012;25(10):1945–9.

62. Ovesen P, Rasmussen S, Kesmodel U. Effect of prepregnancy maternal over-weight and obesity on pregnancy outcome. Obstet Gynecol 2011;118:305–12.

63. Amir LH, Donath S. A systematic review of maternal obesity and breastfeeding intention, initiation and duration. BMC Pregnancy Childbirth 2007;7:9.

64. Mok E, Multon C, Piguel L, et al. Decreased full breastfeeding, altered practices, perceptions, and infant weight change of prepregnant obese women: a need for extra support. Pediatrics 2008;121(5):e1319–24.

65. Rasmussen KM, Kjolhede CL. Prepregnant overweight and obesity diminish the prolactin response to suckling in the first week postpartum. Pediatrics 2004; 113(5):e465–71.

66. Simmons R. Perinatal programming of obesity. Exp Gerontol 2005;40:863–6.

67. Mody S, Han M. Obesity and contraception. Clin Obstet Gynecol 2014;57(3): 501–7.

68. Whitaker RC. Predicting preschooler obesity at birth: the role of maternal obesity in early pregnancy. Pediatrics 2004;114(1):e29–36.

69. Al-safi Z, Polotsky AJ. Obesity and menopause. Best Pract Res Clin Obstet Gy-naecol 2015;29:548–53.

70. Rodstrom K, Bengtsson C, Milsom I, et al. Evidence for a secular trend in meno-pausal age: a population study of women in gothenburg. Menopause 2003;10: 538–43.

71. Reynolds RF, Obermeyer CM. Age at natural menopause in spain and the united states: results from the DAMES project. Am J Hum Biol 2005;17:331–40.

72. Gold EB, Sternfeld B, Kelsey JL, et al. Relation of demographic and lifestyle fac-tors to symptoms in a multi-racial/ethnic population of women 40-55 years of age. Am J Epidemiol 2000;152:463–73.

73. Bromberger JT, Matthews K, Kuller LH, et al. Prospective study of the determi-nants of age at menopause. Am J Epidemiol 1997;145:124–33.

74. Thurston RC, Sowers MR, Sutton-Tyrrell K, et al. Abdominal adiposity and hot flashes among midlife women. Menopause 2008;15:429–34.

75. Alexander C, Cochran CJ, Gallicchio L, et al. Serum leptin levels, hormone levels, and hot flashes in midlife women. Fertil Steril 2010;94:1037–43.

76. Pastore LM, Carter RA, Hulka BS, et al. Self-reported urogenital symptoms in postmenopausal women: women's health initiative. Maturitas 2004;49:292–303.

77. Bleich SN, Pickett-Blakely O, Cooper LA. Physician practice patterns of obesity diagnosis and weight-related counseling. Patient Educ Couns 2011;82(1):123–9.

78. Mokdad AH, Marks JS, Stroup DF, et al. Actual causes of death in the united states, 2000. JAMA 2004;291(10):1238–45.

79. Olson CL, Schumaker HD, Yawn BP. Overweight women delay medical care. Arch Fam Med 1994;3(10):888–92.

80. Pickett-Blakely O, Bleich SN, Cooper LA. Patient-physician gender concordance and weight-related counseling of obese patients. Am J Prev Med 2011;40(6): 616–9.

81. Wardle J, Haase AM, Steptoe A, et al. Gender differences in food choice: the contribution of health beliefs and dieting. Ann Behav Med 2004;27(2):107–16.

82. Ballor DL, Keesey RE. A meta-analysis of the factors affecting exercise-induced changes in body mass, fat mass and fat-free mass in males and females. Int J Obes 1991;15(11):717–26.

83. Sanal E, Ardic F, Kirac S. Effects of aerobic or combined aerobic resistance exercise on body composition in overweight and obese adults: gender differences. A randomized intervention study. Eur J Phys Rehabil Med 2013;49(1):1–11.

84. Buchwald H, Avidor Y, Braunwald E, et al. Bariatric surgery: a systematic review and meta-analysis. JAMA 2004;292(14):1724–37.

85. Stroh C, Weiner R, Wolff S, et al, Obesity Surgery Working Group and Competence Network Obesity. Are there gender-specific aspects in obesity and metabolic surgery? data analysis from the german bariatric surgery registry. Viszeralmedizin 2014;30(2):125–32.

86. Stroh C, Weiner R, Wolff S, et al. Influences of gender on complication rate and outcome after roux-en-Y gastric bypass: data analysis of more than 10,000 operations from the german bariatric surgery registry. Obes Surg 2014;24(10): 1625–33.

87. Nguyen NQ, Game P, Bessell J, et al. Outcomes of roux-en-Y gastric bypass and laparoscopic adjustable gastric banding. World J Gastroenterol 2013;19(36): 6035–43.

Metabolic Bone Disease in Primary Biliary Cirrhosis

Lisa M. Glass, MD[a], Grace Li-Chun Su, MD[b],*

KEYWORDS

- Primary biliary cirrhosis • Metabolic bone disease • Osteoporosis
- Antiresorptive agents

KEY POINTS

- Primary biliary cirrhosis (PBC) is a liver-specific autoimmune disease that primarily affects women (female-to-male ratio, 10:1) between 40 and 60 years of age.
- Metabolic bone disease is a common complication of PBC, affecting 20% to 52% of patients, depending on the duration and severity of liver disease.
- The osteoporosis seen in PBC seems mainly due to low bone formation, although increased bone resorption may contribute.
- Treatment of osteoporosis consists primarily of the antiresorptive agents that are typically used to treat postmenopausal patients with osteoporosis without liver disease. Bisphosphonates appear to be the most promising given their efficacy, as well as the lack of potential adverse side effects that are associated with other agents such as HRT.
- Additional large prospective, long-term studies in patients with PBC are needed in order to determine efficacy in improving bone density as well as reducing fracture risk.

OVERVIEW OF PRIMARY BILIARY CIRRHOSIS

PBC is a liver-specific autoimmune disease that primarily affects women between the ages of 40 and 60 years, although there are rare patients diagnosed in their teens or even into their 90s.[1,2] Although some epidemiologic studies have reported a rising incidence over the past 2 decades, others report stable numbers. A systematic review of data from Europe, North America, and Australia reports an incidence of 0.9 to 5.8 per 100,000 people. Disease prevalence varies from 1.9 to 40.2 per 100,000 people, depending on geographic location, with increased rates of disease in North America and Northern Europe,[3] likely due to earlier recognition of the disease.

The exact pathophysiology of PBC is unknown, but, as with other autoimmune diseases, both genetic and environmental factors are involved. The prevalence of PBC in

[a] Gastroenterology Section, Department of Internal Medicine, VA Ann Arbor Health Care System, University of Michigan Health System, 2215 Fuller Road, Ann Arbor, MI 48105, USA;
[b] Gastroenterology Section, Specialty Care and Access, VA Ann Arbor Health Care System, University of Michigan Medical School, 2215 Fuller Road, Ann Arbor, MI 48105, USA
* Corresponding author. Gastroenterology, Veterans Affairs Medical Center, 111D VAMC 2399, 2215 Fuller Road, Ann Arbor, MI 48105.
E-mail address: gsu@med.umich.edu

Gastroenterol Clin N Am 45 (2016) 333–343
http://dx.doi.org/10.1016/j.gtc.2016.02.009
0889-8553/16/$ – see front matter Published by Elsevier Inc.
gastro.theclinics.com

first-degree relatives is more than 10 times higher than in the general population.[4] Genetic studies have shown an association between the HLA alleles DRB1*08, DR3, and DPB1*0301 and increased risk of disease, whereas DRB1*11 and DRB1*13 confer protection from PBC.[5] The advent of genome-wide association studies have uncovered many potential pathways affected in PBC, including B-cell function, antigen presentation, and T-cell differentiation.[5] Several potential environmental exposures include various bacteria (in particular, Escherichia coli and Mycobacterium gordonae), viruses, and toxic compounds, but none is definitive.[4] PBC is characterized by T-cell–mediated inflammation of the intralobular bile duct epithelium, which leads to their damage and subsequent loss. The resultant cholestasis leads to retention of toxic bile acids and eventual cirrhosis.[4]

Approximately 90% to 95% of patients with PBC are women. As with most other autoimmune diseases, the etiology of such female predominance in PBC is unclear; however, based on more recent genetic research, pathogenesis may include a combination of sex hormone abnormalities and X chromosome instabilities and defects. The X chromosome contains genes that control sex hormone levels and that are critical in maintaining immune tolerance.[6] Furthermore, preliminary data have shown there is an increased frequency of X monosomy in the circulating leukocytes of women with PBC compared with controls and that this frequency increases with patient age.[7] Although the relationship between these associations and disease pathogenesis remains to be fully understood, the findings are intriguing.

Patients can present with fatigue and pruritus or they are diagnosed on further investigation of an elevated alkaline phosphatase found on routine liver chemistries. The serologic hallmark of the disease is an elevated antimitochondrial antibody (AMA), which is present in 95% of PBC cases and in less than 1% of the normal population.[8] Liver biopsy is not always required to make the diagnosis if both alkaline phosphatase and AMA levels are elevated, but it would confirm the diagnosis if laboratory tests are inconclusive as well as stage the extent of liver disease.

The only approved treatment of PBC in the United States is ursodeoxycholic acid (UDCA). Treatment response is associated with increased survival and decreased liver transplantation, especially in long-term follow-up of patients with early-stage disease.[9–12] Proposed beneficial effects of UDCA include its ability to stimulate ductular secretions and to protect against injury from toxic bile acids as well as to downregulate B cells and AMA production.[13] Response to treatment is measured by improvement in alkaline phosphatase and bilirubin.[12] Normalization of liver tests is seen in just over half of patients at 5 years.[9]

BONE DISEASE IN PRIMARY BILIARY CIRRHOSIS
Hepatic Osteodystrophy

The term, hepatic osteodystrophy, refers to metabolic bone disease that can accompany advanced liver disease, in particular cholestatic liver diseases, such as PBC and primary sclerosing cholangitis, and includes both osteomalacia and osteoporosis[14] (Table 1). Both disorders weaken bones and increase the risk of low-trauma fractures, particularly of the vertebrae, proximal femur, and distal forearms. Osteoporosis is a skeletal bone disorder of decreased bone mass with a normal ratio of mineral and osteoid matrix, whereas osteomalacia causes softening of the bone because of defective mineralization of newly formed osteoid, which results in a decreased ratio of mineral to osteoid matrix.[15]

Osteomalacia

Osteomalacia, or decreased bone mineralization, is not as common as osteoporosis in patients with PBC and is usually associated with vitamin D deficiency, which can arise

Table 1
Bone disease in primary biliary cirrhosis

	Definition	Pathogenesis/ Diagnosis	Treatment
Hepatic osteodystrophy	• Metabolic bone disease in advanced liver disease, in particular cholestasis • Includes both osteoporosis and osteomalacia	—	—

Osteomalacia	• Decreased mineralization of newly formed osteoid
	• Decreased ratio of mineral to osteoid matrix
		• Vitamin D, calcium or phosphate deficiency
		• Laboratory abnormalities:
		  ○ Low vitamin D
		  ○ Low phosphate
		  ○ High alkaline phosphatase
		  ○ High PTH
			High-dose vitamin D and calcium supplementation

Osteoporosis	• Decreased cortical bone mass • Normal ratio of mineral to osteoid matrix	• Decreased bone formation • Increased bone resorption • Diagnosed with BMD by DXA: T score ≥ -2.5	See **Table 2**

in the setting of cholestasis and fat malabsorption. Other laboratory findings include low or low-normal calcium and phosphate and high parathyroid hormone (PTH) levels. As with those with osteoporosis, patients can present with pain, fragility fractures, and similar abnormal imaging characteristics. Patients with osteomalacia also can have muscle wasting, weakness, and pain with movement. High PTH with low levels of phosphate and vitamin D are thought to contribute to the myopathy. Definitive diagnosis is made by bone biopsy, but clinical diagnosis is often used when blood work reveals low 25-hydroxyvitamin levels (<20 ng/mL) and high PTH levels. Treatment consists of repletion of 25-hydroxyvitamin D with calcium and high doses of vitamin D_2 or vitamin D_3 at 50,000 IU once to twice per week for 6 to 8 weeks. Ongoing daily supplementation at lower doses should be continued indefinitely because patients with PBC and cholestasis continue to be at risk for recurrent deficiency.[16]

Osteoporosis

Background
Osteoporosis is the most common bone disease and currently affects more than 10 million people in the United States. It is characterized by decreased cortical bone mass as well as deterioration of the trabecular bone architecture, both of which reduce bone strength and increases risk of fracture. Low-trauma or fragility fractures are responsible for more than 400,000 hospitalizations and approximately 200,000 nursing home admissions annually in the United States.[15] Hip fractures, in particular, account for 14% of all fractures and 72% of the fracture costs. They increase 1-year mortality by 10% to 20%; 20% of patients require long-term nursing home care and

only 40% regain independence after a hip fracture.[15] Bone densitometry measures bone mass, which is the best predictor of bone strength. The gold standard of bone mineral density (BMD) measurement technology is dual-energy x-ray absorptiometry (DXA). Because bone density in the general population follows a bell-shaped curve, DXA results are reported as a z score, which is the number of SDs either above or below that of age-matched controls, and the T-score is the number of SDs above or below the mean of a young adult population. The World Health Organization defines osteoporosis in postmenopausal women and men above age 50 years as BMD at the proximal femur or spine that is greater than or equal to 2.5 SDs below the mean normal young adult reference population (T score <−2.5). Osteopenia is defined as a T score between −1 SD and −2.5 SDs. For premenopausal patients and men below the age of 50 years, osteoporosis is defined as a z score of greater than or equal to −2.0 SDs below the mean of an age-matched population.[15]

Osteoporosis is a common complication of PBC that affects between 20% and 52% of patients, depending on the characteristics of the study population (gender, age, and PBC stage) as well as the diagnostic criteria for osteoporosis (based on z score or T score).[17] The incidence of osteoporosis increases as the liver disease progresses; only approximately 20% of patients with advanced PBC have normal BMD.[18] The prevalence of osteoporosis in patients with PBC increases with female gender, age, postmenopausal state, body mass index less than 19 kg/m^2, increased severity of liver disease, and advanced fibrosis on liver biopsy.[19,20] Overall, 7% to 14% of patients with PBC sustain fractures and this risk rises to 20% in patients with end-stage PBC.[21] Because the estrogen deficiency in menopause is a well-known risk factor of osteoporosis and PBC is primarily a disease of postmenopausal women, there has been some speculation about whether PBC specifically increases the risk of osteoporosis.[17] Patients with PBC are 4 times more likely to have osteoporosis and are twice as likely to sustain a fracture compared with age-matched controls, confirming the association between liver disease and osteoporosis.[22,23] More recent data suggest that the overall prevalence decreased from 57% to 26% in PBC patients awaiting transplant from 1985 to 1989 versus 1996 to 2000, respectively, likely related to improved nutrition as well as earlier recognition and treatment of PBC.[18]

Pathogenesis in Primary biliary cirrhosis

Normal bone metabolism consists of continuous remodeling that requires a fine balance between osteosynthesis carried out by osteoblasts and osteoclast-driven bone resorption. This remodeling is largely controlled by a trimolecular complex comprised of osteoprotegerin (OPG), the receptor activator of nuclear factor κB ligand (RANKL), and RANK. RANKL is located on osteoblast membranes and its binding with RANK strongly activates osteoclast activity and therefore bone resorption. OPG, produced by the liver, can bind to RANKL to inhibit the binding of RANK and prevent osteoclast maturation and activation.[24] Bone metabolism changes significantly in women in the perimenopausal period when estrogen levels decline significantly; specifically, estradiol levels fall by 85% to 90%, causing accelerated bone loss of up to 30% in the 6-year to 10-year menopausal transition.[25] Estrogen is known to greatly influence bone metabolism by inhibiting osteoclast activity by increasing the expression of OPG and inducing osteoclast apoptosis.[26]

The exact mechanism of osteoporosis in PBC is not completely understood, but there is evidence that hormone balance, genetics, and cholestasis may contribute. There has been conflicting evidence as to whether PBC-related osteoporosis results from diminished bone formation, which is a low-turnover state, or from increased bone resorption, which is a high-turnover state. The mechanism may differ as the liver disease progresses and there may be gender-related differences in bone metabolism in PBC, making it difficult to clearly define the pathogenesis. For example, bone biopsies in patients with advanced cholestatic liver disease had evidence of decreased bone formation[20,26]; however, 1 study showed that only the women were more likely to also have markers of increased bone resorption, including increased osteoclast numbers and eroded bone surfaces whereas the men did not.[26] This difference cannot necessarily be explained by estrogen effects, because premenopausal women had similarly severe abnormalities as postmenopausal women. Additionally, levels of the liver-derived protein OPG can decrease as liver dysfunction worsens, which can then prevent the inhibition of osteoclast activity and, therefore, increase bone resorption.[17] In theory, calcium or vitamin D deficiencies could develop in the setting of decreased bile salt flow in advanced cholestasis, leading to secondary hyperparathyroidism and, finally, increased osteoclast bone resorption. There are no definitive data, however, to support this given that patients with PBC osteoporosis often have normal levels of 25-hydroxyvitamin D and 1,25-dihydroxyvitamin D[14]; additionally, complete vitamin D repletion did not have a significant impact on BMD in PBC patients with osteoporosis.[27,28]

Alternatively, there is more evidence that bone formation can be diminished, leading to low-turnover osteoporosis. Cirrhosis is associated with the reduction of specific growth factors, such as insulinlike growth factor 1, which impairs osteoblast function and bone formation. Severe cholestasis can allow build-up of lithocholic acid, which inhibits osteoblast activity and can interfere with genetic regulation of bone formation.[29] It can also lead to vitamin K deficiency, which has been shown to impair osteoblast formation and facilitate osteoclast activity in vitro.[30] There is some evidence to suggest that vitamin K repletion can improve BMD, but this study was performed in patients without liver disease.[31]

DIAGNOSIS

Bone densitometry with DXA should be performed at the initial diagnosis of PBC and should be repeated in 1 to 3 years if initial results are normal, depending on the presence of additional risk factors, including BMI less than 19 kg/m^2, heavy alcohol use, tobacco use, early menopause (<age 45 years), glucocorticoid use greater than 3 months, or family history of bone fragility fractures. Routine monitoring of calcium, phosphorus, 25-hydroxyvitamin D, and PTH should be performed every 1 to 2 years.[32]

MANAGEMENT
Prevention of Bone Loss

A reduction in the factors that can facilitate bone loss is important in the prevention of osteoporosis. Tobacco and alcohol cessation are important for many reasons, but this can also help prevent worsening bone disease. Other lifestyle modifications include increased weight-bearing exercises and diet. A 16-year prospective study has recently reported significant improvements in both lumbar spine and femoral neck BMD in early-menopausal osteopenic women who exercised regularly versus controls. These differences increased as follow-up time progressed with year 4 follow-up showing 1.9% to 2.4% and year 16 showing 3.0% to 4.5% increases.[33]

Diets should be well balanced and contain adequate levels of calcium and vitamin D. Daily dietary calcium intake should consist of at least 1200 mg per day to prevent bone loss[15]; 99% of total body calcium is stored in bone; therefore, low serum levels stimulate increased bone resorption to normalize the serum level. The average diet in people older than 50 years contains only approximately 600 mg per day to 700 mg per day; therefore, calcium supplementation is important to ensure adequate intake.

Patients over age 50 years should have between 800 and 1000 units of vitamin D per day, because this is typically sufficient for average people to maintain a 25-hydroxy-vitamin D level above 30 ng/mL.[15] Patients with malabsorption often require higher doses to maintain a normal level.

Data on calcium and vitamin D supplementation having an impact on bone density and fracture risk in the setting of PBC or chronic liver disease in general are limited. There are some data that vitamin D supplementation can at least help prevent bone loss. One trial, which included 76 patients with cirrhosis, reported the effect of calcitriol (1,25-dihydroxyvitamin D) supplementation on BMD over a 12-month to 57-month follow-up. The difference of annual change in BMD was significant, with the treated group having +0.6% versus −2.3% in the control group.[34] Similar results were seen in 34 patients with PBC where calcitriol supplementation resulted in a median annual change in BMD of +0.3% versus −3.1% in the control group.[35]

Treatment

Treatment should be initiated in any patient who presents with a low-trauma fracture or who has definitive osteoporosis with a lumbar spine or femoral neck DXA T score less than −2.5. The data for treatment in the setting of osteopenia, a T score between −1.0 and −2.5, are less clear, but the National Osteoporosis Foundation guidelines recommend treatment initiation in anyone with a 10-year hip fracture risk greater than or equal to 3% or osteoporosis-related fracture risk of greater than or equal to 20%, based on the World Health Organization Fracture Risk Assessment Tool, which uses BMD in addition to patient clinical factors.[36] Furthermore, T scores less than −1.5 are associated with increased fragility fracture risk of the lumbar spine,[37] so it is reasonable to initiate treatment in this setting.

For the most part, osteoporosis in PBC has been treated similarly to postmenopausal osteoporosis because there are few data focused specifically on PBC-related bone disease (**Table 2**).

Antiresorptive Drugs

Drugs that inhibit bone resorption are the mainstay in the treatment of osteoporosis. These agents have studied primarily in postmenopausal women and include bisphosphonates, estrogens, selective estrogen receptor modulators (SERMs), and calcitonin. Bisphosphonates and estrogen have been shown to improve both trabecular and cortical bone and lead to more robust improvement in BMD and reduce the fracture rate in the general population with osteoporosis.[38] Weaker effects have been seen in studies of SERMs and calcitonin.

Bisphosphonates

The bisphosphonates group of drugs includes alendronate, risedronate, zoledronic acid, and ibandronate. A comprehensive systematic review, including 567 trials of various treatments for osteoporosis in all patients with osteoporosis or osteopenia and a fracture, concluded that there is strong evidence that alendronate, risedronate, and zoledronic acid reduce the risk of hip and nonvertebral fractures and that alendronate, risedronate, zoledronic acid, and ibandronate reduce the risk of vertebral fractures in postmenopausal women with osteoporosis.[39] Small studies in PBC have suggested improvement in BMD with bisphosphonate treatment, but short follow-up duration and small study size precluded assessment of fracture risk.[40,41] A comprehensive Cochrane systematic review found that there are no conclusive data showing improved mortality, BMD, or reduced fracture risk with bisphosphonate treatment; furthermore, they deemed most studies included in the analysis to be highly

Table 2
Overview of Food and Drug Administration–approved medications for osteoporosis

	Dose: Prevention	Dose: Treatment	Adverse Effects
Bisphosphonates			
Alendronate	Oral 5 mg daily or 35 mg weekly	Oral 10 mg daily or 70 mg weekly	• Gastrointestinal problems:
Ibandronate	Not indicated	Oral 150 mg monthly Intravenous 3 mg every 3 mo	○ Dyspepsia ○ Esophageal and gastric inflammation
Risedronate	Oral 5 mg daily or 35 mg weekly or 150 mg monthly	Oral 5 mg daily or 35 mg weekly or 150 mg monthly	○ Diarrhea • Musculoskeletal pain
Zoledronic acid	Intravenous 5 mg every 2 y	Intravenous 5 mg every year	• Renal insufficiency • Osteonecrosis of the jaw • Hypocalcemia • Ocular side effects • atypical femur fracture • Acute reaction (intra-venous formulation)
Calcitonin[a]			
Fortical	Not indicated	Intranasal 200 IU daily	• Rhinitis
Miacalcin	Not indicated	Intranasal or subcutaneous 100 IU every other day to daily	• Nasal irritation • Nausea and vomiting • Injection site reac-tions (subcutaneous formulation)
SERM			
Raloxifene	Oral 60 mg daily	Oral 60 mg daily	• Venous thromboembolism • Hot flashes • Flu syndrome
HRT	Various oral or transdermal formulations are available	Not indicated	• Venous thromboembolism • Myocardial infarction • Stroke • Breast cancer

[a] Women who are postmenopausal ≥5 years.

biased.[42] A more recent prospective, randomized controlled trial compared the adherence to and efficacy of a 2-year regimen of the more common once-weekly aldendronate to the newer once-monthly ibandronate in 42 postmenopausal women with PBC and osteoporosis.[43] The primary endpoint of this trial was actually self-reported treatment adherence using the Morisky-Green scale, but change in BMD as measured by DXA every 6 months, liver function, and bone turnover markers were also measured. After 2 years, both treatments resulted in a significant mean increase in BMD at the lumbar spine of 4.5% in the alendronate group and 5.7% in the ibandronate group as well as at the hip, with mean improvements of 2.0% and 1.2%, respectively. Not surprisingly, adherence was significantly better in the monthly ibandronate group. Short follow-up duration did not allow for data on fracture risk.

There is a potential risk of oral bisphosphonate administration in the setting of esophageal varices, given the risk of mucosal erosion in the esophagus or stomach.

It is, therefore, recommended that patients receive parenteral bisphosphonates as an alternative in these high-risk patients.[35]

Hormone replacement therapy

Estrogens have a well-known antiresorptive effect on bone metabolism; although it carries other risks, hormone replacement therapy (HRT) has been shown to improve bone loss and decrease fracture risk. There was concern about HRT causing worsened cholestasis, particularly in preexisting liver disease, but it seems safe[44] and effective at improving BMD in PBC.[45]

Selective estrogen receptor modulators

Raloxifene is an approved SERM available in the United States to treat osteoporosis. This option was developed in response to the growing concerns about the risks of HRT. Overall, the effects of raloxifene are lower than of bisphosphonates and estrogens, but improvements in BMD have been shown. There is 1 pilot study that revealed significant improvement in lumbar BMD after 1 year of therapy in 9 women with PBC but not in age-matched controls. There was no significant effect on femoral neck bone density in either group, however, and no data on fracture risk.[46]

Calcitonin

Calcitonin has weak antiresorptive activity but has shown benefit in postmenopausal and steroid-induced osteopenia. Again, there are scant data in patients with PBC, but an early study looking at 6 months of intranasal calcitonin use in a small cohort of PBC patients showed no significant improvement; however, there was likely insufficient time to see any change.[47] Another small study showed that women with PBC receiving calcium, 1,25-dehydroxyvitamin D, and calcitonin had less bone loss than controls, although the benefit could have been related to the calcium and vitamin D supplementation.[48]

SUMMARY

PBC is a liver-specific autoimmune disease affecting mostly middle-aged women. The pathogenesis is multifactorial and not completely understood, but both genetic and environmental factors are likely involved. There is a 10-fold increased risk of developing the disease in first-degree relatives and there are several proposed environmental triggers, although none has been definitive. PBC is characterized by T-cell–mediated inflammation of the intralobular bile duct epithelium, which leads to their damage and subsequent loss. The resultant cholestasis leads to retention of toxic bile acids and eventual cirrhosis.

Metabolic bone disease, predominantly osteoporosis but also osteomalacia, is a common complication of PBC, with prevalence of osteoporosis ranging between 20% and 52%. The risk of developing osteoporosis increases with histologic severity of liver disease, older age, and duration of cholestasis. The osteoporosis seen in PBC seems mainly due to low bone formation, although increased bone resorption may contribute. The development of osteoporosis confers risk of low-trauma fracture, which adds significant health care cost and increases patient morbidity and mortality.

Prevention of bone disease by avoiding excess alcohol and tobacco and eating a well-balanced diet with adequate calcium and vitamin D are important. Although strong data in the PBC population are lacking, treatment consists primarily of the antiresorptive agents typically used to treat postmenopausal patients with osteoporosis without liver disease. Bisphosphonates are the most promising given their efficacy as well as the lack of potential adverse side effects that are associated with other agents, such as HRT. Additional large, prospective, long-term studies of antiresorptives in patients with PBC are needed to more definitively determine the impact on BMD as well as fracture risk. Additionally, improved understanding of the pathogenesis of PBC-related osteoporosis may result in improved treatment options.

REFERENCES

1. Kaplan MM, Gershwin ME. Primary biliary cirrhosis. N Engl J Med 2005; 353(12):1261.
2. Dahlan Y, Smith L, Simmonds D, et al. Pediatric-onset primary biliary cirrhosis. Gastroenterology 2003;125(5):1476.
3. Boonstra K, Beuers U, Ponsioen CY. Epidemiology of primary sclerosing cholangitis and primary biliary cirrhosis: a systematic review. J Hepatol 2012;56:1181–8.
4. Carey EJ, Ali AH, Lindor KD. Primary biliary cirrhosis. Lancet 2015;386(10003): 1565–75.
5. Bianchi I, Carbone M, Lleo A, et al. Genetics and epigenetics of primary biliary cirrhosis. Semin Liver Dis 2014;34:255–64.
6. Invernizzi P, Miozzo M, Selmi C, et al. X chromosome monosomy: a common mechanism for autoimmune diseases. J Immunol 2005;175(1):575–8.
7. Invernizzi P, Miozzo M, Battezzati PM, et al. Frequency of monosomy X in women with primary biliary cirrhosis. Lancet 2004;363:533–5.
8. Miyakawa H, Tanaka A, Kikuchi K, et al. Detection of antimitochondrial autoantibodies in immunofluorescent AMA-negative patients with primary biliary cirrhosis using recombinant autoantigens. Hepatology 2001;34(2):243.
9. Parés A, Caballería L, Rodés J. Excellent long-term survival in patients with primary biliary cirrhosis and biochemical response to ursodeoxycholic acid. Gastroenterology 2006;130(3):715.
10. Poupon RE, Poupon R, Balkau B. Ursodiol for the long-term treatment of primary biliary cirrhosis. The UDCA-PBC Study Group. N Engl J Med 1994;330(19):1342.
11. Kuiper EM, Hansen BE, de Vries RA, et al. Improved prognosis of patients with primary biliary cirrhosis that have a biochemical response to ursodeoxycholic acid. Gastroenterology 2009;136(4):1281.
12. Lammers WJ, Hirschfield GM, Corpechot C, et al. Development and validation of a scoring system to predict outcomes of patients with primary biliary cirrhosis receiving ursodeoxycholic acid therapy. Gastroenterology 2015;149(7): 1804–12.e4.
13. Poupon R. Ursodeoxycholic acid and bile-acid mimetics as therapeutic agents for cholestatic liver diseases: an overview of their mechanisms of action. Clin Res Hepatol Gastroenterol 2012;36(Suppl 1):S3–12.
14. Leslie WD, Bernstein CN, Leboff MS. AGA technical review on osteoporosis in hepatic disorders. Gastroenterology 2013;125:941–66.
15. US Department of Health and Human Services. Bone health and osteoporosis: a report of the surgeon general. Rockville (MD): US Department of Health and Human Services, Office of the Surgeon General; 2004.
16. Lips P, van Schoor NM, Bravenboer N. Vitamin D-related disorders. In: Rosen CJ, Compston JE, Lian JB, editors. Primer on the metabolic bone diseases and disorders of mineral metabolism. 7th edition. Washington, DC: American Society for Bone and Mineral Research; 2008. p. 329.
17. Pares A, Guanabens N. Osteoporosis in primary biliary cirrhosis: pathogenesis and treatment. Clin Liver Dis 2008;12:407–24.

18. Guichelaar MMJ, Kendall R, Schmoll J, et al. Bone mineral density before and after OLT: long-term follow-up and predictive factors. Liver Transpl 2006;12: 1390–402.

19. Menon J, Angulo P, Weston S, et al. Bone disease in primary biliary cirrhosis: independent indicators and rate of progression. Hepatology 2001;35:316–23.

20. Guanabens N, Pares A, Marinoso L, et al. Factors influencing the development of metabolic bone disease in primary biliary cirrhosis. Am J Gastroenterol 1990;85: 1356–62.

21. Guichelaar M, Hay J, Clark B, et al. Pretransplant bone histomorphometric status of patients with end-stage cholestatic liver disease. J Hepatol 2000;32:54.

22. Guanabens N, Pares A, Ros I, et al. Severity of cholestasis and advanced histological stage but not menopausal status are the major risk factors for osteoporosis in primary biliary cirrhosis. J Hepatol 2005;42:573–7.

23. Solaymani–Dodaran M, Card TR, Aithal GP, et al. Fracture risk in people with primary biliary cirrhosis: a population-based cohort study. Gastroenterology 2006; 131:1752–7.

24. Kohli SS, Kohli VS. Role of RANKL–RANK/osteoprotegerin molecular complex in bone remodeling and its immunopathologic implications. Indian J Endocrinol Metab 2011;15(3):175–81.

25. Drake MT, Clarke BL, Lewiecki EM. The pathophysiology and treatment of osteoporosis. Clin Ther 2015;37(8):1837–50.

26. Guichelaar MMJ, Malincho M, Sibonga J, et al. Bone metabolism in advanced cholestatic liver disease: analysis by bone histomorphometry. Hepatology 2002;36(4):895–903.

27. Herlong H, Recker R. Bone disease in primary biliary cirrhosis: histologic features and response to 25-hydroxyvitamin D. Gastroenterology 1982;83:103–8.

28. Matloff D, Kaplan M, Neer RM, et al. Osteoporosis in primary biliary cirrhosis: effects of 25-hydroxyvitamin D3 treatment. Gastroenterology 1982;83:97–102.

29. Ruiz-Gaspa S, Guanabens N, Enjuanes A, et al. Lithocholic acid downregulates vitamin D effects in human osteoblasts. Eur J Clin Invest 2010;40:25–34.

30. Koshihara Y, Hoshi K, Okawara R, et al. Vitamin K stimulates osteoblastogenesis and inhibits osteoclastogenesis in human bone marrow cell culture. J Endocrinol 2003;176:339–48.

31. Cockayne S, Adamson J, Lanham-New S, et al. Vitamin K and the prevention of fractures. Arch Intern Med 2006;166:1256–61.

32. Pares A, Guanabens N. Treatment of bone disorders in liver disease. J Hepatol 2006;45:445–53.

33. Kemmler W, Engelke K, von Stengel S, et al. Long-term exercise and Bone Mineral density changes in postmenopausal women- are there periods of reduced effectiveness? J Bone Miner Res 2016;31(1):215–22.

34. Shiomi S, Masaki K, Habu D, et al. Calcitriol for bone disease in patients with cirrhosis of the liver. J Gastroenterol Hepatol 1999;14:547–52.

35. Shiomi S, Masaki K, Habu D, et al. Calcitriol for bone loss in patients with primary biliary cirrhosis. J Gastroenterol 1999;34:241–5.

36. NOF's Clinician's Guide to Prevention and Treatment of Osteoporosis. Available at: http://nof.org/files/nof/public/content/file/344/upload/159.pdf. Accessed October 25, 2015.

37. Guanabens N, Cerda D, Monegal A, et al. Low bone mass and severity of cholestasis affect fracture risk in patients with primary biliary cirrhosis. Gastroenterology 2010;138:2348–56.

38. Hay JE, Guichelaar MMJ. Evaluation and management of osteoporosis in liver disease. Clin Liver Dis 2005;9:747–66.
39. Agency for Healthcare Research and Quality. Treatment to prevent osteoporotic fractures: An update. Available at: http://www.effectivehealthcare.ahrq.gov/index.cfm. Accessed October 25, 2015.
40. Guanabens N, Pares A, Ros I, et al. Alendronate is more effective than etidronate for increasing bone mass in osteopenic patients with primary biliary cirrhosis. Am J Gastroenterol 2003;98:2268–71.
41. Zein CO, Jorgensen RA, Clarke B, et al. Alendronate improves bone mineral density in primary biliary cirrhosis: a randomized placebo-controlled trial. Hepatology 2005;42:762–71.
42. Rudic JS, Giljaca V, Krstic MN, et al. Bisphosphonates for osteoporosis in primary biliary cirrhosis. Cochrane Database Syst Rev 2011;(12):CD009144.
43. Guanabens N, Monegal A, Cerdá D, et al. A randomized trial comparing monthly ibandronate and weekly alendronate for osteoporosis in patients with primary biliary cirrhosis. Hepatology 2013;58:2070–8.
44. Menon KVN, Angulo P, Boe GM, et al. Safety and efficacy of estrogen therapy in preventing bone loss in primary biliary cirrhosis. Am J Gastroenterol 2003;98:889–92.
45. Pereira SP, Donohue J, Moniz C, et al. Transdermal hormone replacement therapy improves vertebral bone density in primary biliary cirrhosis: results of a 1-year controlled trial. Aliment Pharmacol Ther 2004;19:563–70.
46. Levy C, Harnois DM, Angulo P, et al. Raloxifene improves bone mass in osteopenic women with primary biliary cirrhosis: results of a pilot study. Liver Int 2005;25:117–21.
47. Floreani A, Chiaramonte M, Giannini S, et al. Longitudinal study on osteodystrophy in primary biliary cirrhosis (PBC) and a pilot study on calcitonin treatment. J Hepatol 1991;12:217–23.
48. Floreani A, Zappala F, Naccarato R, et al. A 3-year pilot study with 1,25-diydroxyvitamin D, calcium, and calcitonin for severe osteodystrophy in primary biliary cirrhosis. J Clin Gastroenterol 1997;24:239–44.

Women with Cirrhosis
Prevalence, Natural History, and Management

Jeanne-Marie Giard, MD, MPH, Norah A. Terrault, MD, MPH*

KEYWORDS

- Women's health • Cirrhosis • Pregnancy • Hepatitis B • Hepatitis C
- Alcoholic Liver Disease • Nonalcoholic Fatty Liver Disease • Portal Hypertension

KEY POINTS

- Cirrhosis is less frequent in women than in men, in large part due to the lower prevalence of hepatitis B, hepatitis C, and alcohol use/abuse in women.
- The most common causes of cirrhosis in women are hepatitis C, autoimmune etiologies, nonalcoholic steatohepatitis, and alcoholic liver disease.
- For most liver diseases, fibrosis progression appears to be slower in premenopausal women than in men, but with rates of progression equalizing in postmenopausal women.
- Women are at lower risk of hepatocellular carcinoma and have better outcomes than men following diagnosis.
- Pregnancy in women with cirrhosis is rare, as fertility is reduced and associated with high risk of complications.

INTRODUCTION

Cirrhosis is an important public health concern in the United States. In a recent analysis of the National Health and Nutrition Examination Survey (NHANES) data conducted between 1999 and 2010, the prevalence of cirrhosis in the United States was approximately 0.27%, corresponding to 633,323 adults.[1] Women represented 27% of those adults. This lower prevalence of cirrhosis in women is closely related to their lower prevalence of hepatitis B virus (HBV) and hepatitis C virus (HCV) infections,[2,3] alcohol dependence,[4] and iron overload. It is still unsettled if nonalcoholic steatohepatitis is more prevalent in women that in men.[5] The most common causes of cirrhosis

No conflict of interest related to this article.
Division of Gastroenterology, Department of Medicine, University of California, San Francisco, 400 Parnassus Avenue, San Francisco, CA 94143, USA
* Corresponding author. 400 Parnassus Avenue, San Francisco, CA 94143.
E-mail address: norah.terrault@ucsf.edu

among women in the United States are HCV, autoimmune etiologies, nonalcoholic steatohepatitis, and alcoholic liver disease[6,7] (**Table 1**).

With increasing focus on a more personalized approach to care, knowledge of sex differences in liver disease prevalence, natural history, and treatment is important to optimize individual long-term outcomes. Additionally, there are unique issues in managing women with advanced stages of fibrosis with regard to conception, pregnancy, and postpartum care.

SEX DIFFERENCES IN THE NATURAL HISTORY OF SPECIFIC LIVER DISEASES

Chronic Hepatitis C

Globally and especially in North America, chronic HCV is a major cause of cirrhosis, hepatocellular carcinoma, and liver-related mortality (**Table 2**).[8,9] The natural history of HCV has consistently been shown to be different in women compared with men. Spontaneous clearance of the virus occurs more frequently among women than men. In a recently published collaboration of 9 prospective cohorts of HCV-infected patients, 37% of women with acute HCV infection cleared the virus, whereas only 21% of men did so.[10] Female sex is also a protective factor for the progression of liver fibrosis in premenopausal but not postmenopausal women with HCV, believed to reflect the protective effect of estrogens. In an analysis of 157 women with HCV (61 premenopausal and 96 postmenopausal), postmenopausal women had higher mean fibrosis scores than premenopausal women (1.87 ± 0.16 vs 1.17 ± 0.10; $P<.01$) and rates of fibrosis progression (119 ± 5 vs $93 \pm 12 \times 10^{-3}$ METAVIR units/y; $P<.05$).[11] Moreover, among postmenopausal women, there was less advanced fibrosis in those who had received hormone replacement therapy compared with those who had not (1.79 ± 0.25 vs 1.93 ± 0.20; $P<.05$) and slower rate of fibrosis progression (99 ± 16 vs $133 \pm 6 \times 10^{-3}$ METAVIR units/y; $P = .02$). In addition to the potential fibrosis-modifying effect of sex hormones, other factors contributing to a lower rate of advanced liver disease in women compared with men include the lower frequency of cofactors associated with accelerated disease progression, like alcohol use and human immunodeficiency virus infection.[12,13] In a study of 376 young Irish women who contracted HCV in 1977 and 1978 from contaminated anti-D immune globulin, only 1.9% had probable or definitive cirrhosis after a follow-up of 17 years.[14] A similar German cohort study of 1980 women who contracted HCV in 1978 to 1979 from contaminated anti-D immune globulin showed that after 25 years, only 9 patients (0.5%) had cirrhosis and 1 hepatocellular carcinoma (HCC) was diagnosed.[15] Comparatively, an analysis of the Electronically Retrieved Cohort of HCV Infected Veterans (92.9% men), in which HCV-positive patients were identified with an initial

Table 1		
Common causes of cirrhosis in women versus men		
Patient Type and Country	**Women[a]**	**Men[a]**
Cirrhosis estimated by population-based study (England)[7]	Alcoholic liver disease Cryptogenic Autoimmune Viral hepatitis	Alcoholic liver disease Cryptogenic Viral hepatitis Autoimmune
Cirrhosis estimated by those on waiting list for transplantation (US)[6]	Viral Autoimmune etiologies Nonalcoholic fatty liver disease Alcoholic liver disease	Viral Alcoholic liver disease Nonalcoholic fatty liver disease Autoimmune etiologies

[a] Listed from most prevalent to less prevalent.

Table 2
Sex variation in natural history of liver diseases

Liver Disease	Disease Progression in Women Compared with Men
Hepatitis C	• More frequent spontaneous clearance[10] • Slower progression to cirrhosis before menopause[11] • Accelerated progression to cirrhosis after menopause[11] • More ribavirin-associated anemia[22,23]
Hepatitis B	• Less flares[27,28] • Less reactivation following HBeAg seroconversion[29]
Alcoholic liver disease	• More hepatic damage for same alcohol quantity[33]
Nonalcoholic steatohepatitis	• Slower progression to cirrhosis before menopause[40] • Accelerated progression to cirrhosis after menopause[40]

negative and subsequent positive test result for HCV antibody, showed that after 10 years of follow-up, 18.4% of patients had developed cirrhosis.[16]

To date, there are no sex differences identified in studies of HCV treatment with direct-acting antiviral (DAA) therapy.[17–21] However, tolerability of ribavirin, a component of some DAA regimens, may be reduced in women due to lower baseline hemoglobin levels.[22,23] The teratogenicity associated with ribavirin should also be considered in every woman of child-bearing age undergoing HCV therapy.

Chronic Hepatitis B Virus

Chronic HBV is an important disease globally, and in the United States approximately 2.2 million infected persons are chronically infected, mostly among those who are foreign born.[24] Women have a lower rate of progression to cirrhosis and HCC then men. In an analysis of 3582 patients with HBV, followed for a mean of 11 years, male sex was associated with a 2.5 increased risk of progression to cirrhosis.[25] Likewise, the incidence of HBV-related HCC is 3 to 6 times higher in men than in women.[26]

As discussed with HCV, those sex differences may be related to a higher prevalence of cofactors for disease progression, including alcohol use, iron overload, and HCV infection. Additionally, natural history studies suggest a higher frequency of HBV flares in men compared with women.[27,28] In a longitudinal study of 217 patients with HB envelope Antigen (HBeAg)-negative HBV and alanine aminotransferase (ALT) levels ≤40 IU/mL (with range of HBV DNA levels) followed for a median of almost 6 years, 24% of the men experienced an acute increase in ALT (≥80 IU/mL) compared with only 7% of women. The sex discrepancy persisted even after adjustment for confounders, including age, HBV DNA level, fibrosis stage and presence of precore and basal core promoter variants.[27] Similarly, another study of acute exacerbation of HBV in HBeAg-positive and HBeAg-negative patients, found that men were more likely to develop exacerbations than women.[28] In keeping with those findings, reactivation of HBV following HBeAg seroconversion was found to happen more often in men than in women in a study of 133 patients in Taiwan.[29] This sex difference is not completely understood but it may contribute to the higher prevalence of HBV-related cirrhosis and hepatocellular carcinoma in men.

Treatment recommendations for HBV do not differ for men versus women, other than the upper limits of a normal ALT are 19 U/L for women and 30 U/L for men.[30] Women who have ALT levels greater than 38 U/L (2 times upper of limit of normal) and persistently elevated HBV DNA levels are potential candidates for antiviral therapy.[30] For women with cirrhosis, antiviral therapy is recommended if HBV viremia is present, regardless of ALT level.

Alcoholic Liver Disease

In a recent systematic review on sex differences in alcohol use, women were found to consume less alcohol than men, to drink less frequently, and to be less likely to be hazardous drinkers.[12] Similarly, recent results of the US National Epidemiologic Survey on Alcohol and Related Conditions (which used DSM-5 criteria) reported a higher lifetime prevalence of alcohol use disorders in men (36.0%) compared with women (22.7%).[31] However, women who drink alcohol develop more liver problems than men who drink alcohol. It is recognized that for a comparable amount of alcohol intake, blood ethanol concentrations are higher in women than men. This is likely explained by 2 physiologic differences. First, women express less gastric alcohol dehydrogenase, an enzyme involved in first-pass metabolism of alcohol.[32] Moreover, women have less fat tissue and less total water than men, hence smaller volume of distribution of alcohol. Multiple studies have found that alcohol-related hepatic damage occurs more rapidly in women than in men. The most frequently referenced study, following 13,285 adults prospectively for 12 years, determined that the level of alcohol intake above which the relative risk of liver damage was significantly greater than 1 was 7 to 13 drinks per week for women and 14 to 27 drinks per week for men.[33] Thus, women should be counseled to keep alcohol intake to less than 1 drink per day or 7 per week. If women have another cause for chronic liver disease, such as HCV or HBV, abstinence is recommended.

The cornerstone of treatment of cirrhosis caused by alcohol is abstinence. Women tend to do better after outpatient treatment and achieve more sustained abstinence then men.[12] In a 20-year prospective study of 393 alcoholic patients who had undergone therapy, women achieved higher abstinence rates (47.2% vs 29.0%, $P = .005$) and had lower mortality (22.4% vs 34.5%, $P = .03$) than men.[34] There was no sex difference in outcomes among 3 studies looking into the treatment of alcohol dependence with pharmacologic agents (acamprosate and naltrexone).[12]

Nonalcoholic Fatty Liver Disease

Nonalcoholic fatty liver disease (NAFLD) appears to be less common in women than in men, although population-based studies with accurate measures of NAFLD are lacking.[35–37] In a study of 328 American patients, 89 (55.3%) of 161 men and 62 (37.1%) of 167 women had evidence of NAFLD on ultrasound. In another study looking into the hepatic triglyceride content of 2287 patients in Texas, using proton magnetic resonance spectroscopy, frequency of hepatic steatosis was 42% in white men and 24% in white women. Black and Hispanic women and men showed approximately the same frequency of hepatic steatosis (45% and 23%, respectively). Among women, advancing age, postmenopausal status, and more features of the metabolic syndrome have been linked with presence of NAFLD.[38]

Whether there are sex differences in the natural history of NAFLD is uncertain. A systematic review of 10 studies evaluating risk factors associated with fibrosis progression in nonalcoholic steatohepatitis (NASH) found that age and hepatic inflammation were predictors of fibrosis, but it did not identify female sex as a significant risk factor.[39] However, in a recent cross-sectional study of 541 patients that examined premenopausal and postmenopausal women and men, greater severity of liver fibrosis was seen in men compared with premenopausal women, but postmenopausal women had comparable degrees of liver fibrosis as men. Adjusted cumulative odds ratio for greater fibrosis severity was 1.4 ($P = .17$) for postmenopausal women and 1.6 (95% confidence interval 1.0–2.5, $P = .03$) for men, compared with premenopausal women.[40] Those findings support the hypothesis that sex hormones influence hepatic fibrosis in NASH, similar to seen in other chronic liver diseases.[11,25] Along those same lines, hormone replacement therapy has been shown to reduce the serum aminotransferase levels in women with NAFLD.[41] The effect of oral contraceptives on NAFLD progression is unclear. In a study of 4338 menstruating women in NHANES III, oral contraceptive users had 50% lower odds of NAFLD (defined as moderate–severe steatosis on ultrasonography) than nonusers, but this association was no longer significant after adjusting for obesity.[42]

WOMEN AND COMPLICATIONS OF CIRRHOSIS
Prognosis

Female sex has been inconsistently associated with mortality in cirrhosis.[43–45] In a systematic review of 68 studies evaluating prognostic factors associated with mortality and that included sex as an explanatory variable, only 9 studies identified sex as one of the top 5 prognostic factors.[45] In 1 of the larger series of 1155 patients with cirrhosis (404 women and 751 men) followed for 6 years, female sex was associated with a reduced risk of mortality in patients with compensated cirrhosis ($P = .003$)[43] but did not influence mortality among decompensated patients. However, other studies have not identified sex as an important factor in predicting mortality in patients with cirrhosis.[46,47] Heterogeneity in treatable causes of cirrhosis, different times to diagnosis, and/or difference in adherence to cirrhosis management may be potential factors influencing outcomes in women versus men with cirrhosis.

In patients with complications of end-stage liver disease, liver transplantation is the treatment of choice. Women have higher wait-list mortality than men, and this disparity is greater in the model of end-stage liver disease (MELD) era.[48] This is, in part, due to creatinine (a component of MELD) underestimating severity of renal dysfunction in women and also because women are shorter than men and smaller grafts are less available.[49–51] In general, posttransplant graft and patient survival do not differ by sex,[52] with the notable exception of HCV: women have more severe recurrent disease, with a 23% higher risk of advanced fibrosis than men after a median of 3 years after liver transplantation.[53] Women are also at higher risk of chronic kidney disease posttransplant (5 years posttransplant, odds ratio 2.5, $P = .004$).[51] The explanation for these sex disparities is unknown.

Portal Hypertension Complications

Rates of portal hypertensive complications are comparable in women and men with cirrhosis. The development and progression of esophageal varices,[54,55] portal hypertensive gastropathy,[56] ascites,[57] spontaneous bacterial peritonitis,[58] and encephalopathy[59] are not affected by sex. A few notable exceptions are gastric antral vascular ectasia (GAVE) and portopulmonary hypertension. Across all patients (those with and without cirrhosis), GAVE tends to be diagnosed more frequently in women than men, an association thought to reflect the higher prevalence of autoimmune diseases in women. However, among patients with cirrhosis, GAVE does not appear to a sex predilection. Portopulmonary hypertension affects 6% of patients with cirrhosis and some,[60] but not all, studies[61,62] report a higher rate of this complication among women. In a multicenter case-control study, female sex was associated with a 2.9-fold higher risk of portopulmonary hypertension ($P = .018$).[60]

Hepatocellular Cancer Risk

Globally, HCC ranks as the fifth most common cancer diagnosed in men and the ninth most common cancer diagnosed in women.[63] Studies consistently report a lower risk of HCC in women than men.[64] In the United States, results from the Surveillance, Epidemiology, and End Results Program indicate an incidence of liver cancer between

2008 and 2012 of 12.7/ 100,000 persons in males and 4.3/100,000 persons in females, for a risk ratio of 2.95. Worldwide, this ratio varies from 1.3 to 3.6.[65] This difference in incidence is partially explained by the reduced female exposure to HBV and HCV, alcohol, and iron overload. However, the decreased risk of HCC in women persists even after controlling for those confounders. The biological explanation for this residual difference in risk is uncertain, but may in part be related to the protective effect of estrogens. In a multicenter case-control study including only women, the risk of HCC was inversely related to the number of full-term pregnancies at age of menopause.[66] Oophorectomy at age younger than 50 years and absence of hormonal replacement therapy were also risks factors for HCC.[66] Testosterone level also seems to play a role in HCC etiology, as some studies in Taiwan have reported a positive association between the level of circulating testosterone and HCC in men.[67,68]

In a large Italian study of 1834 patients (482 women and 1352 men), women with HCC were found to be diagnosed at an older age (age of diagnosis >70 years; women 52%, men 32%), had higher alpha-fetoprotein levels (<20 ng/mL; women 31%, men 40%) and were more likely to have smaller unifocal and well-differentiated HCC than men.[69] Women had a significantly longer survival than men after diagnosis (median 29 vs 24 months, $P = .0001$). However, this survival difference disappeared when only patients undergoing surveillance were considered, which may suggest that women were more compliant with surveillance and, consequently, tumors were detected at an earlier stage, offering more therapeutic opportunities.

INFERTILITY AND CONTRACEPTION

A frequent problem in premenopausal women with cirrhosis is anovulation or irregular ovulation, thought to be secondary to hypothalamic-pituitary dysfunction[70,71] and alteration in hepatic sex hormone metabolism.[72] In a study of women younger than 46 years of age on the waiting list for liver transplantation, 53% reported regular menstrual cycles, 27% irregular and unpredictable bleeding, and 20% amenorrhea.[73] Liver function was not correlated with menstrual patterns. Sexual dysfunction, defined as reduced sex frequency and satisfaction, was more prevalent in women with end-stage liver disease than in men.[74] Increased age and more severe liver disease were related to lower sexual frequency and satisfaction.

Despite decreased fertility, undesired pregnancies can occur and therefore contraception must be discussed with premenopausal women who have cirrhosis (**Table 3**). There were early concerns regarding a potential association between oral contraceptive use and heightened risk of HCC. However, a meta-analysis of observational studies concluded that there was insufficient evidence to establish a relation between oral contraceptives and the risk of HCC.[75] In 2009, the World Health Organization expert Working Group on Family Planning Guidance reviewed published literature on contraception and liver diseases and declared that in women with compensated cirrhosis, there was no restriction on the use of any hormonal contraceptive method, whereas in women with severe, decompensated cirrhosis, the risks usually outweigh the benefits.[76] Intrauterine contraception devices have not been studied in patients with cirrhosis but caution is warranted, as spontaneous bacterial peritonitis associated with an intrauterine device has been reported.[77] Barrier methods can be used, but failure rates of contraception with this method are limiting.[78]

PREGNANCY IN CIRRHOSIS

The incidence of cirrhosis in pregnant women is very low, approximately 1 in 5950 pregnancies.[79] Pregnancies in women with cirrhosis carry higher risks for the mother

Table 3
Contraception methods in women with cirrhosis: pros and cons

Contraception Method	Contraception Failure, %[78,a]	Pros	Cons
Oral contraceptive	0.3–9.0	• No link between oral contraception and hepatocellular carcinoma has been confirmed[75,76] • No formal restriction in patients with compensated cirrhosis[76]	• Not suggested in decompensated cirrhosis[76]
Condom	2–18	• Can be used at any stage of cirrhosis	• Moderate efficacy
Tubal ligation	0.5	• Permanent solution	• Necessitates surgery, not recommended if Child-Pugh B or C cirrhosis
Intrauterine device	0.2	• Highest efficacy • If compensated cirrhosis, insertion should not be associated with increased bleeding risk[85]	• 1 case of reported of intrauterine device–associated spontaneous bacterial peritonitis[77]
barrier methods (sponge, spermicides, diaphragm)	6–28	• Safe in patients with cirrhosis[85]	• Low efficacy

[a] Among patients without cirrhosis. Percentage of women experiencing an unintended pregnancy during the first year of perfect use of contraception and the first year of typical use.

and fetus and a multidisciplinary team that includes a liver specialist and a high-risk obstetrician are essential throughout the pregnancy and postpartum period.

Maternal Outcomes

The most worrisome aspect of pregnancy in women with cirrhosis is the possible exacerbation of portal hypertension and its clinical consequences. The normal physiologic changes associated with pregnancy can contribute to worsening portal hypertension[80] (**Table 4**). Those alterations start to develop as early as the sixth week and peak between the 30th and 34th week of gestation.[81,82] In the most recent review on pregnancy and cirrhosis, the investigators followed 62 pregnancies in 29 women.[83] A significant maternal complication occurred in 6 (10%) of 62 of the pregnancies and included variceal bleeding (n = 3), significant ascites (n = 2), and hepatic encephalopathy (n = 1). Importantly, MELD-predicted risk of maternal complications.[83] Receiver operator curve analysis demonstrated that a MELD score ≥10 predicted, with 83% sensitivity and 83% specificity, which women were likely to have significant, liver-related complications. Although there are no specific guidelines on the management of varices during pregnancy, expert opinion favors an aggressive approach to prophylaxis (**Fig. 1**).[80,82,84–86]

In the case of acute variceal bleed during pregnancy, the endoscopic management is similar to that in nonpregnant patients; that is, variceal band ligation until obliteration. In the acute phase, the concomitant use of octreotide is debatable as it is formally

Table 4
Liver-relevant laboratory and hemodynamic changes during pregnancy

Hemodynamic[82]	Increased blood volume by 30%–50%
	Increased heart rate
	Reduced systemic vascular resistance
Laboratory	Reduced albumin and total protein (dilutional)[92]
	Elevated alkaline phosphatase (placental source)[92]
	Physiologic anemia (dilutional)[93]
	Decreased bilirubin levels and γ-glutamyl transferase (dilutional)[92]
	No significant changes in aspartate aminotransferase, alanine aminotransferase[92]
	Platelets: most studies suggest no changes[94–96]

classified by the Food and Drug Administration as pregnancy category B, but its similarity to vasopressin raises the concerns for splanchnic vasoconstriction, which can result in decreased placental perfusion and an increased risk of placental abruption.[85] Four successful placements of a transjugular intrahepatic portosystemic shunt (TIPS) have been described during pregnancy, all with negligible radiation exposure.[86,87] All women survived and 1 fetus died from premature delivery, but this outcome was not considered to be TIPS-related.

Peri-Partum Management

Labor management is dependent on the degree of portal hypertension. For women with known varices, caesarian delivery has traditionally been suggested, to minimize the risk of variceal bleeding related to excessive straining and increased intravariceal pressure associated with vaginal delivery.[88] However, very few cases of variceal hemorrhage at the time of delivery have been reported.[89] Moreover, caesarian delivery carries risks, including bleeding from injury to abdominal wall collaterals,

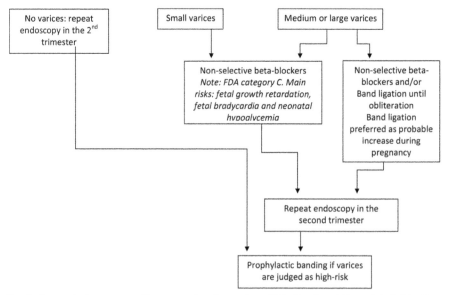

Fig. 1. Suggested preconception screening for varices. FDA, Food and Drug Administration.

postoperative ascites, and poor wound-healing issues. Additionally, as with any operative procedure in a patient with cirrhosis, there is a risk of worsening liver decompensation. Therefore, some experts suggest an attempt at vaginal delivery conducted by a senior obstetrician, with caesarian delivery reserved for obstetric indications.[80,82,90] The second stage of labor should be kept short and excessive fluid overload should be avoided. As for sedation, gentle intravenous labor analgesia can be given, whereas epidural analgesia safety depends on the coagulopathy severity. Postpartum women with portal hypertension should also be vigilantly watched for possible uterine hemorrhage.

Fetal Outcomes

Data are relatively limited, but in a 2015 retrospective cohort of 2,284,218 pregnancies in California, cirrhosis was associated with more risk of preeclampsia, preterm delivery, low birth weight, small for gestational age, and neonatal death.[91]

SUMMARY/DISCUSSION

The most common causes of cirrhosis among women are HCV, nonalcoholic steatohepatitis, and alcoholic liver disease. Women generally have slower rates of fibrosis progression to cirrhosis and lower incidence of HCC than men, at least until the onset of menopause. For those women needing liver transplantation, waiting-list mortality is higher than men, a disparity made greater in the MELD era. Posttransplant outcomes for women are similar to men. Clinicians should have those differences in mind when evaluating a woman with end-stage liver disease, so as to tailor follow-up and management. Contraception should be discussed with premenopausal women with cirrhosis. As for pregnancy-related outcomes, women with cirrhosis women are at higher risk of maternal and fetal complications and patients should be fully informed that despite optimal perinatal care, there remains a substantial risk of complication and this should be strongly considered before deciding on conception.

REFERENCES

1. Scaglione S, Kliethermes S, Cao G, et al. The epidemiology of cirrhosis in the United States: a population-based study. J Clin Gastroenterol 2015;49(8):690–6.

2. Denniston MM, Jiles RB, Drobeniuc J, et al. Chronic hepatitis C virus infection in the United States, National Health and Nutrition Examination Survey 2003 to 2010. Ann Intern Med 2014;160(5):293–300.

3. Ioannou GN. Hepatitis B virus in the United States: infection, exposure, and immunity rates in a nationally representative survey. Ann Intern Med 2011;154(5): 319–28.

4. Hasin DS, Stinson FS, Ogburn E, et al. Prevalence, correlates, disability, and comorbidity of DSM-IV alcohol abuse and dependence in the United States: results from the National Epidemiologic Survey on alcohol and related conditions. Arch Gen Psychiatry 2007;64(7):830–42.

5. Vernon G, Baranova A, Younossi ZM. Systematic review: the epidemiology and natural history of non-alcoholic fatty liver disease and non-alcoholic steatohepatitis in adults. Aliment Pharmacol Ther 2011;34(3):274–85.

6. Lai JC, Terrault NA, Vittinghoff E, et al. Height contributes to the gender difference in wait-list mortality under the MELD-based liver allocation system. Am J Transplant 2010;10(12):2658–64.

7. Ratib S, West J, Crooks CJ, et al. Diagnosis of liver cirrhosis in England, a cohort study, 1998-2009: a comparison with cancer. Am J Gastroenterol 2014;109(2): 190–8.

8. Razavi H, Elkhoury AC, Elbasha E, et al. Chronic hepatitis C virus (HCV) disease burden and cost in the United States. Hepatology 2013;57(6):2164–70.

9. Tholey DM, Ahn J. Impact of Hepatitis C virus infection on hepatocellular carcinoma. Gastroenterol Clin North Am 2015;44(4):761–73.

10. Grebely J, Page K, Sacks-Davis R, et al. The effects of female sex, viral genotype, and IL28B genotype on spontaneous clearance of acute hepatitis C virus infection. Hepatology 2014;59(1):109–20.

11. Di Martino V, Lebray P, Myers RP, et al. Progression of liver fibrosis in women infected with hepatitis C: long-term benefit of estrogen exposure. Hepatology 2004; 40(6):1426–33.

12. Erol A, Karpyak VM. Sex and gender-related differences in alcohol use and its consequences: contemporary knowledge and future research considerations. Drug Alcohol Depend 2015;156:1–13.

13. Centers for Disease Control and Prevention (CDC). HIV infections attributed to male-to-male sexual contact—metropolitan statistical areas, United States and Puerto Rico, 2010. MMWR Morb Mortal Wkly Rep 2012;61(47):962–6.

14. Kenny-Walsh E. Clinical outcomes after hepatitis C infection from contaminated anti-D immune globulin. Irish Hepatology Research Group. N Engl J Med 1999; 340(16):1228–33.

15. Wiese M, Grungreiff K, Guthoff W, et al. Outcome in a hepatitis C (genotype 1b) single source outbreak in Germany–a 25-year multicenter study. J Hepatol 2005; 43(4):590–8.

16. Butt AA, Yan P, Lo Re V 3rd, et al. Liver fibrosis progression in hepatitis C virus infection after seroconversion. JAMA Intern Med 2015;175(2):178–85.

17. Poordad F, Hezode C, Trinh R, et al. ABT-450/r-ombitasvir and dasabuvir with ribavirin for hepatitis C with cirrhosis. N Engl J Med 2014;370(21):1973–82.

18. Afdhal N, Zeuzem S, Kwo P, et al. Ledipasvir and sofosbuvir for untreated HCV genotype 1 infection. N Engl J Med 2014;370(20):1889–98.

19. Lawitz E, Sulkowski MS, Ghalib R, et al. Simeprevir plus sofosbuvir, with or without ribavirin, to treat chronic infection with hepatitis C virus genotype 1 in non-responders to pegylated interferon and ribavirin and treatment-naive patients: the COSMOS randomised study. Lancet 2014;384(9956):1756–65.

20. Jacobson IM, Gordon SC, Kowdley KV, et al. Sofosbuvir for hepatitis C genotype 2 or 3 in patients without treatment options. N Engl J Med 2013;368(20):1867–77.

21. Sulkowski MS, Gardiner DF, Rodriguez-Torres M, et al. Daclatasvir plus sofosbuvir for previously treated or untreated chronic HCV infection. N Engl J Med 2014; 370(3):211–21.

22. Narciso-Schiavon JL, Schiavon Lde L, Carvalho-Filho RJ, et al. Gender influence on treatment of chronic hepatitis C genotype 1. Rev Soc Bras Med Trop 2010; 43(3):217–23.

23. Sulkowski MS, Wasserman R, Brooks L, et al. Changes in haemoglobin during interferon alpha-2b plus ribavirin combination therapy for chronic hepatitis C virus infection. J Viral Hepat 2004;11(3):243–50.

24. Kowdley KV, Wang CC, Welch S, et al. Prevalence of chronic hepatitis B among foreign-born persons living in the United States by country of origin. Hepatology 2012;56(2):422–33.

25. Iloeje UH, Yang HI, Su J, et al. Predicting cirrhosis risk based on the level of circulating hepatitis B viral load. Gastroenterology 2006;130(3):678–86.

26. Fattovich G. Natural history and prognosis of hepatitis B. Semin Liver Dis 2003; 23(1):47–58.
27. Kumar M, Chauhan R, Gupta N, et al. Spontaneous increases in alanine amino-transferase levels in asymptomatic chronic hepatitis B virus-infected patients. Gastroenterology 2009;136(4):1272–80.
28. Lok AS, Lai CL. Acute exacerbations in Chinese patients with chronic hepatitis B virus (HBV) infection. Incidence, predisposing factors and etiology. J Hepatol 1990;10(1):29–34.
29. Chu CM, Liaw YF. Predictive factors for reactivation of hepatitis B following hep-atitis B e antigen seroconversion in chronic hepatitis B. Gastroenterology 2007; 133(5):1458–65.
30. Terrault NA, Bzowej NH, Chang KM, et al. AASLD guidelines for treatment of chronic hepatitis B. Hepatology 2015;63(1):261–83.
31. Grant BF, Goldstein RB, Saha TD, et al. Epidemiology of DSM-5 alcohol use dis-order: results from the National Epidemiologic Survey on Alcohol and Related Conditions III. JAMA Psychiatry 2015;72(8):757–66.
32. Frezza M, di Padova C, Pozzato G, et al. High blood alcohol levels in women. The role of decreased gastric alcohol dehydrogenase activity and first-pass meta-bolism. N Engl J Med 1990;322(2):95–9.
33. Becker U, Deis A, Sorensen TI, et al. Prediction of risk of liver disease by alcohol intake, sex, and age: a prospective population study. Hepatology 1996;23(5): 1025–9.
34. Gual A, Bravo F, Lligona A, et al. Treatment for alcohol dependence in Catalonia: health outcomes and stability of drinking patterns over 20 years in 850 patients. Alcohol Alcohol 2009;44(4):409–15.
35. Williams CD, Stengel J, Asike MI, et al. Prevalence of nonalcoholic fatty liver dis-ease and nonalcoholic steatohepatitis among a largely middle-aged population utilizing ultrasound and liver biopsy: a prospective study. Gastroenterology 2011;140(1):124–31.
36. Browning JD, Szczepaniak LS, Dobbins R, et al. Prevalence of hepatic steatosis in an urban population in the United States: impact of ethnicity. Hepatology 2004; 40(6):1387–95.
37. Lazo M, Hernaez R, Eberhardt MS, et al. Prevalence of nonalcoholic fatty liver dis-ease in the United States: the Third National Health and Nutrition Examination Survey, 1988-1994. Am J Epidemiol 2013;178(1):38–45.
38. Lonardo A, Bellentani S, Argo CK, et al. Epidemiological modifiers of non-alcoholic fatty liver disease: focus on high-risk groups. Dig Liver Dis 2015; 47(12):997–1006.
39. Argo CK, Northup PG, Al-Osaimi AM, et al. Systematic review of risk factors for fibrosis progression in non-alcoholic steatohepatitis. J Hepatol 2009;51(2):371–9.
40. Yang JD, Abdelmalek MF, Pang H, et al. Gender and menopause impact severity of fibrosis among patients with nonalcoholic steatohepatitis. Hepatology 2014; 59(4):1406–14.
41. McKenzie J, Fisher BM, Jaap AJ, et al. Effects of HRT on liver enzyme levels in women with type 2 diabetes: a randomized placebo-controlled trial. Clin Endocri-nol 2006;65(1):40–4.
42. Liu SH, Lazo M, Koteish A, et al. Oral contraceptive pill use is associated with reduced odds of nonalcoholic fatty liver disease in menstruating women: results from NHANES III. J Gastroenterol 2013;48(10):1151–9.
43. D'Amico G, Morabito A, Pagliaro L, et al. Survival and prognostic indicators in compensated and decompensated cirrhosis. Dig Dis Sci 1986;31(5):468–75.

44. Gines P, Quintero E, Arroyo V, et al. Compensated cirrhosis: natural history and prognostic factors. Hepatology 1987;7(1):122–8.
45. D'Amico G, Garcia-Tsao G, Pagliaro L. Natural history and prognostic indicators of survival in cirrhosis: a systematic review of 118 studies. J Hepatol 2006;44(1): 217–31.
46. Zoli M, Cordiani MR, Marchesini G, et al. Prognostic indicators in compensated cirrhosis. Am J Gastroenterol 1991;86(10):1508–13.
47. Llach J, Gines P, Arroyo V, et al. Prognostic value of arterial pressure, endogenous vasoactive systems, and renal function in cirrhotic patients admitted to the hospital for the treatment of ascites. Gastroenterology 1988;94(2):482–7.
48. Mathur AK, Schaubel DE, Gong Q, et al. Sex-based disparities in liver transplant rates in the United States. Am J Transplant 2011;11(7):1435–43.
49. Sharma P, Schaubel DE, Messersmith EE, et al. Factors that affect deceased donor liver transplantation rates in the United States in addition to the model for end-stage liver disease score. Liver Transpl 2012;18(12):1456–63.
50. Huo SC, Huo TI, Lin HC, et al. Is the corrected-creatinine model for end-stage liver disease a feasible strategy to adjust gender difference in organ allocation for liver transplantation? Transplantation 2007;84(11):1406–12.
51. Fussner LA, Charlton MR, Heimbach JK, et al. The impact of gender and NASH on chronic kidney disease before and after liver transplantation. Liver Int 2014; 34(8):1259–66.
52. Sarkar M, Watt KD, Terrault N, et al. Outcomes in liver transplantation: does sex matter? J Hepatol 2015;62(4):946–55.
53. Lai JC, Verna EC, Brown RS Jr, et al. Hepatitis C virus-infected women have a higher risk of advanced fibrosis and graft loss after liver transplantation than men. Hepatology 2011;54(2):418–24.
54. Merli M, Nicolini G, Angeloni S, et al. Incidence and natural history of small esophageal varices in cirrhotic patients. J Hepatol 2003;38(3):266–72.
55. Bruno S, Crosignani A, Facciotto C, et al. Sustained virologic response prevents the development of esophageal varices in compensated, Child-Pugh class A hepatitis C virus-induced cirrhosis. A 12-year prospective follow-up study. Hepatology 2010;51(6):2069–76.
56. Kumar A, Mishra SR, Sharma P, et al. Clinical, laboratory, and hemodynamic parameters in portal hypertensive gastropathy: a study of 254 cirrhotics. J Clin Gastroenterol 2010;44(4):294–300.
57. Berzigotti A, Garcia-Tsao G, Bosch J, et al. Obesity is an independent risk factor for clinical decompensation in patients with cirrhosis. Hepatology 2011;54(2): 555–61.
58. Obstein KL, Campbell MS, Reddy KR, et al. Association between model for end-stage liver disease and spontaneous bacterial peritonitis. Am J Gastroenterol 2007;102(12):2732–6.
59. Jepsen P, Watson H, Andersen PK, et al. Diabetes as a risk factor for hepatic encephalopathy in cirrhosis patients. J Hepatol 2015;63(5):1133–8.
60. Kawut SM, Krowka MJ, Trotter JF, et al. Clinical risk factors for portopulmonary hypertension. Hepatology 2008;48(1):196–203.
61. Chen HS, Xing SR, Xu WG, et al. Portopulmonary hypertension in cirrhotic patients: prevalence, clinical features and risk factors. Exp Ther Med 2013;5(3): 819–24.
62. Benjaminov FS, Prentice M, Sniderman KW, et al. Portopulmonary hypertension in decompensated cirrhosis with refractory ascites. Gut 2003;52(9):1355–62.

63. Torre LA, Bray F, Siegel RL, et al. Global cancer statistics, 2012. CA Cancer J Clin 2015;65(2):87–108.
64. El-Serag HB, Rudolph KL. Hepatocellular carcinoma: epidemiology and molecular carcinogenesis. Gastroenterology 2007;132(7):2557–76.
65. Bosch FX, Ribes J, Cleries R, et al. Epidemiology of hepatocellular carcinoma. Clin Liver Dis 2005;9(2):191–211, v.
66. Yu MW, Chang HC, Chang SC, et al. Role of reproductive factors in hepatocellular carcinoma: impact on hepatitis B- and C-related risk. Hepatology 2003;38(6): 1393–400.
67. Yu MW, Chen CJ. Elevated serum testosterone levels and risk of hepatocellular carcinoma. Cancer Res 1993;53(4):790–4.
68. Yu MW, Yang YC, Yang SY, et al. Hormonal markers and hepatitis B virus-related hepatocellular carcinoma risk: a nested case-control study among men. J Natl Cancer Inst 2001;93(21):1644–51.
69. Farinati F, Sergio A, Giacomin A, et al. Is female sex a significant favorable prognostic factor in hepatocellular carcinoma? Eur J Gastroenterol Hepatol 2009; 21(10):1212–8.
70. Cundy TF, Butler J, Pope RM, et al. Amenorrhoea in women with non-alcoholic chronic liver disease. Gut 1991;32(2):202–6.
71. Bell H, Raknerud N, Falch JA, et al. Inappropriately low levels of gonadotrophins in amenorrhoeic women with alcoholic and non-alcoholic cirrhosis. Eur J Endocrinol 1995;132(4):444–9.
72. Burra P, De Martin E, Gitto S, et al. Influence of age and gender before and after liver transplantation. Liver Transpl 2013;19(2):122–34.
73. Mass K, Quint EH, Punch MR, et al. Gynecological and reproductive function after liver transplantation. Transplantation 1996;62(4):476–9.
74. Sorrell JH, Brown JR. Sexual functioning in patients with end-stage liver disease before and after transplantation. Liver Transpl 2006;12(10):1473–7.
75. Maheshwari S, Sarraj A, Kramer J, et al. Oral contraception and the risk of hepatocellular carcinoma. J Hepatol 2007;47(4):506–13.
76. Kapp N. WHO provider brief on hormonal contraception and liver disease. Contraception 2009;80(4):325–6.
77. Brinson RR, Kolts BE, Monif GR. Spontaneous bacterial peritonitis associated with an intrauterine device. J Clin Gastroenterol 1986;8(1):82–4.
78. Trussell J. Contraceptive failure in the United States. Contraception 2011;83(5): 397–404.
79. Aggarwal N, Sawnhey H, Suril V, et al. Pregnancy and cirrhosis of the liver. Aust N Z J Obstet Gynaecol 1999;39(4):503–6.
80. Aggarwal N, Negi N, Aggarwal A, et al. Pregnancy with portal hypertension. J Clin Exp Hepatol 2014;4(2):163–71.
81. Pritchard JA. Changes in the blood volume during pregnancy and delivery. Anesthesiology 1965;26:393–9.
82. Sandhu BS, Sanyal AJ. Pregnancy and liver disease. Gastroenterol Clin North Am 2003;32(1):407–36, ix.
83. Westbrook RH, Yeoman AD, O'Grady JG, et al. Model for end-stage liver disease score predicts outcome in cirrhotic patients during pregnancy. Clin Gastroenterol Hepatol 2011;9(8):694–9.
84. Zeeman GG, Moise KJ Jr. Prophylactic banding of severe esophageal varices associated with liver cirrhosis in pregnancy. Obstet Gynecol 1999;94(5 Pt 2):842.
85. Allen AM, Hay JE. Review article: the management of cirrhosis in women. Aliment Pharmacol Ther 2014;40(10):1146–54.

86. Tan J, Surti B, Saab S. Pregnancy and cirrhosis. Liver Transpl 2008;14(8): 1081–91.
87. Pillai AK, Joseph AM, Reddick M, et al. Intravascular US-guided transjugular intrahepatic portosystemic shunt creation in a second-trimester pregnancy to prophylactically decompress abdominal wall varices before cesarean section. J Vasc Interv Radiol 2014;25(3):481–3.
88. Matin A, Sass DA. Liver disease in pregnancy. Gastroenterol Clin North Am 2011; 40(2):335–53, viii.
89. Bissonnette J, Durand F, de Raucourt E, et al. Pregnancy and vascular liver disease. J Clin Exp Hepatol 2015;5(1):41–50.
90. Aggarwal N, Sawhney H, Vasishta K, et al. Non-cirrhotic portal hypertension in pregnancy. Int J Gynaecol Obstet 2001;72(1):1–7.
91. Puljic A, Salati J, Doss A, et al. Outcomes of pregnancies complicated by liver cirrhosis, portal hypertension, or esophageal varices. J Matern Fetal Neonatal Med 2016;29(3):506–9.
92. Bacq Y, Zarka O, Brechot JF, et al. Liver function tests in normal pregnancy: a prospective study of 103 pregnant women and 103 matched controls. Hepatology 1996;23(5):1030–4.
93. Whittaker PG, Macphail S, Lind T. Serial hematologic changes and pregnancy outcome. Obstet Gynecol 1996;88(1):33–9.
94. Sill PR, Lind T, Walker W. Platelet values during normal pregnancy. Br J Obstet Gynaecol 1985;92(5):480–3.
95. Tygart SG, McRoyan DK, Spinnato JA, et al. Longitudinal study of platelet indices during normal pregnancy. Am J Obstet Gynecol 1986;154(4):883–7.
96. Ahmed Y, van Iddekinge B, Paul C, et al. Retrospective analysis of platelet numbers and volumes in normal pregnancy and in pre-eclampsia. Br J Obstet Gynaecol 1993;100(3):216–20.

Hepatitis B in the Female Population

Erica Cohen, MD[a], Tram T. Tran, MD[b],*

KEYWORDS

- Hepatitis B • Liver • Pregnancy • Transmission

KEY POINTS

- Hepatitis B is preventable with vaccination, but mother-to-child transmission (MTCT) is still a common mode of transmission worldwide.
- Treatment of hepatitis B in chronically infected women can suppress the virus, but cure is still elusive.
- Prevention of MTCT using judicious antiviral therapy in selected individuals can be considered.

INTRODUCTION

Chronic hepatitis B virus (HBV) infection is a leading global cause of chronic liver disease with the potential to result in cirrhosis, liver failure, and/or hepatocellular carcinoma (HCC) in as many as 15% to 40% of patients.[1,2] It is estimated that 2 billion people worldwide have been infected with HBV, 350 to 400 million of whom are chronically infected. Despite the availability of an effective and safe vaccine, 50 million new cases continue to be diagnosed annually with the largest burden of incident cases due to mother-to-child transmission (MTCT). In the United States, previously reported estimates of chronic HBV infection have recently been modified to 2.2 million when accounting for foreign-born individuals from regions with high endemic rates of seropositivity.[2,3]

Chronic hepatitis B infection in the female population has implications not just for the individual but for her children as well. This article discusses the natural history of hepatitis B and how it plays an important role in HBV transmission, current strategies and new strategies to control HBV and reduce transmission, and the updated guidelines for the management of HBV.

Exposure and infection in hepatitis B is age dependent. Infection in the very young, particularly in infancy, results in high rates of chronic HBV infection. Conversely,

Disclosures: None.
[a] Division of Gastroenterology, Cedars Sinai Medical Center, 8730 Alden Dr, Los Angeles, CA 90025, USA; [b] Liver Transplant, Cedars Sinai Medical Center, 8900 Beverly Boulevard, Los Angeles, CA 90048, USA
* Corresponding author.
E-mail address: Tram.Tran@cshs.org

infection in the adult population is associated with relatively low rates of chronic infection. Although exposure to hepatitis B in adults may result in an acute syndrome, viral clearance is more common (**Fig. 1**).

Chronic hepatitis B progresses through 4 distinct phases as described in **Table 1**. First, the host acquires immune tolerance. The second phase is characterized by immune activity/clearance. In the third phase the host enters into an inactive carrier state. Finally, the fourth phase is characterized by reactivation/HBeAg chronic hepatitis B.[4] Phase duration is variable, and fluctuation between phases is frequent. Therefore, determining the true natural history of HBV in an individual patient is rather challenging. Correctly determining the phase of infection in which that patient lies is critical in optimizing management.

IMMUNE-TOLERANT PHASE

In the earliest phase of a perinatally infected individual, immune tolerance is the norm with little immune response raised by the host against the virus. Thus, very high virus levels are typical, whereas little inflammation is found on liver biopsy and ALT is persistently normal. The probability of hepatitis B e antigen (HBeAg) loss and seroconversion, which are immune-related events, is low.

The viral mechanism of the immune-tolerant state has not been fully elucidated. HBV-specific T-cell hyporesponsiveness causing energy, deletion, and expansion of regulatory T cells may all be contributing to the immune-tolerance phase.[5] Vertical transmission leading to fetal infection is postulated to occur by transplacental maternal HBeAg induction of T-cell intolerance to HBV core antigen and HBeAg in the neonate.[6] As neonates do not have immunoglobulin M (IgM) antibodies to hepatitis B core antigen (HBcAg), a primary response cannot be mounted.[7]

The utilization of an appropriate cutoff for normal alanine transaminase (ALT) values is important as it can affect treatment decisions. It is known that age, body mass index, and metabolic factors all impact ALT levels.[8] Lai and colleagues[9] evaluated liver biopsies in patients with Chronic hepatitis B (CHB) with normal ALT values ($\leq$40 IU/L at the institutional laboratory) as well as patients with elevated values. In those with

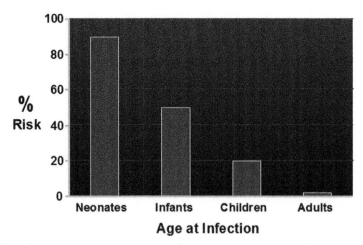

Fig. 1. Risk of chronic infection. (*Adapted from* McMahon BJ, Alward WL, Hall DB, et al. Acute hepatitis B virus infection: relation of age to the clinical expression of disease and subsequent development of the carrier state. J Infect Dis 1985;151:599–603; with permission.)

Table 1
Phases of hepatitis B virus infection

Phase	HBeAg	HBV DNA	ALT	Liver Histology	Optimal Treatment Times
Immune tolerant	Positive	Elevated: ≥1 million IU/mL	Normal	Minimal inflammation and fibrosis	–
HBeAg-positive immune active	Positive	≥20,000 IU/mL	Elevated: >2× ULN	Moderate to severe inflammation or fibrosis	+
Inactive CHB	Negative	Low or undetectable	Normal	Minimal inflammation, variable fibrosis	–
HbeAg-negative reactivation phase	Negative	Elevated: ≥2000 IU/mL	Elevated	Moderate to severe inflammation or fibrosis	+

Abbreviations: ALT, alanine transaminase; HbeAg, hepatitis B e antigen; ULN, upper limit of normal.

persistently normal ALT levels, 34% had grade 2 to 4 inflammation and 18% had stage 2 to 4 fibrosis. Patients in this cohort tended to be of an older age, highlighting that even with normal ALT values a liver biopsy may be useful in older patients with long-standing disease. In a large retrospective analysis of 6835 healthy blood donors, Prati and colleagues[10] reported that the normal limit of ALT should be 30 IU/mL for men and 19 IU/mL for women: this is the current upper limit of normal (ULN) recommended in clinical practice irrespective of institutional laboratory limits. The key to determining true immune tolerance is close long-term follow-up. Therefore, ALT levels should be tested every 6 months for adults with immune-tolerant CHB to monitor the transition to immune active or inactive carrier states.[11]

In general, antiviral therapy is not recommended in this subset of pediatric or adult patients, as achieving treatment end points is unlikely.[4] If HBV has been acquired perinatally or in early childhood, the immune-tolerant phase is long, typically lasting 2 or 3 decades; in contrast, it may be absent or very short in adult-acquired HBV. It is recommended to consider initiation of antiviral therapy in adults if they are older than 40 years with normal ALT and elevated HBV DNA of 1,000,000 IU/mL or greater and a liver biopsy demonstrating significant necroinflammation or fibrosis. Additionally, clinicians should take into account fluctuating ALT levels and whether there is a family history of cirrhosis or HCC into decision management considerations.

IMMUNE-ACTIVE PHASE

After a variable period of immune tolerance, immune activity may begin, in which patients show evidence of elevated ALT levels, fluctuating viremia, and liver biopsies consistent with inflammation and injury. If the immune activity is successful, immune clearance occurs with HBeAg loss and development of anti-HBe, a transition to inactive carrier status. If clearance fails to occur, the liver damage may ensue potentially leading to cirrhosis and increased risk for HCC. The immune-active state is an appropriate time to initiate antiviral therapy, as there is a greater risk of progression of liver disease. Elevated baseline ALT, 2 to 5 times the ULN, and moderate to high inflammation on biopsy are associated with higher likelihood of achieving the intermediate outcomes with treatment (HBeAg seroconversion and HBV DNA <2000 IU/mL after treatment). The American Association for the Study of Liver Disease (AASLD) recommends indefinite therapy in HBeAg-negative immune-active CHB unless there is a compelling reason to stop. Noninvasive tests, such as transient elastography, may be helpful in ruling out cirrhosis but are less accurate in evaluating fibrosis.

If the ALT is elevated but not greater than 2 times the ULN, or HBV DNA is less than the threshold of greater than 2000 IU/mL, additional factors should be included in the treatment decision. Again, risk factors for more severe disease include older age (>40 years), family history of HCC, male sex, and extrahepatic manifestations of CHB. Treatment of HBV with antivirals does not eliminate the risk of HCC, and those at risk should continue surveillance.

INACTIVE CARRIER

In the inactive-carrier phase, the immune system has effectively cleared the HBeAg and an anti-HBe becomes present. HBV DNA levels are low and ALT levels have normalized. Liver histology is variable depending on previous liver injury during the immune-active phase. Unless advanced liver disease has developed during the preceding immune-clearance phase, the inactive-carrier phase confers a favorable prognosis, with improvements in liver histology and a halt of disease progression. Guidelines recommend close monitoring rather than treatment of people in this state. Patients in this phase typically have a low risk of disease progression; however, a cohort of 146 inactive carriers was followed for 23 years and 43 patients had increases in ALT levels greater than normal, one had spontaneous reactivation to the HBeAg-negative state, and 2 developed HCC.[12] This finding highlights the importance of continued monitoring for disease activity and HCC progression.

Resolved CHB infection is defined by clearance of hepatitis B surface antigen (HBsAg) with acquisition of HBsAg antibody. Approximately 0.5% of those with inactive CHB will clear HBsAg yearly, which is considered a functional cure, a state as close to remission as possible. However, if this occurs late in life (after ~40 years of age), the prolonged immune response may still allow liver disease to progress. Low levels of HBV DNA are transiently detected in the serum in the minority of persons achieving seroclearance. Clearance of HBsAg, whether spontaneous or following antiviral therapy, reduces the risk of hepatic decompensation and improves survival.[13]

Among persons who undergo spontaneous HBeAg seroconversion, 67% to 80% will continue to remain in the inactive CHB phase. Approximately 4% to 20% of inactive carriers will revert back to HBeAg positivity, with the highest rates in men, genotype C–infected patients, and those achieving HBeAg seroconversion after 40 years of age.[4]

REACTIVATION/HEPATITIS B E ANTIGEN–NEGATIVE CHB

Even after HBeAg seroconversion and entrance into a quiescent HBV inactive-carrier state, a subset of patients may enter a disease state of viral reactivation. This disease state may happen after being in the inactive-carrier state for several years. Similar to the inactive-carrier state, this phase is notable for an absence of HBeAg due to a precore stop codon mutation that becomes dominant, whereas the wild-type e antigen is eliminated.[14] These subset of patients have a 2-fold risk of progressing to cirrhosis and/or HCC versus those with HBeAg-positive infection.[15] HBsAg levels may also help differentiate between inactive carriers and chronic active HBeAg negative infection. Inactive carriers have lower HBsAg levels (<1000 U/mL have 87.9% positive predictive value and 96.7% negative predictive value for patients with HBV DNA <2000 IU/mL).[16]

This clinical entity highlights the dynamic natural history of HBV with variable duration, severity, and reversibility from one stage to another.

CURRENT RECOMMENDATIONS FOR THERAPY

The primary goal of therapy is to decrease morbidity and mortality related to CHB. Current available therapies provide the opportunity for an *immunologic cure* defined by HBsAg loss and sustained HBV DNA suppression. A *virological cure,* defined as viral eradication, including the covalently closed circular DNA remains an unattainable goal.

There are 6 therapeutic agents approved for the treatment of adults with CHB in the United States. Head-to-head trials of antiviral therapies fail to show superiority in one medication versus another in achieving risk reduction in liver-related complications. Peg-interferon (Peg-IFN), tenofovir, and entecavir are preferred therapies because of the lack of resistance with long-term usage. Peg-IFN has more side effects than nucleos(t)ide analogue (NAs) therapy. NAs have a good safety profile overall, including use in patients with decompensated cirrhosis and transplant recipients,[17] and side effects are infrequent (**Table 2**).

The AASLD recommends that HBeAg-positive adults without cirrhosis with CHB who seroconvert to anti-HBe on therapy discontinue NAs after a period of treatment consolidation involving treatment of at least 12 months with normal ALT levels and undetectable serum HBV DNA. It remains unclear if a longer treatment duration would further decrease rates of virological relapse. An alternative approach is to treat until HBsAg loss, but this may be not feasible because of the medication cost and need for long-term follow-up. It is unknown whether outcomes, such as HCC, cirrhosis, or decompensation, are different in persons who discontinue therapy after HBeAg seroconversion versus those continuing until HBsAg loss. However, HbeAg-positive adults with cirrhosis should remain on therapy indefinitely because of concerns for potential clinical deterioration and death unless there is a strong contraindication.

SEX DIFFERENCES IN HEPATOCELLULAR CARCINOMA RISK WITH HEPATITIS B VIRUS

There are a variety of host, viral, and environmental factors that contribute to the risk of progression to cirrhosis and HCC.[18] Although HBV DNA levels, ALT, and HBeAg status are important predictors of progression to cirrhosis, HBeAg status, HBV DNA levels (>2000 IU/mL), and cirrhosis itself are the primary determinants of HCC risk.[19]

An intriguing universal epidemiologic characteristic of HCC is the male predominance, with a male/female ratio range of 1.5 to 11:1 from a variety of analyses.[18] Not only is the incidence of HCC increased in men but they also experience higher HCC-related mortality than women.[18] Conversely, rates of spontaneous survival and postresection survival are higher in the female population.[20] These differences, however, disappear after menopause, with increased cirrhotic and HCC cases occurring in older women,[21] in both patients with HBV and patients with hepatitis C virus.

Multiple studies indicate that the sex differences in HBV infection begin as early as the development of chronic hepatitis,[22] implying that causative factors may contribute early in the carcinogenic progress. Male sex has been identified as a risk factor for reactivation of HBV in inactive carriers and increased risk of progression to fibrosis, both of which confer higher risk of progression to cirrhosis and HCC.[23] One long-term study found that women achieve a higher percentage of seroconversion of HBeAg and HBsAg than men.[24] One proposed mechanism for these differences is that women may have more active immune responses against HBV infection than

Table 2
Approved antiviral therapies for hepatitis B virus

Drug and Dosage	Indication	Pregnancy Category	Potential Side Effects	Monitoring on Treatment
Peg-IFN 2a (180 µg weekly)	HBV (HBeAg positive or negative), compensated disease, viral replication, liver inflammation	C[c]	Flulike symptoms, fatigue, depression, cytopenias, autoimmune disorders	1. CBC (every 1–3 mo) 2. TSH (every 3 mo) 3. Clinical monitoring: infectious, neuropsychiatric, autoimmune, ischemic complications
Lamivudine (100 mg daily)	Chronic HBV with viral replication and liver inflammation	C[c]	Pancreatitis, lactic acidosis	1. Lactic acid or amylase if indicated
Telbivudine (600 mg daily)	Chronic HBV with viral replication, transaminitis, or active histology	B[b]	Myopathy, creatine kinase elevations	1. Creatine kinase if symptomatic
Entecavir (0.5/1.0 mg daily[a])	Chronic HBV with active viral replication	C[c]	Lactic acidosis	1. Lactic acid if clinical concern
Adefovir (10 mg daily)	Chronic HBV	C[c]	Acute renal failure, Fanconi syndrome, nephrogenic diabetes insipidus, lactic acidosis	1. Creatinine clearance at baseline, creatinine clearance, phosphate, urine glucose, and protein at least annually 2. Bone density study at baseline and during treatment if risk for osteopenia 3. Lactic acid levels if clinical concern
Tenofovir (300 mg daily)	Chronic HBV	B[b]	Nephropathy, Fanconi syndrome, osteomalacia, lactic acidosis	1. Creatinine clearance at baseline, creatinine clearance, phosphate, urine glucose, and protein at least annually 2. Bone density study at baseline and during treatment if risk for osteopenia 3. Lactic acid levels if clinical concern

Abbreviations: CBC, complete blood count; TSH, thyroid-stimulating hormone.
[a] Entecavir 1 mg if lamivudine or telbivudine experienced or decompensated cirrhosis.
[b] Animal reproduction studies have shown an adverse effect on the fetus, and there are no adequate and well-controlled studies in humans; but potential benefits may warrant use of the drug in pregnant women despite potential risks.
[c] Animal reproduction studies have failed to demonstrate a risk to the fetus, and there are no adequate and well-controlled studies in pregnant women.

men. Supporting this hypothesis, one study showed that the chronic HBsAg carrier rate was lower in women than men vaccinated at birth and followed into adulthood.[25]

Although sex-specific differences in behavior (tobacco use, alcohol consumption) may be at play, a growing body of literature suggest sex steroid hormones, both androgen and estrogen, may function as regulatory factors in conjunction with viral factors in the progression of HCC. Epidemiologic and animal studies suggest that androgens may stimulate carcinogenesis, whereas estrogen is protective. Knockout androgen receptor (AR) expression in mice hepatocytes delayed the development of N′-N;-dietylnitrosamine–induced HCC suggesting the AR pathway enhances development of HCC.[26] Likewise, a viral protein Hepatitis B Virus X protein (HBx) can enhance transcriptional activity of AR through its effects on the c-Src and GSK-3B kinase pathways.[27] In this mouse model, estrogen protected hepatocytes from malignant transformation via downregulation of interleukin 6 release from Kupffer cells.[28] Interestingly, women with HCC were found to overexpress miR-18a, which blocks the tumor protective function of estrogen.[29] In clinical studies, early oophorectomy (at <50 years of age) was identified as a risk factor for HCC, whereas postmenopausal hormone replacement therapy was shown to be protective.[30]

To date, the mechanism in sex disparity of HCC in HBV infection remains controversial. Although several studies identified distinct roles of both androgen and estrogen sex hormone pathways in the development of HCC, clinical applications have yet to be identified.

A WOMAN OF CHILDBEARING AGE: SHOULD SHE BE TREATED?

Women of childbearing age infected with HBV present an interesting clinical dilemma given the risk of chronic liver disease, flares during pregnancy and in the peripartum period, as well as the concern for fetal transmission. If a woman of childbearing age presents with chronic HBV and is not pregnant, the aim of management is to determine the disease severity by HBV DNA level, HBeAg status, and evidence of livery injury by ALT level and/or liver histology. Most often women of childbearing age are in the immune-tolerant phase and, according to the AASLD's practice guidelines, are not candidates for antiviral therapy.

Women presenting for evaluation with chronic HBV who are planning pregnancy in the immediate future should not be started on antiviral therapy because of concerns regarding fetal exposure to these drugs in early pregnancy. Nucleoside or nucleotide antiviral therapy has the potential to promote mitochondrial toxicity and is of unclear benefit in young patients without evidence of advanced liver disease.[30] In the setting of highly active disease or more advanced liver injury, however, the clinical risk to benefit assessment may favor initiating therapy and continuation throughout the pregnancy course. Peg-IFN, which, unlike the oral HBV therapies, has a defined treatment duration of 1 year, may be a viable option to offer women who are candidates for therapy. They must be willing to wait more than 18 months to complete therapy before conception but have a better chance at HBsAg loss with interferon.

Those who have been started on antiviral therapy for chronic HBV and then become pregnant require a careful evaluation, weighing the risks of antiviral discontinuation against fetal exposure early in pregnancy. It is helpful to consider the severity of underlying liver disease on initiation of therapy. The highest risks of HBV-associated decompensation in pregnancy are seen in those with underlying cirrhosis. In a retrospective review of 399 mothers with cirrhosis, 15% experienced severe flare with 1.8% risk of mortality for mothers and 5.2% risk of fetal mortality.[31] One small series of women (n = 12) who discontinued therapy during pregnancy reported viral rebound in 67% of patients and a 5-fold increase in ALT levels observed in 50% of patients.[32] Spontaneous recovery was observed in all cases but highlights the potential risk of discontinuing therapy in a pregnant woman who has advanced fibrosis even without overt cirrhosis.

Typically, women of childbearing age are not candidates for antiviral therapy owing to early disease. However, patients with high viremia who are planning to get pregnant may benefit from antiviral therapy not for their own disease but to reduce the risk of perinatal transmission (**Fig. 2**).

TREATMENT IN PREGNANCY

The purpose of initiating antiviral therapy in pregnant women with chronic HBV is to reduce rates of MTCT, the leading cause of chronic HBV infection worldwide.

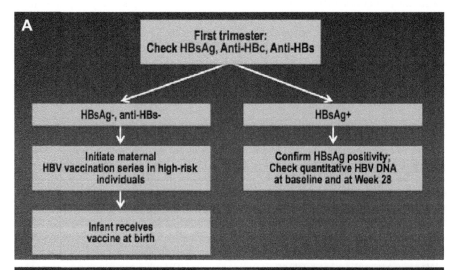

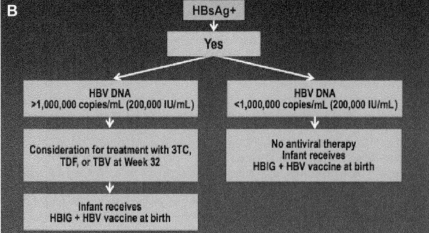

Fig. 2. (*A, B*) Suggested management of HBV infection during pregnancy in first trimester. HBIG, hepatitis B immunoglobulin; TBV, telbivudine; TDF, tenofovir.

Standard active-passive immunoprophylaxis with Hepatitis B immunoglobulin (HBIG) and hepatitis B vaccination administered within 12 hours of birth followed by 2 additional doses of vaccine within 6 to 12 months was traditionally thought to prevent transmission in almost all offspring of HBsAg-positive mothers. However, a recent literature review noted active-passive immunoprophylaxis fails to prevent transmission in up to 30% of children.[32] High maternal viremia is associated with the highest risk for HBV transmission in pregnancy and failure of immunoprophylaxis. There is conflicting evidence surrounding the effect the mode of delivery has on MTCT. A recent Chinese meta-analysis suggests that elective cesarean delivery may reduce perinatal HBV transmission; however, limitations were noted in this study and it needs further validation.[33]

Several trials support the safety and efficacy of antiviral therapy initiated in late pregnancy for reduction of MTCT among women with high risk of immunoprophylaxis failure (HBV DNA >10^7 log copies per milliliter). Han and colleagues[34] conducted a prospective trial comparing telbivudine 600 mg daily versus no treatment in highly viremic mothers (HBV DNA >10^7 log copies per milliliter). All infants received standard immunoprophylaxis. The mean viral load decreased to 2.44 log 10 copies per milliliter in the treatment arm before delivery. The MTCT rate was 0% with telbivudine compared with 8% without therapy. There were no differences in perinatal complications or congenital abnormalities[35] between groups. Another multicenter trial followed 58 women with HBV DNA >10^7 log copies per milliliter starting tenofovir dipivoxil at 32 weeks' gestation and compared them with 52 women treated with lamivudine and 20 untreated controls. MTCT was reduced to 0% in the lamivudine cohort and 2% in the tenofovir cohort versus 20% in untreated controls. There were no differences in infant or obstetric outcomes.[36]

Many new mothers may hesitate to initiate antiviral therapy because of concerns for the medication effects in their children. One recent study compared 74 infants exposed to tenofovir in late pregnancy versus 69 unexposed infants and assessed their bone mineral content (BMC). There were no differences in mean gestational age (38.2 vs 38.1 weeks in tenofovir vs controls, respectively), mean length (−0.41 vs −0.18), or weight (−0.71 vs −0.48) Z scores. The mean (standard deviation) BMC of tenofovir-exposed infants was 12% lower than for unexposed infants (56.0 [11.8] vs 63.8 [16.6] g; $P = .002$). The adjusted mean BMC was 5.3 g lower (95% confidence interval, −9.5, −1.2; $P = .013$) in the tenofovir-exposed infants.[37] Pan and colleagues more recently described a multicenter randomized controlled study in which tenofovir disoproxil fumarate initiated between 30 to 32 weeks reduced perinatal transmission in highly viremic mothers without an increased risk of adverse events to their infants.[37] Although new studies are encouraging, until more data emerges, the use of antivirals during pregnancy requires an in depth discussion of the risks and benefits of antiviral therapy with pregnant patients.

Updated recommendations by the AASLD recommend a viral cut off of 2×10^5 IU/mL[38] as there is still a 3% to 5% risk of transmission even at this level. First-line therapies include tenofovir and telbivudine (Food and Drug Administration pregnancy category B), but lamivudine can also be considered. Long-term data regarding tenofovir and BMD remain unclear. The end point for antiviral therapy to reduce MTCT risk is immediately in the postpartum period unless treatment continuation is indicated for the clinical benefit of the mother. The risk of transmission during breastfeeding is low in infants receiving immunoprophylaxis, although it is still recommended in those who do not. It has been shown that oral NAs are excreted in low levels in breast milk. There are limited data on the effect of these medications on infants.[39]

SUMMARY/DISCUSSION

CHB infection is an important cause of morbidity and mortality worldwide because of progression to cirrhosis and HCC. The natural history of the virus is highly variable with respect to disease severity and duration necessitating persistent close monitoring. Optimal timing for initiation of antiviral therapy is during the immune-active or reactivation phases aiming to suppress HBV DNA and decrease ongoing liver inflammation. Current available therapies can suppress viral DNA but cannot eradicate the virus and often require prolonged treatment duration.

Hepatitis B infection status is important for women, especially those of childbearing age. Antiviral therapy is not typically recommended in women planning on conceiving because of possible fetal harm from early exposure to these medications. Conversely, treatment is now recommended by the AASLD in pregnant women with very high viral levels greater than 200,000 IU/mL. A thorough discussion of the risks versus benefits of the therapy must be explained. Emerging data suggest a possible effect on BMC in tenofovir-exposed pregnant women, which is balanced by a 10% risk of chronic infection with an incurable virus. Pregnant women with HBV, regardless of treatment status, should be monitored for flares. Breastfeeding is permitted in the postpartum setting. Lastly, important sex differences exist with respect to progression to cirrhosis and HCC in hepatitis B–infected patients. Estrogen may play a protective role in the progression to cirrhosis and HCC in women, whereas male androgen pathways may stimulate this progression. Knowledge of these pathways has yet to translate into clinical applications, and routine screening for disease progression is recommended.

REFERENCES

1. World Health Organization: Hepatitis B. World Health Organization fact sheet 204. 2000. Available at: http://www.who.int/mediacentre/factsheets/fs204/en/. Accessed April, 2016.
2. GBD 2013 Mortality and Causes of Death Collaborators. Global, regional, and national age-sex specific all-cause and cause-specific mortality for 240 causes of death, 1990-2013: a systematic analysis for the Global Burden of Disease Study 2013. Lancet 2015;385(9963):117–71.
3. Kowdley KV, Wang CC, Welch S, et al. Prevalence of chronic hepatitis B among foreign born persons living in the United States by country of origin. Hepatology 2012;56(2):422–33.
4. Terrault NA, Bzowej NH, Chang K-M, et al. AASLD guidelines for treatment of chronic hepatitis B. Hepatology 2016;63:261–83.
5. Carey I, D'Antiga L, Bansal S, et al. Immune and viral profile from tolerance to hepatitis B surface antigen clearance: a longitudinal study of vertically hepatitis B virus-infected children on combined therapy. J Virol 2011;85:2416–28.
6. Lin HH, Lee TY, Chen DS, et al. Transplacental leakage of HBeAg-positive maternal blood as the most likely route in causing intrauterine infection with hepatitis B virus. J Pediatr 1987;111:877–81.
7. Lazizi Y, Badur S, Perk Y, et al. Selective unresponsiveness to HBsAg vaccine in newborns related with an in utero passage of hepatitis B virus DNA. Vaccine 1997;15:1095–100.
8. Lee JK, Shim JH, Lee HC, et al. Estimation of the healthy upper limits for serum alanine aminotransferase in Asian populations with normal liver histology. Hepatology 2010;51:1577–83.

9. Lai M, Hyatt BJ, Nasser I, et al. The clinical significance of persistently normal ALT in chronic hepatitis B infection. J Hepatol 2007;47:760–7.

10. Prati D, Taioli E, Zanella A, et al. Updated definitions of healthy ranges for serum alanine aminotransferase levels. Ann Intern Med 2002;137:1–10.

11. Tong MJ, Trieu J. Hepatitis B inactive carriers: clinical course and outcomes. J Dig Dis 2013;14:311–7.

12. Kim GA, Lee HC, Kim MJ, et al. Incidence of hepatocellular carcinoma after HBsAg seroclearance in chronic hepatitis B patients: a need for surveillance. J Hepatol 2015;62:1092–9.

13. Hadziyannis SJ, Vassilopoulos D. Hepatitis B e antigen-negative chronic hepatitis B. Hepatology 2001;34:617–24.

14. Fattovich G, Bortolotti F, Donato F. Natural history of chronic hepatitis B: special emphasis on disease progression and prognostic factors. J Hepatol 2008;48: 335–52.

15. Chu CM, Lin CC, Chen YC, et al. Basal core promoter mutation is associated with progression to cirrhosis rather than hepatocellular carcinoma in chronic hepatitis B virus infection. Br J Cancer 2012;107:2010–5.

16. Fontana RJ. Side effects of long-term oral antiviral therapy for hepatitis B. Hepatology 2009;49(Suppl 5):S185–95.

17. Chen PJ, Chen DS. Hepatitis B virus infection and hepatocellular carcinoma: molecular genetics and clinical perspectives. Semin Liver Dis 1999;19:253–62.

18. Aravalli RN, Steer CJ, Cressman EN. Molecular mechanisms of hepatocellular carcinoma. Hepatology 2008;48:2047–63.

19. Ng IO, Ng M, Fan ST. Better survival in women with resected hepatocellular carcinoma is not related to tumor proliferation or expression of hormone receptors. Am J Gastroenterol 1997;92:1355–8.

20. Shimizu I, Ito S. Protection of estrogens against the progression of chronic liver disease. Hepatol Res 2007;37:239–47.

21. Chu CM, Liaw YF, Sheen IS, et al. Sex difference in chronic hepatitis B virus infection: an appraisal based on the status of hepatitis B e antigen and antibody. Hepatology 1983;3:947–50.

22. Chu CM, Liaw YF. Predictive factors for reactivation of hepatitis B following hepatitis B e antigen seroconversion in chronic hepatitis B. Gastroenterology 2007; 133:1458–65.

23. Alward WL, McMahon BJ, Hall DB, et al. The long term serological course of asymptomatic hepatitis B virus carriers and the development of primary hepatocellular carcinoma. J Infect Dis 1985;151:604–9.

24. Su FH, Chen JD, Cheng SH, et al. Seroprevalence of hepatitis-B infection amongst Taiwanese university students 18 years following the commencement of a national hepatitis-B vaccination program. J Med Virol 2007;79:138–43, 41, 42, 59, 62, 44.

25. Ma WL, Hsu CL, Wu MH, et al. Androgen receptor is a new potential therapeutic target for the treatment of hepatocellular carcinoma. Gastroenterology 2008;135: 947–55.

26. Chiu CM, Yeh SH, Chen PJ, et al. Hepatitis B virus X protein enhances androgen receptor responsive gene expression depending on androgen level. Proc Natl Acad Sci U S A 2007;104:2571–8.

27. Mantovani A, Allavena P, Sica A, et al. Cancer-related inflammation. Nature 2008; 454:436–44.

28. Karin M. Nuclear factor-B in cancer development and progression. Nature 2006; 441:431–6.

29. Yu MW, Chang HC, Chang SC, et al. Role of reproductive factors in hepatocellular carcinoma: impact on hepatitis B- and C-related risk. Hepatology 2003;38: 1393–400.
30. Lok AS, McMahon BJ. AASLD practice guideline update chronic HBV. Hepatology 2009;50:1–36.
31. Shaheen A, Myers RP. The outcomes of pregnancy in patients with cirrhosis: a population based study. Liver Int 2010;30:275–83.
32. Pan CQ, Duan ZP, Bhamidimarri KR, et al. An algorithm for risk assessment and intervention of mother to child transmission of hepatitis B virus. Clin Gastroenterol Hepatol 2012;10:452–9.
33. Lee SD, Lo KJ, Tsai YT, et al. Role of caesarean section in prevention of mother-infant transmission of hepatitis B. Lancet 1988;2:833–4.
34. Han GR, Jiang HX, Yue X, et al. Efficacy and safety of telbivudeine treatment: an open label prospective study in pregnant women for the prevention of perinatal transmission of HBV infection. J Viral Hepat 2015;22(9):754–62.
35. Pan CQ, Zou H-B, Chen Y, et al. Cesarean section reduces perinatal transmission of HBV infection from hepatitis B surface antigen-positive women to their infants. Clin Gastroenterol Hepatol 2013;11(10):1349–55.
36. Pan CQ, Han GR, Jiang HX, et al. Telbivudine prevents vertical transmission from HBeAg-positive women with chronic hepatitis B. Clin Gastroenterol Hepatol 2012; 10(5):520–6.
37. Available at: http://www.natap.org/2015/AASLD/AASLD_153.htm. Accessed April, 2016.
38. Greenup AJ, Tan PK, Nguyen V, et al. Efficacy and safety of tenofovir disoproxil fumarate in pregnancy to prevent perinatal transmission of hepatitis B virus. J Hepatol 2014;61(3):502–7.
39. Protection against viral hepatitis. Recommendations of Immunization Practices Advisory Committee (ACIP). MMWR Recomm Rep 1990;39(RR-2):1–26. WHO Update No 22, Nov 1996.

View from the Top: Perspectives on Women in Gastroenterology from Society Leaders

Colleen M. Schmitt, MD, MHS[a], John I. Allen, MD, MBA[b],*

KEYWORDS

- Women in medicine • Women in gastroenterology • Leadership
- Gastroenterology practice • Gender and promotion • Diversity initiatives

KEY POINTS

- An increasing percentage of gastroenterologists in the United States are women and they are in demand in both academic and community practices.
- Requests for women gastroenterologists by patients continues to increase.
- Specific initiatives by the American Gastroenterological Association, American Society of Gastrointestinal Endoscopy foster growth of women's careers and provide opportunities to work into leadership roles.

INTRODUCTION: BARRIERS TO ENTRY AND THE LEAKY PIPELINE

Choosing gastroenterology as a career was a natural choice for the 2 authors of this article. Our decisions were driven in part by our belief that, as gastroenterologists, we would impact patient's lives, be intellectually challenged as we care for people with complex diseases and that we would be able to use exciting and emerging endoscopic tools to alleviate suffering, prevent cancer, and cure disease. We envisioned a satisfying lifestyle that was compatible with family priorities. The 2 authors, however, faced different landscapes and encountered unique challenges based in part on their different genders. Those differences are the subject of this joint publication, written from the viewpoint of 2 immediate past presidents of gastroenterology societies.

Currently, there are approximately 13,000 active US-based gastroenterologists with the vast majority engaged in direct patient care.[1] Although women comprise one-third of active physicians in all specialties, the proportion of women in gastroenterology still

Conflicts of Interest: None.
[a] Galen Medical Group, 2200 East 3rd Street, Suite 200, Chattanooga, TN 37404, USA; [b] Section of Digestive Diseases, Department of Medicine, Yale University School of Medicine, 40 Temple Street, Suite 1A, New Haven, CT 06510, USA
* Corresponding author.
E-mail address: john.i.allen@yale.edu

Gastroenterol Clin N Am 45 (2016) 371–388
http://dx.doi.org/10.1016/j.gtc.2016.02.012
0889-8553/16/$ – see front matter © 2016 Elsevier Inc. All rights reserved.

is only 15%, ranking among the lowest for specialty choice among women physicians. Reasons for this gender gap are varied and complex.[2] One key factor influencing how women physicians choose a career is the definition of what constitutes a "suitable" lifestyle, which is often defined by senior physicians who are almost all men. Even more complex are factors that lead women physicians to exit from careers at times when men are focused on advancing their careers and are stepping into leadership roles (**Box 1**).[2,3]

We all begin our careers with ambition; however, this ambition can fade or be eclipsed by competing priorities. For example, women still provide a disproportionate share of childcare and housework at every career level, even those in the younger generations, among women professionals and in families where both partners work full time.[3,4] As a result of these and other factors discussed later in this paper, advancement opportunities decline or disappear over a career span more often in women than in men.[5] A major focus of this article discusses how medical societies such as the American Society for Gastrointestinal Endoscopy (ASGE) and the American Gastroenterological Association (AGA) must provide leadership and a proactive approach to understanding and reducing external barriers encountered by women in our specialty.

WHY WOMEN IN GASTROENTEROLOGY MATTER

Increasing the proportion of women in gastroenterology is important for our patients, our practices, and our profession. For many patients, their experience, comfort, overall satisfaction, and adherence to medical therapy all may be improved when they have the option of working with a woman physician.[6] Women tend to seek health care on a more regular basis compared with men and are the health care "executive" for many families because they are the primary managers of children's care and make most health care decisions for the family.[7] Further, women make 85% of household purchasing decisions, thus commanding significant economic clout and make up one-half of all earners in the United States. In many large metro areas, they are as (or more) educated and earn a higher income compared with their male partners.[8] Thus women as patients, primary caregivers for children and elderly, and earners are key drivers of important health care decisions, including physician selection and management decisions.[4,7]

Numerous studies have documented women's preference for the gender of medical providers, particularly when it comes to endoscopy.[9–15] In fact, some women may decline colonoscopy unless guaranteed a female provider,[9] and this preference may be increasing for office visits as well as endoscopic procedures.[12] We are likely to see such preference trends increase for the following reasons:

- The Medicare population will become younger and more diverse as the baby boomer generation ages into Medicare.[16]
- Preference for same gender physician increases with younger patient age, current employment, no previous history of colonoscopy, and having a female primary provider.[9,11]
- There are strong gender preferences among certain ethnic and cultural groups and these groups are increasing as a proportion of our practices.[13–15]

Diversity invites stimulating, creative problem solving and innovation. Workforce diversity thus increases the richness and heuristic range for patient care, practice innovation, and science. The specialty of gastroenterology particularly lends to a collaborative and team-based approach. These are attributes more commonly found among women leaders, who are well-equipped with skills that are widely recognized

Box 1
Factors contributing to career obstacles for women in gastroenterology

Structural factors

- Lack of networking opportunities that informally create and fertilize catalyst and mentor connections.
- Lack of mentors and sponsors.
- Amounts and types of support.
- Positions in education and training that are less likely to lead to research productivity.
- Time constraints of training.
- Impact of training on decisions regarding pregnancy and family expansion.
- Child care-related responsibilities.
- Elder care-related responsibilities.
- Other responsibilities regarding household management.

Cultural factors

- Gender stereotyping that may inform choice of career focus.
- Networking opportunities.
- Differences in performance expectations and leadership skills.
- Lack of female role models in positions of visibility, influence, and leadership.
- Perceived inconsistency with work–life balance.

Individual mindsets

- Personal control decisions.
- Lack of job satisfaction.
- Lack of self-confidence.
- Decreased ambition over time.
- Uncertain career clarity.

Institutional mindsets

- Insidious or subtle biases about subspecialization or procedural training.
- Hiring decisions or assignments that intentionally or unintentionally convey bias.
- Differences in promotion decisions based on gender.
- Differences in publication acceptance, funding, or other objective measures of success, based on gender.
- Failure in accountability.
- Inflexibility in traditional work hour expectations.
- Absence of programs that promote work–life balance.

Data from Schmitt CM. Flute or tuba: women and publishing success in top gastroenterology journals. Gastrointest Endosc 2015;81:1448–50; and Barsh J, Lee L. Unlocking the full potential of women at work. Washington, DC: McKinsey & Company; 2012. Available at: http://www.mckinsey.com/client_service/organization/latest_thinking/unlocking_the_full_potential. Accessed October 3, 2015.

as requirements for successful leaders: intellectual stimulation, inspiration, participatory decision making, and setting expectations/rewards.[5] Recognizing the leadership potential of women helps to capitalize on the intellectual capacity of our entire workforce.

WOMEN IN GASTROENTEROLOGY

The first record of a woman physician dates to about 2730 BC during the reign of a queen in Egypt. Women were included in the famous medical school at Heliopolis and even Cleopatra was trained in the healing arts.[17] Over the ensuing 3 centuries, however, women's inclusion as medical practitioners grew slowly, impeded by religious and societal prejudices and codified in numerous legal statutes. In the United States, the first woman to earn a medical degree was Elizabeth Blackwell, who graduated from Geneva Medical College in 1849.[18] For those wishing to read personal reflections on the rewards and challenges of women becoming physicians, we refer you to the book *This Side of Doctoring: Reflections from Women in Medicine*, edited by Chin.[19]

In the last 3 decades, the number of women entering medical school has grown substantially, reflecting a trend in many areas of academia, business, and medicine.[20,21] In the 1960s, only 5.5% of medical graduates were women but by 2006 that figure had increased to 48.6%.[22] Even though the percentage of women in general internal medicine residencies has increased, women did not pursue subspecialty practice until later, an issue that was emphasized in a 1986 policy paper prepared for the Department of Health and Human Services.[22] Traditionally, procedure-oriented specialties, such as gastroenterology, were male dominated. Inherent training and cultural biases favored men at both the entry point and throughout career advancement. Factors contributing to career barriers for women in gastroenterology are listed in **Box 1**.

Dr Gail Hecht (the second woman president of the AGA) pointed out, in an editorial published in *Gastroenterology*, that only 16% of first-year gastroenterology fellows were women in the academic year 1996/1997.[20] In the ensuing decade, the percentage of women in gastroenterology doubled, whereas the percentage of women in another procedure-oriented specialty (cardiology) remained the same (**Fig. 1**). We believe that this difference reflects the focused efforts of the major gastroenterology societies to recruit women into gastroenterology fellowship positions, despite a shift in the specialty to becoming more procedure dominant.

Although the proportion of women entering subspecialty fields increased, advancing to positions of leadership remained a challenge. As one of this article's co-authors (CS) stated, "Although the pipeline into our specialty appears robust, like other areas of academia, business and medicine, there has not been a commensurate increase in the proportion of women into positions of seniority, such as advancement into associate or full professor, or into positions of leadership, such as department chair or dean."[2]

Numerous authors, dating back to the 1970s, have studied the gender bias that occurs in a variety of academic and business careers. Barriers to the ascension of women to leadership positions have collectively been termed the "glass ceiling."[22-24] The term "glass" was coined to reflect the subtle and frequently invisible qualities of the barrier; something not rooted in legitimate limitations but rather on discrimination or bias. A clear bias (and one evident in the medical field) is a "status quo bias."[22] This occurs when companies (or academic departments) are performing well and headed by men. In these situations, there is no perceived need to change the historic pattern of male leadership. Researchers have demonstrated that when male leaders drive a company into crisis, a switch to female leadership often occurs. However,

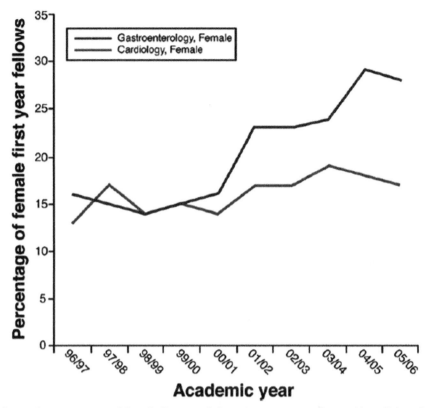

Fig. 1. The percentage of female first-year fellows in gastroenterology and cardiology between 1996/1997 and 2005/2006. (*From* Barsh J, Lee L. Unlocking the full potential of women at work. Washington, DC: McKinsey & Company; 2012. Available at: http://www. mckinsey.com/client_service/organization/latest_thinking/unlocking_the_full_potential. Accessed October 3, 2015.)

when someone (woman or man) ascends to leadership during a crisis, the chance of failure is high. If the leader in this situation is a woman, companies often remove the new leader and revert to more familiar patterns (male leaders). This phenomenon has been termed "the glass cliff."[23]

Glass ceilings and glass cliffs have been evident to women gastroenterologists and scientists.[2,25–28] We are grateful that a robust pool of excellent women physicians and scientists, with training and accomplishments equal to their male counterparts, now enter our specialty. Yet, we continue to observe a decreasing proportion of women at upper levels of gastroenterology in both private practices and academia. There are few women who lead the large independent gastroenterology groups that now are common in the United States. Similarly, there has not been a comparable increase in women at the level of division or department chair, full professor, or dean.[2]

One measure of academic success is publications, especially in top tier journals. Women's success in publishing was studied by Long and colleagues[25] and published in *Gastrointestinal Endoscopy* this year. They found that the proportion of women who are publishing as first or senior authors in the top gastroenterology journals has tripled over the last 20 years, illustrating the fact that gender balance is a recent phenomenon. They also found that women tended to publish in areas of basic science and were less likely to publish endoscopy-related articles. In addition, women tended to publish fewer editorials (usually an invited paper) than would be expected considering the proportion of women in our field. Finally, there were more women first authors when women were in the senior author position, highlighting the importance of mentorship and sponsorship.[25] Jagsi and colleagues[26] noted similar trends when they reviewed women's contributions to prominent general medical journals. Substantial research indicates that research productivity does not explain differences in career success.[27] Research data such as these will help to inform us about patterns of subtle bias and potentially effective interventions to augment the contribution of women in our field.

Gender equity in digestive disease biomedical sciences has been a topic of publication for years. P. Kay Lund discussed these issues in a 2001 editorial, when she was the lone female associate editor for *Gastroenterology*.[28] She acknowledged the high representation of women in training and junior faculty positions, but emphasized the disproportionate attrition of women during their ascent to higher ranks. Then, women comprised only 11% of academic professors (data from the Association of American Medical Colleges), 12% of division chiefs, and 7.5% of department chairs. She cited The Project Access study (see reference in the editorial) that showed disparity in career advancement for women in a well-controlled group of matched male and female postdoctoral fellows where neither marriage nor children were statistically different between genders. Other research pointed to gender bias in grant success as well.[29] Lund concluded that a lack of mentoring played a key role in attrition of women from academic ranks, a point she emphasized again in a recent publication.[28] Both Lund and authors Henning and Estes[30] have offered personal hints for women to ponder as they develop a career plan and interact with academic colleagues.

WOMEN AS LEADERS: AMERICAN SOCIETY FOR GASTROINTESTINAL ENDOSCOPY AND AMERICAN GASTROENTEROLOGICAL ASSOCIATION COMMITMENTS

Some authors have speculated that women approach recognition and reward differently from men.[31] Women typically await recognition, approach work with the notion that the quality of their endeavors will be recognized without self-promotion, and tend to minimize their own contributions in an area of expertise.[3,32,33] Women may be risk averse to learning new skills and may step away from roles that can be required for professional advancement.[33,34] They accept roles that have personal meaning and some level of autonomy, such as clinical educator or staffing clinical offices, but these roles are less likely to lead to peak career opportunities, such as becoming department head or a society president.[3,34]

Whatever the reasons for diminished numbers of women in peak leadership roles, one only needs to look to our gastroenterology societies to understand the consequences. In more than 340 combined years of history, the 4 major gastroenterology and hepatology societies have elected only 12 women presidents (including 3 pending terms) and most occurred in the last decade (**Box 2**). Leadership roles finally are attracting more women owing in part to those who have been able to break through the glass ceiling. The first woman to become President of the AGA was Sara Jordan, PhD, MD, who served 2 terms between 1942 and 1944. This remarkable woman rose to the highest ranks in the AGA when its membership numbered 187.[35] The next female president was elected 70 years later. Gail Hecht, MD, MS, served in 2010 and Sheila Crowe, MD, will become president in 2017. The ASGE will see 4 women as presidents over a 26-year span: Barbara Frank, MD (1991), Grace Elta, MD (2008), Colleen Schmitt, MD, MHS (2014), and Karen Woods, MD, whose term begins

Box 2
The Distribution of Female Presidents among the 4 Major gastroenterology and Hepatology Societies

American Society for Gastrointestinal Endoscopy

- Founded 1941
- 14,000 members
- 4 female presidents

American College of Gastroenterology

- Founded 1932
- 12,000 members
- 3 female presidents

American Gastroenterological Association

- Founded 1897
- 16,000 members
- 3 female presidents

American Association for the Study of Liver Diseases

- Founded 1950
- 9,500 members
- 2 female presidents

in 2017. One of the authors (CS) was the first female president to represent community practice among any major gastroenterology or hepatology society.

Since the 1990s, there have been focused and concerted efforts to enhance the roles of women in science, technology, engineering, and math at entry levels through leadership roles. Numerous national organizations have been created to help address the needs of women in science. The Association for Women in Science (available: http://www.awis.org) is the largest organization for women in science, technology, engineering, and math according to their website. The current governing board reads like a "Who's Who" of science and industry. Other similar organizations are reviewed by Hamilton and colleagues.[29] Reasons that proactive efforts are needed to attract and promote women into leadership roles relate directly to continuing barriers to career advancement as summarized in **Box 1**.

The ASGE and AGA have long advocated for diversity and gender equity in both community practices and academic settings. Successful advancement of women in medicine should follow a path similar to companies with successful initiatives and our organizations must embrace and support this endeavor.[3,34,36–38] However, without a continuing strong focus on inclusiveness and change, one that alters the historical trend line, gender parity at the leadership level will not occur for decades to come.[36,37] Sheryl Sandberg (Chief Operating Officer of Facebook Inc and Founder of Leanin.Org) noted the same delay and timeframe for women occupying the "C" Suite of corporate America.[38] A number of approaches can be adopted to support women in gastroenterology careers. An example of the focused approaches implemented by the ASGE are illustrated in **Fig. 2**.

By the early 1990s, there were women with vision and foresight who developed an aggressive structure to increase the proportion of women in all levels of

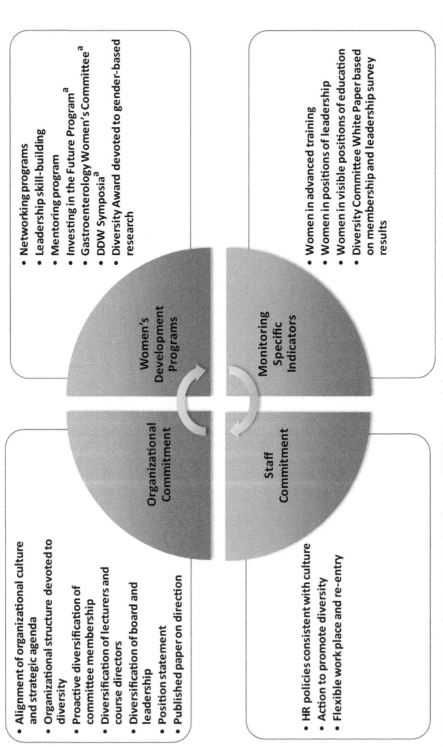

Fig. 2. American Society of Gastrointestinal Endoscopy (ASGE) Approach for Development and Support of Women in Gastroenterology. [a] Denote collaborative efforts with other societies. DDW, Digestive Diseases Week; HR, human resources.

gastroenterology from training to leadership. The Gastroenterology Women's Coalition was formed with Dr Joanne A. P. Wilson as a founding member. Dr Wilson would become the secretary of the AGA Governing Board in 1998, the first woman and first African American to hold that post. Later, a coalition of several gastroenterology societies formed the Gastroenterology Women's Committee. Subsequently, each society, including the ASGE and AGA, have created internal committee structures to be active, creative, and influential resources for our women members.

The Women's Committees of the ASGE and AGA, each have evaluated and supported issues related to women and the conceptual underpinnings of these efforts is illustrated in **Fig. 3**. Both the AGA and ASGE initiated mentor programs that connect senior or experienced members with junior clinicians, faculty, or trainees in an effort to advance their careers. The AGA developed the annual Women's Leadership Conference. At this conference, there is an "early career" track and an "experienced," track each enhancing networking opportunities. The ASGE has committed to helping women and minorities to develop skills for a thriving career that are not taught in the current medical curriculum. The ASGE Leadership and Education Development program has successfully conducted 2 year-long programs with nomination for the third group underway. The success of these programs is driven by a number of factors, including the relevance of the topics with education provided by content experts in their respective disciplines of negotiation, team development, and project management.

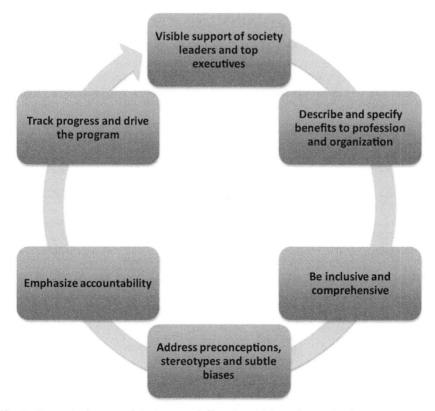

Fig. 3. Conceptual approach to improved diversity within and organization.

Both societies have joined together to identify and highlight gastroenterology as a career for young minorities who are considering medical training, helping to empower gastroenterology as a career choice early for these students through the Investing in the Future Program. The ASGE has devoted a prestigious award given annually for research that includes gender-relevant issues and the AGA secured a multiyear R21 National Institute of Health grant devoted to minority and diversity programs and development.

The AGA and ASGE both have implemented stringent requirements to balance faculty in all programs, and have tracked these trends year to year. We have noted increased participation of women as faculty lecturers, reviewers, and course directors. Participation by women at ASGE-sponsored courses exceeds the proportion of women in the general membership.[39] Participation in the governance and committee work is considered prestigious and enhances professional advancement. We have also examined this important metric, and found that the trend of women participation in the ASGE committees exceeds the proportion of women members.[40]

Within the AGA infrastructure, women currently (as of 2015) chair 8 of the 15 major AGA committees and a woman chairs the prestigious AGA Scientific Council. Considering the 3 major journals of the AGA, 8 of 31 members of the *Gastroenterology* editorial board are women, 1 of 12 for *Clinical Gastroenterology and Hepatology*, and 1 of 3 for *Cellular and Molecular Gastroenterology and Hepatology*.

Despite concerted efforts to increase the proportion of women in key positions within our organizations, there are clear historic and current gaps for which there are no logical explanations. Legacy gender disparity becomes evident when one reviews winners of the major scientific and clinical awards given by the AGA. These data are summarized in **Table 1**. We are encouraged by the current AGA recruitment of women into leadership training and research awards as illustrated in **Fig. 4**.

Both the ASGE and AGA have explicit commitments to break down barriers to gender equity and maintain appropriate diversity balance in clinical and research careers, and on society committees, governing boards and executive leadership

| Table 1 | | | | |
| Major AGA awards: History and purpose | | | | |
Award	Purpose	Beginning Date	Total Winners	Women
Julius Friedenwald	Highest award Contribution to AGA/GI	1941	77	1
William Beaumont	Senior Scientist Research Contribution	1976	24	0
Distinguished Achievement Basic Science	Senior Investigator Basic Science Research	1968	33	1
Distinguished Clinician	Academic and Community Practice	1996	70	4
Distinguished Educator	Contribution to Education and Training	1994	25	2
Distinguished Mentor	Mentorship of Young Trainees and Faculty	2005	13	1
Research Service Award	Advance Science and Research	2006	8	1
Total	—	—	250	10 (4%)

Abbreviation: AGA, American Gastroenterological Association.

41 percent of AGA research grants went to women scientists in 2015.

50 percent of AGA's Inaugural Class of Future Leaders are women

150 women physicians participate annually in AGA's Annual Women in GI Luncheon at DDW.

Fig. 4. American Gastroenterological Association (AGA) programs and grants supporting women. DDW, Digestive Diseases Week.

positions. These commitments are included in a position statement (ASGE) and the new 5-year strategic plan (AGA).

The ASGE's diversity position statement reads as follows:

The American Society for Gastrointestinal Endoscopy values and recognizes the importance of embracing diversity and its impact on strengthening our members' ability to provide excellent care to all patient populations, regardless of their background. The Society is committed to enhancing diversity by educating and training culturally competent gastroenterologists, as well as providing leadership opportunities to all members regardless of gender, age, religion, racial/ethnic group, sexual orientation, and disability status.

The AGA's strategic plan (2015–2020) states that we will: "Strive for diversity at all levels within the association, including governance, committee structure, staffing and program development. Diversity is an inclusive concept that encompasses race, ethnicity, national origin, religion, gender, age, sexual orientation and disability."

COMMUNITY PRACTICE

Private practice remains a popular choice for women in gastroenterology; however, there are currently fewer than 2000 female gastroenterologists providing clinical care in the United States for more than 44 million patients.[1] In a recent survey of more than 20,000 physicians (30% medical specialties, such as gastroenterology), women were evenly divided in their type of practice: 27% of women were a practice owner, partner, or associate, 32% were employed by a hospital, 26% were employed by a medical group, and 15% described their practice as "other" (such as military). Women physicians are more likely to be employed than male physicians (59% vs 50%), and younger and female physicians, specialists in particular, reported a more positive attitude about employment.[41] In another survey, only 42% of women were likely to be practice owners, compared with 55% of men, whereas 52% of women were likely to be employed compared with 39% of men.[42] These observations have important ramifications for parity in earnings for women gastroenterologists (see discussion later in this paper).

Women gastroenterologists average 50 hours for their workweek according to a recent survey.[41] Physician clinical skills are only part of current job requirements because practices require substantial administrative and regulatory oversight, attention to business development, and management of ancillary services such as anesthesia, pathology, and infusion. Women bring unique attributes to practice and many now contribute to a multidisciplinary approach for women's health.

Women join private practices for many reasons, including an interest in clinical medicine, a desire to manage their own business, an appreciation of excellent financial compensation, and the potential to have a flexible schedule or even part-time work.[43,44] Women are highly sought after as clinicians, particularly in specialties such as gastroenterology, where physician gender choice may be preferential. One of us (CS) reviewed private practice social media and websites and noted unique and interesting ways that women highlight their expertise, as follows:

- Unique perspectives on common symptoms such as constipation, bloating, reflux, rectal bleeding, incontinence;
- For gender-influenced diseases or disorders such as irritable bowel syndrome, inflammatory bowel disease, pelvic floor dysfunction, primary biliary cirrhosis, autoimmune hepatitis, obesity, and fatty liver;
- With screening colonoscopy;
- With management approaches such as nutrition, biofeedback;

- For pregnancy-related disorders such as hyperemesis gravidarum and acute fatty liver;
- Using alternative or complimentary care such as acupuncture; and
- For fertility-related disorders.

Independent community practices are transforming in response to health care reform. Many physicians now seek employment models within large health systems, although there remain large numbers of graduating trainees that choose independent practice. Although an employed model of practice may be perceived as having more financial security, fewer administrative responsibilities, and a more predictable work schedule compared with independent practice, trade-offs are evident.[42,45] Potential downsides include a lack of autonomy in management, personnel, and business decision making, plus health system-imposed rules and productivity metrics. One in 5 employed physicians still expresses dissatisfaction with work–life balance.[45]

When contemplating entering into a professional agreement, several critical factors unique to women must be considered, especially contract clauses that cover a career trajectory in the context of maternity leave or family responsibilities. In addition, women should specifically discuss pay equity and equal resource allocation compared with their male counterparts. Employment arrangements have been identified as an important factor contributing to the gender gap in earnings.[42] An attorney who specializes in physician contracts should assist and provide consultation. We advise careful research for the pay scale at least by group size and location relevant for any position, and ensure that women understand the governance of the group, how practice decisions are made, what production, financial and quality metrics are to be used, a practice's peer review process, adjudication of disputes, and how ancillary services are defined and compensated.

The current trend in physician practice consolidation may be favorable for women and younger generations of the workforce. In addition to potential benefits for physicians who enjoy this type of practice setting, larger group practices may allow particular upsides for women gastroenterologists, including:

- Dedicated hospitalists to provide inpatient care,
- More opportunities to concentrate on specialization or subspecialization,
- Ability to focus nonclinical practice interests,
- Increased likelihood of successful multispecialty approach to women's care,
- Improved options for flexible scheduling,
- Decreased call exposure and group coverage, and
- Shared responsibility for resource-intensive patients.

In many practice settings, women are rising to midlevel leadership roles, but still are less likely to be a division chief, department chair, or the managing partner of an independent gastroenterology practice.[44,46] Within the largest national gastroenterology "trade association" representing more than 1300 gastroenterologists among 56 independent gastroenterology practices, 15% of the practice members are women who do not self-describe as managing partner, and none are officers of the organization. There is 1 woman among 55 board members. Of nearly 200 hundred women, 6% self-describe as medical director for a center, hold teaching positions, or serve as section chief (compiled by CS; available: http://www.dhpassociation.org). This observation serves to illustrate the time constraints experienced by women trying to balance a busy clinical practice and other responsibilities, or other factors.

We believe that women leadership is crucial for the "business" of medicine as health care evolves. Women are successful change agents and can be engaged leaders.

As the demographic of the physician workforce changes, there are opportunities to enhance the workplace environment and help both women gastroenterologists and our practices to prosper. Women are more likely than men to enact policies favorable to women's and children's health; and women executive leadership is consistently associated with a positive return on investment.[5,47] In a workplace survey, work–life balance was listed as a challenge for 70% of men and 62% of women; thus, informative and practical support for enhancing this aspect of our career should be a priority.[43] Women possess the necessary skills to be effective team leaders, and to provide health care in an era where patient engagement is considered critically important in the overall health care experience.

Most women attendees at practice management courses are nurses, practice administrators, or industry representatives. The vast majority of women in leadership or leadership development programs come from academic settings. In private practices, where revenue derives only from face-to-face patient encounters, women encounter resistance when they request time away from billable practice, whether they seek to enhance leadership skills or attend to family matters. But as the growth of women in the physician workforce increases, it is crucially important for women to rise to positions of leadership and influence if the current situation within gastroenterology is to change.

FUTURE IMPERATIVES AND SUMMARY

As medicine evolves, we are seeing enormous changes in expectations from patients, providers, purchases, and payers of health care. Now is the time for women to be actively recruited into leadership positions. We believe the following actions are needed[2,29,30,37,44,46]:

- Insist that women be considered for leadership positions and advocate for young women to consider gastroenterology as a career choice.
- Point out that certain leadership skills important in medical practice are those where women excel.
- Study and understand the impact of promotion, publication and salary increases on successful advancement.
- Work to increase mentoring, sponsoring, and networking opportunities.
- Be aware of gender-related differences in expectations and social norms that contribute in subtle ways to a glass ceiling or glass cliff.

With regard to specific support that should be part of academic sections, health system employment, and community practices include the following.

Flexible Schedules

Full-time, part-time, or per diem opportunities depending on phase of life will help women to more fully participate in work-related responsibilities and home and caregiver responsibilities without penalizing either position. Because women rank the option of part-time work as an important factor in moving from academia into private practice, this change could also help to stem the flow of bright individuals leaving a valuable career at the height of their most productive years. Providers and patients alike value clinical availability outside of traditional work times.

Reentry Strategies

As a procedure-heavy specialty, reentry into the workforce requires special consideration. We should determine ways for both women and men to take leaves of absence to participate in parenting or other caregiver responsibilities, and then reenter the workforce. As physicians retire, we must determine ways to preserve or even magnify the existing workforce.

Position Sharing

Intrapractice arrangements can allow a woman to see consultations 1 day, and a partner to provide a necessary procedure on another day, or vice versa. This strategy also contributes to more workplace flexibility.

Professional Development

Attendance at practice management courses, participation in high-level committees, and visible women leaders are needed to move women further down the pipeline, thus encouraging more women to enter the pipeline of gastroenterology as a career choice. As practices adopt more flexible work environments, consideration is needed for appropriate adjustments in income, malpractice premiums, maintenance of certification and licensure requirements, employment benefits, and academic promotion. Some adjustments will require shifts in traditional thinking and approach, and some of these are substantial (such as time out from training). Flexibility in career advancement must account for time outs owing to maternity and paternity related issues, and later, for elder care. Attaining leadership skills for vital aspects of career building are essential.

Structural Support

Onsite daycare is common for hospital employees, who have traditionally been female. One obvious challenge for maintaining a thriving workforce among dual career physician families is childcare, sick care, and elder care that is available, dependable, and flexible.

Our practices will be impacted by the increasing proportion of women providers entering medicine as we note a decline in the proportion of male providers. Current research suggests that women physicians continue to make less money than their male counterparts, no matter what the practice setting.[48] This pay gap has been attributed incorrectly to the belief that women are more likely to work part time or work fewer hours compared with men, but the difference in earnings persists even after adjusting for covariates, including specialty, research productivity as measured by publication number and funding, academic rank, working status of the domestic partner, and number of hours worked per week.[49,50] Fundamental to discussions about women in our specialty is ensuring transparency and fairness in decisions regarding both earnings and promotion.

As we developed this article, both authors (recent presidents of the AGA and ASGE) reflected on the responsibilities of clinicians who have achieved leadership roles in our medical societies, academia and private practice. We believe that the most important role of current leaders with respect to gender bias is 2-fold. First, to understand and address the reasons for residual barriers to entry and promotion, and second to develop programs to support the talents and aspirations of women as they progress through their careers in gastroenterology. Women should not be afforded "special" considerations, but do demand and deserve equal opportunity and the final shattering of glass ceilings and cliffs.

REFERENCES

1. Association of American Medical Colleges. Center for Workforce Studies. 2014 Physician Specialty Data Book. 2014. Available at: https://members.aamc.org/

eweb/upload/Physician%20Specialty%20Databook%202014.pdf.   Accessed
October 2, 2015.

2. Schmitt CM. Flute or tuba: women and publishing success in top gastroenterology journals. Gastrointest Endosc 2015;81:1448–50.

3. Barsh J, Lee L. Unlocking the full potential of women at work. Washington, DC: McKinsey & Company; 2012. Available at: http://www.mckinsey.com/client_service/
organization/latest_thinking/unlocking_the_full_potential. Accessed October 3,
2015.

4. Jolly S, Griffith KA, DeCastro R, et al. Gender differences in time spent
on parenting and domestic responsibilities by high-achieving young physician-
researchers. Ann Intern Med 2014;160:344–53.

5. Women in the Workplace 2015. Washington, DC: LeanIn.org and McKinsey & Company; 2015. Available at: http://womenintheworkplace.com/ui/pdfs/Women_in_the_
Workplace_2015.pdf?v=5. Accessed October 3, 2015.

6. Reid RO, Friedberg MW, Adams JL, et al. Associations between physician characteristics and quality of care. Arch Intern Med 2010;170:1442–9.

7. Ranji U, Salganicoff A. Kaiser Family Foundation. Women's Health Care Chart-
book. Key findings from the Kaiser Women's Health Survey. 2011. Available at:
https://kaiserfamilyfoundation.files.wordpress.com/2013/01/8164.pdf. Accessed
October 25, 2015.

8. Luscombe B. Woman power: the rise of the sheconomy. Available at: http://content.
time.com/time/magazine/article/0,9171,2030913-3,00.html. Accessed October 3,
2015.

9. Menees SB, Inadomi JM, Korsnes S, et al. Women patients' preference for
women physicians is a barrier to colon cancer screening. Gastrointest Endosc
2005;62:219–23.

10. Schneider A, Kanagariajan J, Anjelly D, et al. Importance of gender, socioeconomic status, and history of abuse on patient preference for endoscopist. Am J
Gastroenterol 2009;104:340–8.

11. Lee SY, Yu SK, Kim JH, et al. Link between a preference for women colonoscopists and social status in Korean women. Gastrointest Endosc 2008;67:273–7.

12. Shah DK, Karasek V, Gerkin RD, et al. Sex preferences for colonoscopists and GI
physicians among patients and health care professionals. Gastrointest Endosc
2011;74:122–7.

13. Varia A, Patel MK, Tanikella R, et al. Gender preference for the endoscopist
among Hispanics: the results of a prospective study. J Immigr Minor Health
2014;16:990–3.

14. Lahat A, Assouline-Davan Y, Katz LH, et al. The preference for an endoscopist
specific sex: a link between ethnic origin, religious belief, socioeconomic status,
and procedure type. Patient Prefer Adherence 2013;7:897–903.

15. McLean M, Al Yahyaei F, Al Mansoori M, et al. Muslim women's physician preference: beyond obstetrics and gynecology. Health Care Women Int 2012;33:
849–76.

16. Medicare Payment Advisory Commission. Report to the Congress: Medicare and
the health care delivery system. The next generation of Medicare beneficiaries.
2015. Available at: http://www.medpac.gov/documents/reports/chapter-2-the-
next-generation-of-medicare-beneficiaries-(june-2015-report).pdf?sfvrsn=0. Accessed October 3, 2015.

17. Austin M. History of women in medicine; a symposium early period. Bull Med Libr
Assoc 1956;44:12–5.

18. National Library of Medicine Exposition "Changing the Face of Medicine". Available at: https://www.nlm.nih.gov/changingthefaceofmedicine/exhibition/. Accessed October 1, 2015.
19. Chin EL, editor. This side of doctoring: reflections from women in medicine. Thousand Oaks (CA): Sage Publications; 2002.
20. Hecht G. Women in gastroenterology: exciting times and trends. Gastroenterology 2008;134:913–4.
21. Bowman M, Gross ML. Overview of research on women in medicine – issues for public policymakers. Public Health Rep 1986;101:513–21.
22. Bruckmuller S, Branscombe NR. How women end up on the "glass cliff". Harv Bus Rev 2011;89(1–2):26.
23. Kulich C. Glass ceiling/glass cliff. In: Flood PC, Freeney Y, editors. Wiley encyclopedia of management, organizational behavior, vol. 11, 3rd edition. Hoboken (NJ): John Wiley and Sons; 2015. p. 1–2.
24. Kanter RM. Men and women of the corporation. New York: Harper & Row; 1977.
25. Long MT, Leszcznski A, Thompson KD, et al. Female authorship in major academic gastroenterology journals; a look over 20 years. Gastrointest Endosc 2015;81:1440–7.
26. Jagsi R, Guancial EA, Worobey CC, et al. The "gender gap" in authorship of academic medical literature – a 35-year perspective. N Engl J Med 2006;355: 281–7.
27. Enestvedt B, Diamond S, Thomas C, et al. Gender differences in research productivity, academic rank, and career duration among U.S. academic gastroenterology faculty. Am J Gastroenterol 2014;109(S2):2174.
28. Lund PK. Gender equity in biomedical science: comments from a lone female associate editor. Gastroenterology 2001;121:243–4.
29. Hamilton KE, Tetreault MP, Lund PK. Opportunities and challenges for women PhD investigators in gastrointestinal research. Gastroenterology 2013;145: 266–71.
30. Henning SJ, Estes MK. Women in science: hints for success. Gastroenterology 2015;149:10–3.
31. Frei R. Gastroenterology & Endoscopy News. Pioneering female gastroenterologists have paved the way for younger women. 2008. Available at: http://www.gastroendonews.com/viewarticle.aspx?d_id=187&a_id=10203. Accessed October 10, 2015.
32. Babcock L, Laschever S. Women don't ask. New York: Bantam Books; 2007.
33. Sandberg S. Lean in. women, work, and the will to lead. New York: Alfred A. Knopf; 2013.
34. Johns ML. Breaking the glass ceiling: structural, cultural, and organizational barriers preventing women from achieving senior and executive positions. Perspect Health Inf Manag 2013;10:1e.
35. Hecht G. 2010 AGA Presidential Address. Gastroenterology 2010;139:e15–7.
36. U.S. Department of Labor. Good for Business: Making full use of the nation's human capital. A fact-finding report of the Federal Glass Ceiling Commission Washington, D.C. 1995. Available at: http://www.dol.gov/oasam/programs/history/reich/reports/ceiling.pdf. Accesssed October 3, 2015.
37. Women Matter 2012. Making the Breakthrough. McKinsey & Company; 2012. Available at: http://www.mckinsey.com/client_service/organization/latest_thinking/women_matter. Accessed October 4, 2015.
38. Sandberg S. When women get stuck, corporate America gets stuck. Wall St J 2015;R3.

39. Enestvedt BK, Calderwood AH, Schmitt CM, et al. The gender distribution of ASGE-sponsored program faculty. Gastrointest Endosc 2015;81(5S):AB166.
40. Calderwood AH, Enestvedt BK, Devivo R, et al. Women do ask and receive: an evaluation of the gender representation of requests for ASGE committee assignments. Gastrointest Endosc 2015;81(5S):AB331.
41. The Physician's Foundation. 2014 Survey of America's Physicians. 2014. Available at: http://www.physiciansfoundation.org/uploads/default/2014_Physicians_Foundation_Biennial_Physician_Survey_Report.pdf. Accessed October 3, 2015.
42. Kane CK. Policy research perspectives. Updated data on physician practice arrangements: Inching toward hospital ownership. Chicago (IL): American Medical Association; 2015.
43. Gerson LB, Twomey K, Hecht G, et al. Does gender affect career satisfaction and advancement in gastroenterology? Results of an AGA Institute-sponsored survey. New York: Gastroenterology 2007;132:1598–606.
44. Cajigal S, Weiss G, Silva N. Women as Physician Leaders. New York: MedScape; 2015. Available at: http://www.medscape.com/features/slideshow/public/femaleleadershipreport2015#page=1. Accessed October 3, 2015.
45. Kane L. Employed doctors report: are they better off? Medscape; 2014. Available at: http://www.medscape.com/features/slideshow/public/employed-doctors#1. Accessed October 3, 2015.
46. Joliff L, Leadly J, Coakley E, et al. Women in U.S. academic medicine and science: statistics and benchmarking report 2011–2012. Washington, DC: Association of American Medical Colleges; 2012. Available at: https://www.aamc.org/download/415556/data/2011-2012wimsstatsreport.pdf. Accessed October 25, 2015.
47. Downs JA, Reif LK, Hokororo A, et al. Increasing women in leadership in global health. Acad Med 2014;89:1103–7.
48. Lo Sasso AT, Richards MR, Chou CF, et al. The $16,819 pay gap for newly trained physicians: the unexplained trend of men earning more than women. Health Aff (Millwood) 2011;30:193–201.
49. Jagsi R, Griffith KA, Stewart A, et al. Gender differences in the salaries of physician researchers. JAMA 2012;307:2410–7.
50. Jagsi R, Griffith KA, Stewart A, et al. Gender differences in salary in a recent cohort of early-career physician-researchers. Acad Med 2013;88:1689–99.

Index

Note: Page numbers of article titles are in **boldface** type.

A

Adalimumab, for IBD, 289, 291–292
Adefovir, for hepatitis B, 364
Adiponectin, obesity and, 319
Alcoholic liver disease, 348
Alendronate, for osteoporosis, 338–340
Alosetron, for IBS, 194
American Gastroenterological Association, 376–382
American Society for Gastrointestinal Endoscopy, 376–382
Aminosalicylates, for IBD, 288–290
Amoxicillin/clavulanate, for IBD, 290, 295
Anal sphincter
    augmentation of, for fecal incontinence, 225
    magnetic, 228
Anal wicking, for fecal incontinence, 222–223
Anorectal manometry, for chronic constipation, 209
Antacids, for GERD, 274–275
Antegrade continence enema, for fecal incontinence, 227
Antibiotics, for IBS, 191, 194
Antidepressants, for IBS, 195–197
Antimitochondrial antibody, in primary biliary cirrhosis, 334
Antispasmodics, for IBS, 194
Anxiety, in IBD, 306
Azathioprine, for IBD, 289–291

B

Balloon expulsion test, for chronic constipation, 209
Balsalazide, for IBD, 289
Bariatric surgery, for obesity, 326
Behçet disease, 304
Bile acid-binding agents, for IBS, 194
Biofeedback, for fecal incontinence, 224–225
Birth defects, in obesity, 325
Bisacodyl, for constipation, 277, 279
Bisphosphonates, for osteoporosis, 338–340
Body image, in IBD, 307
Bone disease. *See also* Osteoporosis.
    in primary biliary cirrhosis, 334–340
Breastfeeding, in IBD, 295
Budesonide, for IBD, 290, 294
Bulking agents

Gastroenterol Clin N Am 45 (2016) 389–398
http://dx.doi.org/10.1016/S0889-8553(16)30029-2
0889-8553/16/$ – see front matter

Moving?

Make sure your subscription moves with you!

To notify us of your new address, find your **Clinics Account Number** (located on your mailing label above your name), and contact customer service at:

Email: journalscustomerservice-usa@elsevier.com

800-654-2452 (subscribers in the U.S. & Canada)
314-447-8871 (subscribers outside of the U.S. & Canada)

Fax number: 314-447-8029

Elsevier Health Sciences Division
Subscription Customer Service
3251 Riverport Lane
Maryland Heights, MO 63043

*To ensure uninterrupted delivery of your subscription, please notify us at least 4 weeks in advance of move.

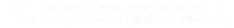